Tennis Mastery

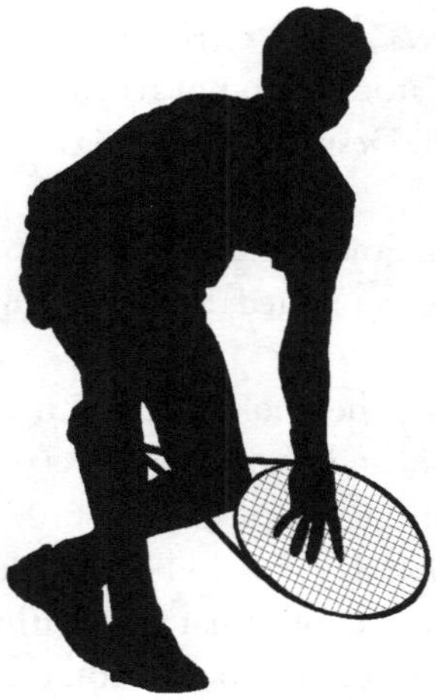

Praise for Tennis Mastery

Since its initial release in 2004, *Tennis Mastery* has received accolades and praise from all corners of the world. Below are samplings of these sentiments, expressed by those who have used *Tennis Mastery* to improve their own game or that of their students or children.

Comments: I was a 3.0 for 5 years straight despite being young, physically fit, and having a lot of athletic ability. I bought *Tennis Mastery* and read about David Smith's methodologies and did what I could to live by them while being self-taught. I went from a computer-rated 3.0 to computer-rated 4.0 in one year, and attribute most of that to Dave Smith for giving me the knowledge to know how to train myself. **From**: Raiden, Tenniswarehouse message board. 12/08

Comments: David Smith's *Tennis Mastery* is as complete a tennis manual as I've ever read. I would be failing in my duty as a tennis educator if I do not recommend it to tennis players of all levels...from the beginner to the aspiring pro. **From**: Dr. Desmond Oon, Master Pro, USPTA. 8/08 Former Davis Cup coach, Singapore

Comments: Just want to give Mr. Smith, the thumbs up on his eponymous book. This is the best general tennis reference book that I have encountered, as it covers every aspect of the game in great depth. **From**: A.T., 11/07

Comments: I just finished reading the book for the 5th time and loaned it to a 3.0 friend of mine. I find it to be a magnificent teaching tool and recommend everyone adding this book to their library. Reading this book was an epiphany of sorts for me. **From**: Drew, 06/07

Comments: This is a brilliant book that should be required reading for any coach of the game. What I love about the book is that he uses pictures of actual pros hitting the ball and he shows you what they have in common. It's hard to believe, but most tennis books don't do this. There really is a lifetime of tennis wisdom packed into *Tennis Mastery*. It's one of the most comprehensive tennis technique books ever published. **From**: Jeff, 05/07

Comments: To be read again and again; a lot of clear indications to enhance tennis playing. I would really advise it to anybody who is interested in a rational step forward. **From**: Pierpaolo, Rome, Italy. 4/07

Tennis Mastery is a must read. People do get stuck with poor mechanics and weak grips. They just never progress beyond the 3.0 stage. I see it every day and I know they could play so much better. I would highly recommend it. **From**: ED, 03/07

Comments: I have read several tennis instructional books, and I think *Tennis Mastery* is the best by far. It covers every stroke, with very good illustrations. I would say his book is a must read for true students of tennis. **From**: Stroke, 03/07

Comments: This book is a gem, probably the most important and insightful tennis publication to appear since Gallwey's masterpiece of the 1970s [Inner Game of Tennis]. It surely hits home for the many of us who have stagnated our game in the 3.5 mediocrity about which you write. **From**: Roy, Virgina, USA. 11/05

Comments: I bought *Tennis Mastery* this past year and have really enjoyed it. This book has terrific tips, especially the "Advanced Foundation" principles. **From**: Josh A. 9/05

Comments: Well, I totally loved it! I always wanted to learn how to hit with both hands off of both sides, and this is the first books that actually show you how to do it! This is about the most excited that I have been since reading "Winning Ugly". This is a very, very interesting and engaging book! Smith has a very engaging writing style! I give an A! I think that you will enjoy it. **From**: John from TW Message Board 06/05

Comments: As a section editor for a professional academic journal, I have rarely seen a better or more sincerely written book. **From**: Ned, St. George Utah, USA. 03/05

Comments: A real eye-opener! This book will change the way tennis has been taught. It provides clarity for the pro and the student. **From**: Mike, Garden Grove, CA, USA. 03/05

Comments: I have never found a source of tennis instruction that combines superb information while at the same time be a truly enjoyable read as *TENNIS MASTERY* is! **From**: Anthony, Canada. 03/05

David Smith's

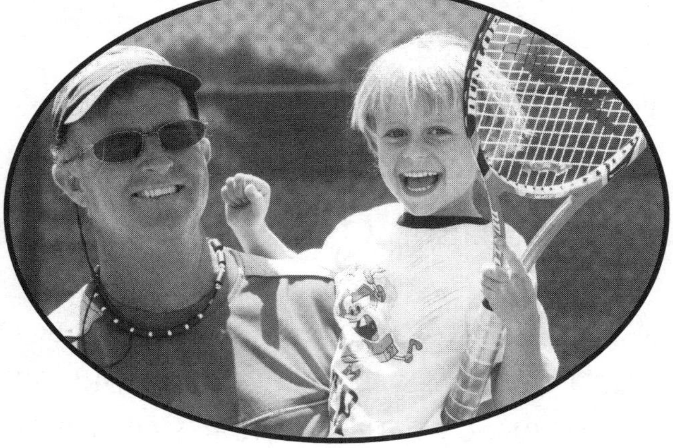

Tennis Mastery

The MOST Complete Guide to Learning, Developing and Mastering the Sport of Tennis

St. George, Utah
2010

First Edition 2004

Reprinted with corrections and a new foreword
by Desmond Oon November, 2010

ISBN: 9-780-97490260-9

Produced by Manahawkin Printing
www.booksprintedhere.com
Printed in The United States of America

This book is dedicated to my wife Dr. Kerri Smith and our two beautiful children Kyla Marie and Keaton Bruce.

*

May they grow up to enjoy this great game as much as their father does and as their grandfather did!

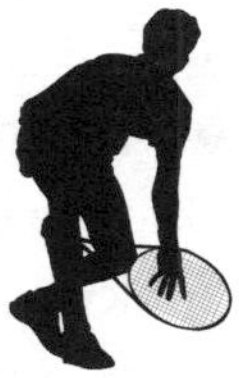

Acknowledgements

I must first recognize Kim Shanley (Publisher and President) and Jay Margolies (Managing Editor) of www.tennisone.com for their incredible web site related to tennis information and education. For any tennis player seeking the "truth" about tennis, this Internet Site provides the most honest and objective representation of what is actually happening in tennis. What can you say about a place you can actually view over 700 video clips of top players in action or some 400 tennis lessons by such recognized tennis instructors as Nick Bollettieri, Allen Fox, Robert Landsdorp, Dennis Van der Meer and many others? Where many questionable authors of tennis only "say" what to do, TennisONE.com shows you what is actually happening. TennisONE has provided many of the pictures used in *Tennis Mastery.* My deep appreciation goes to Kim and Jay for their permission to use these pictures.

Speaking of pictures, all of the pro pictures used in this text have been taken by Gregory Swendsen of TennisONE.com. (Except those identified by other photographers.) It was critical to the understanding of the many conceptual ideas and philosophies I presented to be augmented by quality pictures. I was blessed with a great number of exceptional shots to choose from. A very special thanks also goes out to John Yandell, (Research Director of the Advanced Tennis Research Project and former CEO of TennisONE.com), for his support of this book. His own research and publications have, in my opinion, opened more eyes to true tennis advancement than that of so-called guru-based tennis instructors.

It is with great appreciation and respect that Desmond Oon, an exceptional and incredibly respected teaching professional, (a "teaching pro's Professional"!), agreed to write the foreword to this revised edition of Tennis Mastery. His words have added depth and meaning to my own text.

I also want to thank Mike Letcher, fellow coach, fellow professional, exceptional player and talented instructor, for his some twenty years of friendship and dedication to the game of tennis. Mike has been an inspiration to me on many levels.

Thank you to Scott Adams who assisted me for many of the years I was writing this book. Scott also is featured as the model form for the majority of the teaching pictures within *Tennis Mastery.* With his ability to recognize the power of the Advanced Foundation and sharing it within the training many of our players, Scott discovered the importance of this concept with me. Also, thanks to my currant assistants, Tim Finger, Wayne Bullock, Richard Wigley, Victor Strange and Jason Whittington, talented and knowledgeable instructors in their own right. The insight and encouragement they have shared with me and with our students have helped make everyone a better person and player.

Thanks to Jeff Brose, a former student, a fellow coach, an exceptional player, and one who is blessed with a highly intuitive nature; his knowledge of the game as well as the written word was helpful throughout the production of this book.

A special thanks to Helene Krupa, a person who has stepped up to the plate many times in helping prepare and edit many pages of this book. Our many conversations helped me formulate my thoughts more clearly. She provided me her objective insights time and time again. Also, an equally special thanks to Mike Krupa, Helene's husband and owner of Manahawkin Printing Company, who has provided me with the directional leadership in the printing processes of this book.

Thanks to Virginia "Ginny" Naifeh, my mother-in-law and editor extraordinaire! Her encouragement and proofreading of most of this book has improved its quality and readability! Taking the time to read the more than 200 pages of draft documents and advise me in various grammatical and conception-orientated phrasing was going beyond the call of a "mother-in-law's" duty!

I would especially like to thank all my 3500+ students, past and present, which have allowed me the privilege to perfect my teaching philosophy over the past 30 years. From my juniors to my adult players, from California to Arizona and finally to Utah, without these "proving grounds," and without the dedication by you to these principles, this book would not be possible. It is hoped that an untold number of future tennis players will benefit through the understanding of the Advanced Foundation, a principle that all my students helped me develop.

Thanks to some of my students who are also featured in several of the photographs within this book. These include: Allie Bergin, Stephanie Caplin, Ellen Kastler, Julie Skalla, A.J. Bartlett, Jeremy Atkin, Nate Awohi, and Carlos Morgan.

Perhaps the true catalyst for me wanting to write this book was my father, the late Bruce Smith. An inspiration to thousands of students, my dad was one of the finest tennis coaches in the country. You don't win over 400 team league matches with only one loss over a 14-year period without some almost mythical sense of how to create champions! My drive to write this book was always propelled by his voice somewhere in the back of my brain, always telling me to do what is necessary. And special thanks to my mother, Donna Winchester, a stalwart proponent of everything I have ever done!

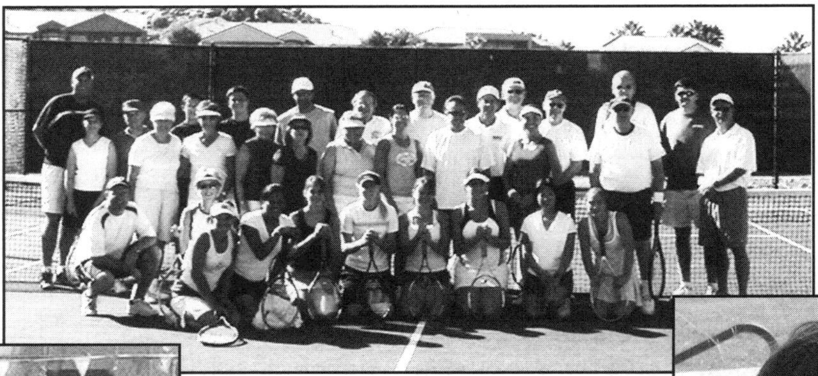

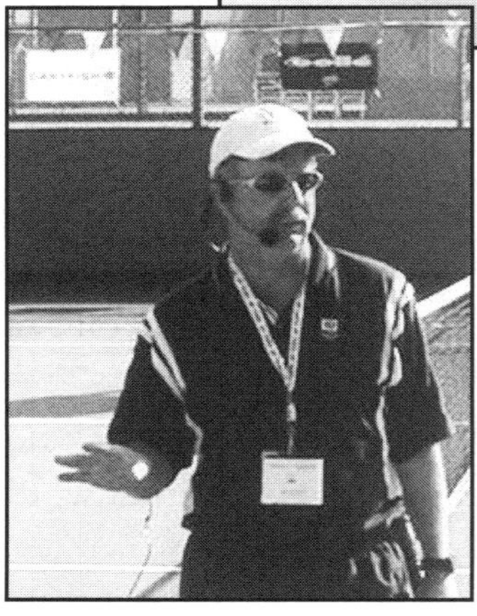

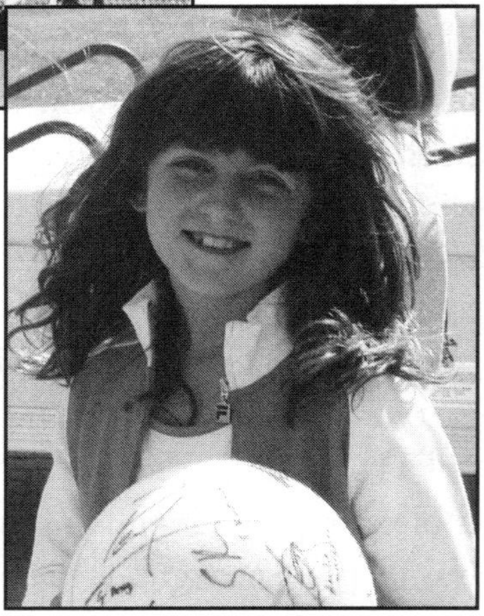

From speaking at conventions, (left), to developing and programming successful club and group programs, (above), to training and helping kids of all ages develop a love for tennis, (right), I've enjoyed over 35 years within the tennis industry.

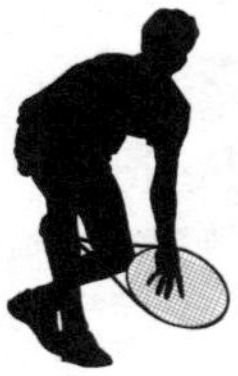

Table of Contents

Section Two: The Strategies of Hitting

Section 3: The Strategies of Playing

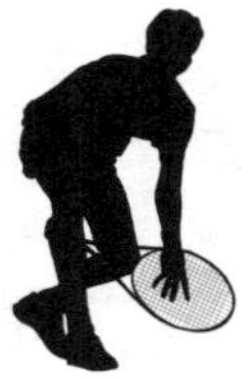

Foreword

By Desmond Oon

I feel privileged to have been given the opportunity to write this foreword. I am humbled by this experience yet feel the importance of the content of this book should not be missed by any individual interested in becoming a skilled tennis player.

As a student of the game, I love reading tennis books. Even as I come to the close of my fifth decade as a teaching pro, I continue to read. Some of the books I have read were entertaining but lacked substance. Others were very instructional, maybe a little rigid and certainly bordered on being boring. David Smith's *Tennis Mastery* is both entertaining and educational. This balance makes reading that much more enjoyable, and perhaps more important, a text where the subject matter will be absorbed and employed.

Once in a generation, a tennis book emerges that sets us talking and singing praises. In the 1970s, Timothy Gallwey's *Inner Game of Tennis* captured our imagination, introducing us to new concepts in training the mind. It has become a classic. In the 1990's, we saw Brad Gilbert's *Winning Ugly*, become a mainstay of tennis literature and substance. Another classic. I believe that Tennis Mastery is destined to become a classic for a new generation of players and students of the game.

So many good things can be said about this book. It qualifies as a manual, a compendium and a midget-sized encyclopedia all rolled into one. Only David Smith with his almost 40 years of tennis experience, and bolstered by his rare journalistic talent, could have penned a book of such monumental stature.

Those who have read it call it a treasure trove of ideas, tips, techniques and wisdom. Others have labeled it, "A measure for tennis literature," "An epiphany," and "A gem"… I cannot agree more.

Tennis is not a game of "perfect". We acknowledge this. Our game is always in the "work under construction" mode. We continue to fine tune our game towards mastery. Our game evolves *ad infinitum.* Yet, I've found while other resources gloss over the concept of true tennis progressions, *Tennis Mastery* points out, with clear and sound research, those methods that create player stagnation; The book then offers David Smith's proven methods that create a path for continued player progression in rich, dynamic instructional prose augmented with hundreds of pictures.

Speaking of pictures, David's use of hundreds of professional pictures within these pages, depicting the concepts of which he speaks, is an incredible resource. It is hard to believe that most books don't do this. *Tennis Mastery* does it in spades!

It behooves all players, whatever your level of play, to pay attention to the content of this book. Read it with relish. It is so well organized that you can feel that you have a personal master keeping pace with you, guiding you and reaching out to you in your tennis evolution.

Playing skilled tennis takes two distinctive elements: Dedication to the principles of practice and proper understanding and instruction to make that dedication worth the effort. *Tennis Mastery* gives every single student of the game the confidence of knowing the process will result in the desired outcome. I fully believe that David Smith's work is something that will result in a new generation—and future generations—of tennis players, reaching their full potential and even exceeding their own expectations.

Desmond Oon, Ph.D.
Master Professional, USPTA
Author of Can Eastern Wisdom Improve Your Tennis?
And, Soft Tennis: Mysteries of the Game Revealed
Founder: Center for MindBody Tennis
Contact: docoon@pacbell.net

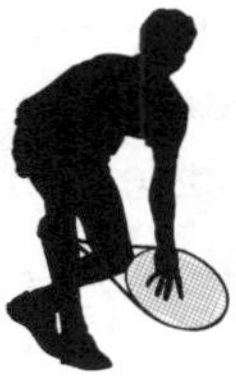

Introduction

Since the 2004 release of my First Edition of *Tennis Mastery*, I have been amazed at the outpouring of responses to the book. Perhaps most revealing is the level of sales the book has sustained over the five years that the book has been available. Tennis Mastery continues to be a top selling tennis book, and, in some distribution points, it has been THE biggest selling tennis book among the selections offered for over five years!

This response was certainly one of the goals of writing the book, however, one never knows how a book will be perceived nor received by the public and professionals of the sport being written until, of course, the book is read and talked about.

What made Tennis Mastery so different or successful?

Most would agree that it is the philosophy of learning the game within my "Advanced Foundation" that so many digested and instantly recognized as not just a 'common sense' approach to learning the game, but a contrast to the ways in which tennis had been taught, (in books, DVD's, tapes, Web Sites, or on the court), where so many millions of able-bodied tennis players failed to reach their potential in the sport they so desperately wished to do so in.

Tennis Mastery struck a nerve. Where hundreds of books and thousands of teaching professionals were teaching tennis from a transitory philosophy, (teaching methods that would HAVE to change later on for the student to progress to higher skill levels), *Tennis Mastery* not only refuted this methodology, but provided clear indications of why such methods are inherently flawed.

Different Methodologies: Different Outcomes

Tennis, like any sport, can be learned through many methods. At the simplest or most rudimentary, a player can pick up a tennis racquet and, through trial and error, figure out ways to hit a ball over the net. Within a number of swings, a player can learn the relative timing of hitting a ball, learn the relative angle of the racquet face to hit the ball—not-to-high or not-to-low, and learn how hard to hit the ball so that it goes over the net but not over the fence! Yet, this "self-discovery" fails nearly every time to produce players into becoming highly skilled. Unless the player can observe skilled tennis strokes, and then emulate them on the court, the level of competency of simply trial and error will be mediocre at best. The reason for this is because skilled tennis strokes are initially seldom comfortable nor are they natural. Players are often confused when watching pros: the pros make tennis seem almost effortless, or at least, the make it look very natural. Well, professional gymnasts, piano players, ice skaters, and magicians all make their sport or activity look effortless or natural. Yet not one of these activities, nor others like them, are ever accomplished without significant and dedicated and specific types of practice, and none of them are mastered quickly…even by so-called prodigies who may pick up elements quickly and with less effort than the general public.

Ironically, many players and students of the game often refer to those who are very skilled at tennis as being "gifted" or blessed with some inherent ability that allowed such high skill levels to emerge.

This assumption is blatantly false.

In my 35-Plus years of teaching tennis, I've taught so many players who seemed just the opposite, players who simply lacked any initial quality or athleticism that would lead any observer to believing that they had any chance of becoming skilled—let alone competitive—tennis players. Yet, many of these students would go on to become highly skilled, ranked, as well as earn incredible winning records on the court.

Likewise, I've come across many "gifted" athletes who were taught—or tried to self-teach themselves—using inferior or mediocre methods…and, as a result, stagnated at incredibly low levels compared to their potential!

This experience taught me long ago in my teaching career that it was seldom the level of coordination or athleticism which would determine a players' ability to reach skilled levels of play.

In addition, while DESIRE was a defining element in terms of player's becoming skilled, it, in and of itself, won't necessarily make a skilled player either. For example, I've seen thousands of players who spent countless hours hitting tens of thousands of balls thinking that through such determination (of hitting hour upon hour), they could become skilled players too. However, in most of these cases, the player was intent on hitting ball after ball instead of focusing on developing proper strokes. In most cases, the player was only getting better at being bad. While they certainly improved the ability to hit balls where they were aiming, and even hitting balls harder within some level of control through such repetition, the bottom line is that they were not developing, nor mastering, stroke patterns that would allow the player to progress to their optimal potential, or what I call hitting more effective shots more consistently.

This potential is defined by four key elements:

- Athleticism
- Opportunity
- Desire
- Education

I've discussed Athleticism and Desire already. However, of these four determining elements, it is the last one, EDUCATION, is the most critical for players who want to not only reach skilled levels of tennis, but also reach their "true tennis potential." Certainly if a player does not have the desire to go out and practice, or possesses the minimal athleticism to hit a moving tennis ball with a moving tennis racket, or have a court to go out and play and practice on, the level of achievement will certainly be rather low. However, a player can indeed have these three 'ingredients' yet still fail miserably in reaching high levels of skilled play, or more accurately, reach their potential if they don't have accurate understanding of what skilled tennis is and knows what the best methods are in which to achieve them. This is what is meant by "Education" as it applies to potential.

I often see parents tossing tennis balls to their little children, believing that through simple attrition, the kid will somehow develop tennis strokes. Sure, in time anyone will improve the timing in which to make contact with a moving ball. But replication of improper stroke patterns will never result in the sudden acquisition of skilled tennis strokes! But, yet, there seems to be this belief that if I hit enough shots on the ball machine, against the hitting wall, or with a hitting partner, I will eventually become an ATP Tour Professional! Don't bet on it! Chances are, you will at best reach a level of mediocrity and then stagnate there for life!

For if a player truly wishes to become the most skilled level within their true potential, then the strokes and shots a player is working on must address patterns that will not only lead to more advanced play, but they must AVOID patterns that will prohibit the long-term progression and mastery of what the player is capable of doing. (Again, addressing TRUE Player Potential.)

Tennis Mastery is written to help players, a) first learn and understand this dilemma, and b) learn what patterns and methodologies will help them achieve the skill levels they desire, and c) discover the progressions that will allow them to master those patterns and methods in such a way that the player owns them for life. Nothing is more frustrating than knowing one is capable of achievement—but never achieving that which one knows they are capable of.

I hope you find great clarity and insight to this and all elements of this great game of Tennis within these pages!

David W. Smith,
January, 2010

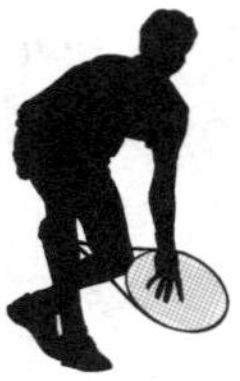

PREFACE

Are you a tennis player who has been stuck at the same level for years? Perhaps even decades? Are you a beginner who does NOT want to become stuck at levels below your potential? If so, you are not alone! There are millions of players who seem to almost spontaneously reach specific levels, usually the 3.0 or 3.5 NTRP levels, then remain entrenched there for the rest of their life. Regardless of your current tennis level, from beginners to the highly skilled, the following question must be asked and then answered correctly: Why do some players move past such levels of play while others must reluctantly resign themselves as mediocre players for life? Surprisingly, the answer is not a lack of athleticism or even a lack of playing experience as many have surmised. Player progression—or lack thereof—can be traced to something more defining and, in my opinion, something that is far more revealing than genetics or opportunity.

About half-way through my nearly 30 years of teaching tennis I became increasingly uncomfortable with the many disparities in the philosophies and methodologies of teaching tennis. Quite frankly, I was concerned that so many below-average tennis players existed, most of whom had been playing the game for many years! This revelation made me question the way tennis was being taught through the various learning mediums: books, videos, and on-court tennis lessons. My observations of thousands of players and how they progressed in tennis-related skills, (or didn't progress!) made me take a very close look at how these players were being introduced to the game. I began an obsessive quest to find answers to four distinct questions:

1. *Why do so many players get stuck at specific NTRP levels (usually the 3.0 or 3.5 levels), and never move on?*
2. *Why do so many players continue to take lessons, read books and watch videos, yet fail to improve?*
3. *Why do so many of these stagnant players still use form associated with beginners even as they continue to play for years?*
4. *Why have so many players quit playing tennis?*

As a physical education instructor and tennis teaching professional, I became interested specifically in the way tennis was being taught compared to virtually all other sports. As I read more books on tennis and listened to fellow professionals in the tennis industry, it became apparent that many in the current tennis-teaching establishment did not necessarily train students in the same teaching philosophy as professionals in other sport did.

The most telling rationale for this discrepancy was the fact that tennis today is being taught "transitionally". Beginning players, when first introduced to the game, often are taught specific introductory techniques that are recognized as ones that must be changed if the player ever hopes to reach any skilled levels. Examples of these transitory methods include basic grips and stroke patterns on the serve and volley that are nothing like that which skilled players use. Such methods are designed to get players "playing tennis" as soon as possible, and yet, the student is instructed that such methods will need to be changed at some point. This process, while simple in its approach, has led to masses of underdeveloped players.

Through books, videos, and professional instruction millions of players have adopted this method of learning or have had it prescribed to them. While such methods can result initially in perceived levels of success by many players, such achievements are not only quite mediocre, but, worse yet, they are almost completely detrimental to any subsequent advancement by the individual. (Which explains why the student is urged to change at some point by the teaching medium!) In a nutshell, such "easy" methods prohibit or, at best, discourage sustainable progression toward recognizable skilled play.

Few sports are taught with such disregard for generally recognized "skilled" methods, methods that will provide the greatest opportunity for player advancement. I know of no other sport where the pedagogy promotes immediate gratification (or "fun" as is often the initial goal!) rather than promoting patterns of learning that are recognized as necessary for developing skilled players.

During the past few decades, there has been a significant shift both by authors of tennis texts and by on-court tennis instructors. Today, many of those of the "tennis authority" favor teaching methods that clearly avoid frustration and that favor the student's immediate ego. "Keep it fun!" This has been the rallying cry of many teaching professionals concerned primarily with not discouraging kids and adults when introducing these students to the game. Unfortunately, proper instruction, (those methods necessary for true player development and progression) frequently takes a back seat to this "fun" concept. In fact, in many tennis environments, "fun" is often all that matters!

But is this really fun?

What I have found is that such a philosophy, one designed to keep students interested through a fun-over-skill methodology, ultimately has had the opposite effect. Most players recognize when they are not progressing or improving. Chasing sprayed balls all over the court, or dinking balls over the net in order to "play tennis," seldom stays fun for anyone…at least not to anyone who wishes to continue his or her improvement!

Much like the criticism of public education, this "dumbing down" of tennis education—providing for the appeasement of egos and avoiding frustration at all costs—has generated millions of mediocre players and millions more who end up quitting the game.

Hitting styles that are initially more manageable and/or comfortable seldom are considered skillful, nor do they lend themselves to progressively more advanced play. The simple avoidance of those techniques that are critical for improvement (but may be perceived as more challenging) is, in my opinion, the main reason why over 20 million tennis players have abandoned the game. (According to various accounts, over the past 30 years, an estimated 22 million tennis players quit playing tennis!) One of the most repeated reasons players quit is: "I just never seem to get better."

Tennis Mastery explores these concepts, both in terms of philosophy as well as methodology. Discover for yourself this examination of tennis and its teachings from a truly coherent and logical point of view. For, if indeed, you are taking the time to read this or any book on tennis, it is safe to assume that you are looking to become a better tennis player. And if this assumption is correct, than it is perhaps even safer to say that you are not looking for a quick fix or some short-lived instant gratification. Instead, you are probably in the market for clear and concise directions. Those directions should be not only directions you can trust, but certainly directions worth your time and effort. I have found that highly skilled tennis is an achievable goal for almost everyone. No one should experience frustration or limited achievement because they were taught a flawed methodology. Through this book you will avoid the common pitfalls that a great number of these frustrated former—and current—players experience while trying to learn the game.

In writing Tennis Mastery, my initial motive was simply to provide tennis enthusiasts with proven tennis methods in which they could accomplish what almost all of the more than 3000 players I have worked with had done: excel at tennis. At the onset of writing Tennis Mastery I didn't believe I was necessarily breaking any new ground or creating something revolutionary through this process. However, during the course of passing on what I had discovered in my 29 years of teaching tennis, I encountered several ideologies which made me question how tennis had been taught and presented to the public in the form of lessons, instructional books, and videos. These questions led to research. And my research led to what you are about to read.

TENNIS METHODS –
VALIDITY THROUGH CRITICAL EVALUATION

In Section One of *Tennis Mastery*, "The Strategies of Learning," I address the issue of why there are so many mediocre tennis players. Roughly, three out of four tennis players reside at the 3.0 – 3.5 NTRP levels. This translates into approximately 9 million tennis players playing tennis at these levels! According to the NTRP scale, these players are considered to be average or below average.

It wasn't the high number of players that exist at these levels that necessarily concerned me. What concerned me was the fact that the vast majority of these players had been playing tennis for years, if not decades! A large portion of these players play regularly, attend clinics, lessons, camps and workshops, or purchase books or videos on tennis, all in an attempt to improve themselves. Yet, even as so many capable players are desperately trying to improve, few of them move out of this level of mediocrity.

I began to question why this was so.

Of the nearly 100 books I personally own on tennis, not one of these books recognizes this phenomenon of player stagnation. Logically, if authors don't recognize the existence of such an occurrence, they certainly can't identify or address issues that contribute to it. Within these pages I will both identify and address the very issues that contribute to this significant problem.

It is in this sense that *Tennis Mastery* is indeed revolutionary.

Tennis Mastery reaches not only beyond this controversial realm of tennis teaching methodology, it clearly redefines the evaluation principles that have been used for decades in determining the validity of specific tennis methods. Obviously, if certain tennis teaching methods are resulting in millions of players languishing at mediocre levels, then players, teachers, and authors must reexamine—and reevaluate—how tennis is being taught. The first step in this endeavor is to examine what evaluation processes are being used in establishing the validity of all tennis teaching and learning methods.

Let me illustrate what I mean by redefining the evaluation concept. Back in 1975, a broadcast featuring W. Timothy Gallwey's best selling *Inner Tennis* was shown on national television. Gallwey demonstrated his Inner Tennis method of learning by teaching a fifty-year-old woman who had never played tennis how to play a "decent" game in only twenty minutes. This was considered quite revolutionary at that time. However, the validity of Gallwey's method is being measured by what I consider "incomplete evaluation".

Gallwey's results raise an important question: did the woman learn a method that would insure steady improvement, (within her means or desire), or did it only offer the momentary gratification of hitting the ball over the net? In other words, does his method offer sustained player improvement or will this woman continue using simple methods of hitting the ball over the net for years using essentially the same technique she was taught in her twenty minute lesson? Simply put, will this woman get better?

This illustration shows that not only do we need to define how we evaluate tennis teaching methods, we need to define what we mean by validity as well. If the results of certain tennis methods produce only immediate success as opposed to long term improvement (and thus greater potential success), then it is clear that those methods are only valid within the context of short-term gratification. If a player who is taking lessons is only seeking immediate gratification and could care less about their tennis-playing future, then those methods that produce only short-term achievements would indeed be valid (and could be evaluated as successful within this criterion as well). However, if those same methods fail to produce continuous improvement and progressive development within a player's ability, they would certainly not be valid in terms of long-term gratification. If we are seeking to provide methods that provide the greatest long-term progression and player potential, we then must evaluate any process of learning within this framework of validity—and not anything short of that.

To determine if any one particular teaching method is undeniably valid within the context of long-term gratification, the method must provide for continued improvement by the student within the means of that student. If we are considering Gallwey's method successful because the woman being taught was able to hit the ball over the net in the general direction in which she was aiming, we are missing a much bigger picture. Would we still consider his method successful if the woman continued to play tennis for twenty years and was unable to do much more than she did in her twenty-minute lesson? Obviously not. However, if the woman took the knowledge and skills gained from such a lesson and was able to improve steadily towards highly recognized tennis skills, then I would evaluate Gallwey's methods as not only successful, but also truly revolutionary!

Something more than just immediate gratification must be used to measure the validity of any teaching method. These processes or methods of instruction, which only focus on producing immediate gratification, have perpetuated a host of charlatan instructors and authors who promise everything from quick fixes to perfect backhands in less than thirty minutes! I don't mean to insinuate these people intentionally have tried to deceive the tennis playing public. However, either through ignorance, arrogance, incomplete research, poor interpretation of investigative results, limited on-court teaching experience, or simply turning a blind-eye to statistical results, many tennis "authorities" have cost hundreds of thousands of players, if not millions, the possible opportunity to play significantly better tennis through such fallible teaching methods. Why? Because they used methods that provided only short-term gratification. They failed to provide long-term progressive improvement within the context of their teaching methods.

Certainly, players need to feel a sense of improvement and accomplishment throughout the learning process. However, we must be very careful of how we satisfy our human need for such gratification through methodologies that sacrifice our long-term success—and greater satisfaction—of becoming a skilled tennis player. (If that is what we are looking to become.)

With all this said, it is not to be construed that books such as Gallwey's *Inner Game of Tennis*, and other notable tennis texts, are void of valuable information. On the contrary, it is my intention to provide you with such a clear understanding of tennis that you will gain a great deal more out of such books after you have read *Tennis Mastery*.

A BETTER WAY TO LEARN

Section Two of *Tennis Mastery* deals with the very essence of hitting a tennis ball. My methodology is unique and, perhaps, revolutionary in its presentation. I wanted to provide players with more than just conceptual phrasing and instructional tips. When I reviewed all the books I had on tennis, they all offered what I call "big picture" information. Tennis is best learned when players can associate specific body positions within the context of each stroke. This same process is used in teaching the world's finest golfers and it is a process that I have used to train thousands of beginners into becoming truly skilled tennis players. I use what I call "Key Position Points" to illustrate and identify specific body parts and their location in relation to several physical components: the body, the racket, the ball, and the court. When players learn this process, they not only are able to identify these same key positions when they hit the ball, they can identify these same positions when they watch quality players playing tennis as well. Tennis is no longer a "blur" on television to observers who learn these methods. When watching the pros, you will be able to discern these same key position points in their game after your understanding of *Tennis Mastery*.

In relation to simple everyday movements and movements we associate with mediocre tennis form, quality tennis strokes are quite complex. Consider a complete beginner, who knows nothing about tennis, attempting to hit a ball while standing at the net. Typically, such a player will hold the racket in front of them like a policeman attempting to stop traffic. They face the oncoming ball with their body square to the net, and push the racket at the ball in the intended direction—not exactly what we associate with accomplished form! Obviously, players who have had experience in other sports that utilize mechanics similar to proper tennis form will probably be more refined than in this example. In any case, such a novice player will continue to execute volleys in essentially this same fashion unless something makes this player realize there is a better way. This discovery can be accomplished through trial and error, (if the player recognizes inadequacies in his form), or it can be through a learning process such as that offered through tennis lessons, books, or videos. Or, players can oftentimes discover proper form from watching good tennis players playing tennis. For every student the quality of the results of such a learning process is obviously dependent upon the quality of the information received or perceived. For example, a player who looks for and is able to identify key positions and mechanics by the pros on television will have a much greater chance of emulating these moves when they take to the courts. One of the problems when beginners take group lessons with other beginners is they have little to emulate in terms of proper strokes. I have found that when beginners are put in a group lesson with better players, the beginner improves at a faster rate than those who are only in a group of other beginners do. The reason for this is simple: they are seeing how others, who have some of the aspects of skilled strokes, hit the ball over and over in drills. The beginners see what tennis actually "looks" like!

Once we are provided quality information, there are other variables that will also have a bearing on these results. Is the player willing to apply the information offered? Is the player willing to practice? Does the player understand how the techniques will help them? As you can see, learning tennis is definitely a partnership between student and instructional entity. If the instructional information is indeed correct, the student must take ownership and responsibility in using and working within those techniques.

Perhaps most importantly, the student must be confident that the information being given is not only appropriate, but it must also be accurate. In other words, the student must be secure that the techniques taught and being practiced will produce the greatest potential for the desired results. The techniques I am offering throughout the technique portion of this book are based on my Advanced Foundation concept and progressive principles procured through nearly thirty years of testing. These concepts will provide you with the confidence of knowing that mediocrity is not an option! One thing is promised: you will not be taught methods that will need to be changed as you progress!

If a player knows for certain that the methods they are learning will insure progressive development, (as opposed to transitory methods that must be abandoned at some point), they generally attack learning more aggressively. Nothing is more deflating to an individual than the prospect of having to learn a new method after spending significant time learning an inferior method first!

STRATEGY OF PLAYING: FROM BASIC TO WORLD-CLASS... A CONTINUOUS EVOLUTION

Section Three is the application of the strokes and mechanics you have learned: The Strategy of Playing. A player must be able to take the proper hitting form learned and be able to apply it to the game itself. From the most basic of strategy, such as getting the ball over the net and in the court, to the highest levels of advanced play, tennis players will need tools to ingrain the execution of effective and strategic shots in competition.

Tennis is a game. As such, when players become more accomplished in their ability to hit the ball, the game takes on new and more complex strategies. Imagine how the simplistic strategy of a beginner who is just concerned with getting the ball over the net compares with that of advanced players who are capable of hitting every shot in the book! Drop shots, passing shots, topspin lobs, angle volleys, kick serves, and penetrating groundstrokes all add to the increasingly complex patterns of strategy players will need to address when other aspects of their game have improved. (And when they play better opponents!)

Included in these strategies are methods that allow players to perform at their best in competition. As players begin executing higher levels of shot-making skills, the risk of making mistakes grows proportionately. These risks sometimes transform a player's ability to think, to react, and to execute correctly. We use words like mental, choke, zone, unconscious, tank, and others to describe the mental condition and the results from mental strengths and weaknesses players exhibit in the heat of competition. Becoming a champion in any sport requires a conditioned mind as well as body. Tennis is certainly no exception.

THE EVOLUTION OF TENNIS – INTRODUCTION TO CHANGE

It is an important concept in the learning of tennis that all students understand both the historical changes that have transformed the modern game of tennis, as well as the origin of these changes. The "when" is not as important as the "why" in terms of true stroke development. However, if we are talking about true *player development*, it serves appropriately to understand just how the "when" is indeed connected to the "why."

The game has gone through many evolutionary changes, especially in the last thirty years. Taking the knowledge developed from the understanding of these changes onto the practice court and eventually into the competitive arena will help all players reach ultimate levels of performance.

Since this book deals with the controversial realm of tennis teaching philosophies and methodologies, I would be remiss not to discuss the concept of change and the source or inspiration that have contributed to these changes over time. In fact, the evolution of tennis is the perfect preface to a book that proposes significant change in the learning processes associated with tennis teaching. I hope you not only agree, but will find the following an interesting and enlightening beginning to playing far better tennis.

The Evolution of Tennis
ANALYZING THE CONCEPTS THAT HAVE TRANSFORMED TENNIS INTO TODAY'S MODERN GAME

Within fine arts the rhetorical question "does art imitate life or does life imitate art?" is often made in reference to discussing life situations. A similar question can initiate dialogue among those of us in the tennis world:

> *"Does the evolution of tennis imitate individual style or does individual style imitate tennis evolution?"*

In other words, has the game of tennis evolved due to the influence of individuals, or have evolutionary changes over time influenced the play of individuals?

Historical "Road Map"

I think most of us would agree that both sentiments have collectively contributed to the game's influence. And if both aspects of this evolutionary question ring true, then it would be both interesting and informative to analyze how each concept has indeed, contributed to the modern game of tennis. (And perhaps at the same time, provide us with a historical "road map" to what we hope will guide us to better play ourselves!)

Certainly, tennis has changed over the generations of play. That statement is a given. The question of how, or more specifically, why changes have taken place is subject to a wide range of circumstances, personal interpretation, and opinion. However, interpretations and opinions are usually based on observable facts. (At least objective interpretations and opinions are!) Thus, it is important to look for foundations in tennis lore that can substantiate stakes of claimed opinions and conclusions.

Can certain strategies of play, from hitting techniques to actual strategic disciplines, be directly attributed specifically to any individuals? If imitation is the ultimate form of flattery, it stands to reason that those who are admired would generate multitudes of participants who would strive to mimic these champions. In golf, the commercially driven phrase "I AM Tiger Woods" hammers home this point emphatically! However, there are instances where the game's evolution prevents or discourages players from following in the footsteps of recognized champions. An example of this can be seen in the methodology of all-time great Pete Sampras. Even as he was labeled as a "modern day Jack Kramer," there are few players emulating Pete's serve-and-volley strategy. Certainly we can identify a few: Australian Patrick Rafter and Briton's Tim Henman come to mind. Yet, these players were not necessarily followers of Sampras…for the most part, they were adversaries in the same era as Sampras. Currently, American Taylor Dent is emerging as a true Serve and Volley player in today's modern game. Few players have emerged as true "net-attackers" as these champions were characterized a short time ago.

Certainly, if such champions of the game generated few followers, what are some of the other driving forces shaping the sport of tennis today? What has shaped the sport in the past?

It is true that tennis has seen substantial changes over time. These changes include shifts in general stroke methodology preference and dominance (from one-handed backhands to two, slice groundstrokes to topspin, touch and finesse to power) to changes in playing strategies (from chip-and-charge to serve-and-volley to baseline supremacy). In addition, changes in manufacturing technology—from shoe improvements to innovative racket construction and design — have added to the mix of tennis change.

The question again is why have such changes occurred?

Part 1: Evolution of Tennis Strokes

Arguably the greatest observable change in tennis has been the pervasive shift from the use of one-handed backhands to two. In fact, I can't think of another sport that has seen such a radical change in a major technical component. Perhaps the closest comparisons I can relate it to would be the crossover grip now used by many while putting in golf or the historical Fosbury Flop innovation for high jumping developed back in 1969 by Dick Fosbury. (Fig 1)

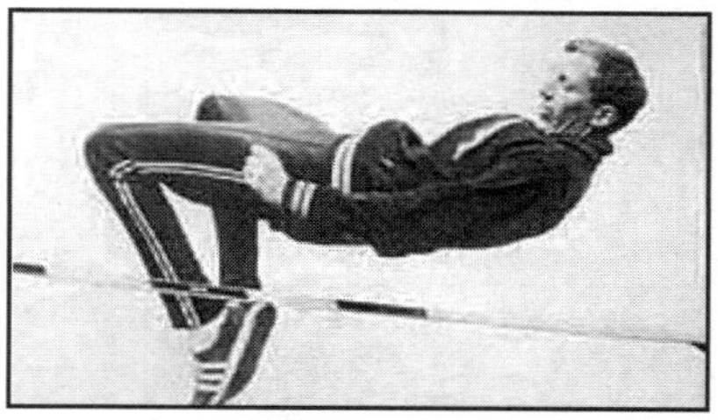

Figure 1
Dick Fosbury literally changed the direction of high jumping in the late 1960's.

It is interesting in studying the evolution of the two-handed backhand that prior to the early 1970's the stroke did not gain any significant attention. It took nearly 100 years—from the time tennis was invented in 1874 until the early 1970's—before the stroke even began gaining acceptance! Considering that other sports that utilize two-handed swing patterns—namely golf, baseball, cricket and hockey—have been around essentially for as long as tennis, it is amazing that top players did not emerge with the shot until the 1970's. (I suppose that the influence of badminton and that sport's wrist-induced, single-handed swing patterns played a role in stroke development early in the history of tennis.)

Those leading the transformation of the two-handed backhand use include Bjorn Borg and Jimmy Connors on the men's side, Chris Evert and Tracy Austin on the women's side. However, it would take essentially another three decades before the two-handed backhand would be seen as a dominant choice of both men and women's pro tours. Of course, historically it stands to reason that if very few players used the stroke in the first place, even fewer pros would be inclined to teach the stroke to beginners. Today, most all players who take lessons are introduced to the two-handed backhand due to the now-recognized inherent qualities that two hands create when learning the stroke. And with so many role models executing the shot today it is easy to see how the current trend is continually being fueled!

Perhaps what triggered this transformation of the backhand was the recognized need for greater topspin. Interestingly, however, Borg adapted his backhand from the slap shot he used in playing hockey as a child and Evert was never encouraged to hit two-handed from her father/coach, and teaching pro, Jimmy Evert! It would seem that in both of these cases, neither player developed the two-handed backhand through any purposeful motive except circumstance! However, if topspin was indeed a factor, than ultimately we can look back to the development of Rod Laver's heavy topspin groundstrokes as a precursor to such a backhand. Although Laver hit a one-handed backhand, his formidable use of topspin on both sides inspired the use of such spin in the subsequent strokes of those who followed. Bud Collins, in his book *Bud Collins' Tennis Encyclopedia*, said this about Laver's influence: "Although others had used topspin, Laver may have inspired a wave of heavy-hitting topspin practitioners of the 1970's such as Bjorn Borg and

Guillermo Vilas. The stroke became basic after Laver."

If the identification of topspin was a desirable attribute for players looking for greater stroke effectiveness, then certainly science, and more specifically physics, have played a part in our evolutionary continuum. Consciously or otherwise, players—beginning with Laver, perhaps—began exploring ways to induce greater power through added topspin. This exploration certainly can explain the rise of more topspin-orientated grips such as semi-western and full western grips on the forehand and the use of the Eastern backhand grip for one-handed backhands. (Plus the influx of two-handed backhands as stated above.) Recognizing that greater topspin not only created greater downward arc of a tennis ball into the court on groundstrokes and thus more potential controllable power, players began to utilize this same spin to create greater angles on their groundstrokes, opening up geometric opportunities on the court like never before. Inside-out forehands and backhands, severe crosscourt angles, and dipping angled passing shots are now a regular commodity among most top players.

Conversely, if there were any shots that have remained un-compromised and essentially unchanged in terms of form, power, effectiveness and control over the historical context of tennis strokes, it would have to be the forehand and backhand slice. Unlike its topspin counterpart, there are limitations based on physical laws of motion that preclude the slice from being hit beyond these certain physical restrictions. In other words, the slice stroke can only be hit so hard before it can't possibly land in the opponent's court. On the other hand, topspin, in theory, can be hit harder and harder as long as the amount of topspin counters the forward velocity of the ball. Many of the past champions of tennis have acknowledged that this demarcation between groundstroke technique represents the greatest historical change in tennis. It is easy to examine this very fact. Watch pros today when they hit the slice. You will NEVER see a pro attempt to hit the slice with the amount of force exerted as they often do with a topspin groundstroke!

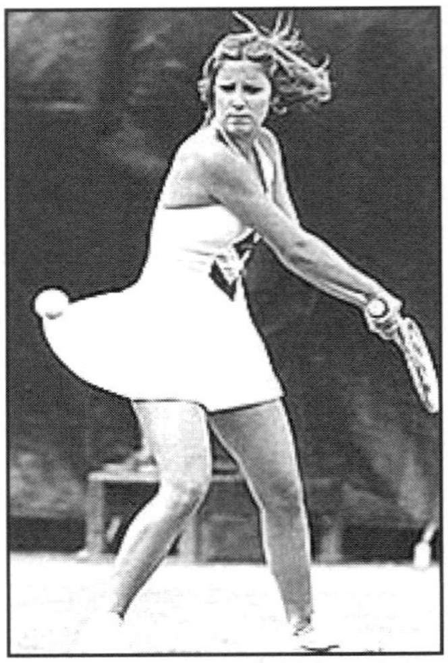

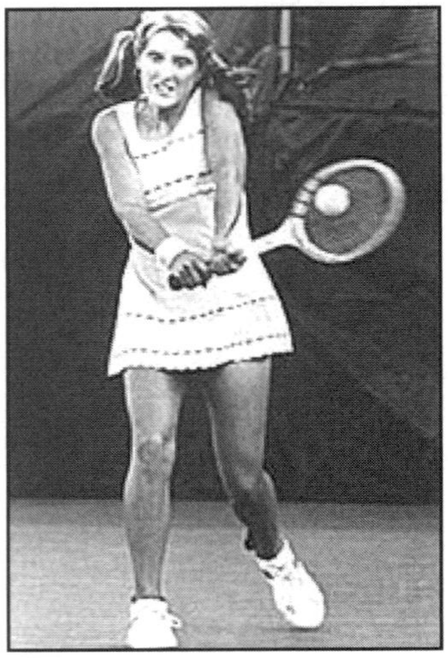

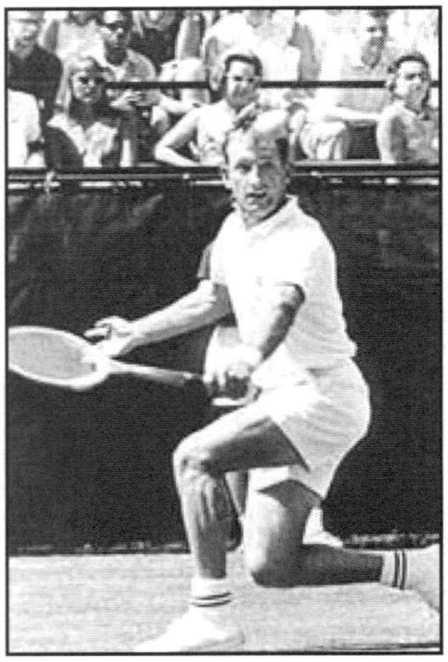

Figures 2, 3 & 4
Chris Evert, Tracy Austin and Rod Laver were all instrumental in creating significant changes in the modern game.

Perhaps more than any stroke, the serve has witnessed changes in speed and effectiveness more recently due to the advent of technologically advanced equipment. Although there have been past notable tennis champions who possessed relatively powerful serves, (Bill Tilden, Pancho Gonzalez, and Lew Hoad of historical significance, and Stan Smith and Roscoe Tanner a short generation ago), there seems to be much greater service dominance by a plethora of players in today's modern game. Presently, we even see women professionals serving at 120 miles per hour…a feat unimaginable twenty years ago! It raises the question of just how good the players of the past could have served if they were afforded today's space-age rackets. Obviously, greater strength training, conditioning and, perhaps conquering psychological speed barriers, have contributed to the increases of speed we have seen in the modern serve as well.

Finally, the two-handed forehand is making similar revolutionary strides in popularity that the two-handed backhand experienced back in the 1970's. Certainly not as prevalent yet, (because of the still-favorable mechanics for many players executing decent topspin with only one hand), the two-handed forehand is growing in popularity especially among the junior ranks. Even as Pancho Segura showed what a weapon it could be back in the 1940's, it didn't raise any eyebrows until the 1990's when Monica Seles utilized the stroke in becoming the number one women's player in the world in 1991. Even then, it seemed more of a fluke occurrence, with few players, especially men, trying the shot. Even today, few tennis instructors know how to teach the shot with confidence, precision and proper mechanics. However, similar to the historical rise of the two-handed backhand, the two-handed forehand is gaining acceptance. With American Jan Michael Gambill and France's Fabrice Santoro demonstrating its use on the men's professional tour and Monica Seles' continued longevity on the women's tour, the two-handed forehand is destined to make its intelligible mark on the evolving game of tennis. Today, significant crops of talented juniors are using the stroke with international success.

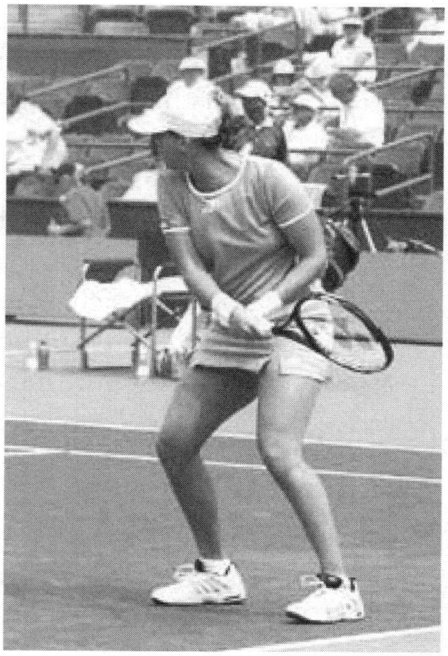

Figure 5
Monica Seles showed that the two-handed forehand could be a weapon on the professional tour.

In addition to evolutionary changes in strokes, the game has seen almost equally extraordinary changes in strategy.

Part 2: The Evolution of Tennis Strategies

Like it or not, the game of tennis has changed over its historical course. Some say for the better, others say for the worse. Certainly the game's general popularity has seen several highs and lows over time. Some rationalize that the game's shifting popularity is based on many of these evolutionary changes...namely, changes in power and, consequently, changes in strategy. Specifically, there seems to be a split among tennis enthusiasts. On one side, there are those who favor the "old school" strategies, strategies that were predominately centered on slices, finesse shots, approach shots and volleys. On the other side are those who favor the more modern game of powerful serves and groundstrokes interlaced with volleys, drops and angles.

I have received passionate pleas from individuals favoring a return to "traditional" strategies of the game, namely chip-and-charge offensive game plans or serve-and-volley strategies. The greatest complaint I have heard expressed is the lack of interesting points, especially in men's tennis. Certainly, over the course of the last ten or fifteen years men's tennis has evolved into a serve-fest, with many points being determined quickly, usually with a potent serve and an occasional volley or groundstroke winner or forced error. However, over the last couple years it appears that the effectiveness of the return-of-serve has caught up to that of the serve, allowing the game to evolve back into points that include rallies, exciting ones at that! Indeed, even on fast surfaces such as the grass at Wimbledon, rallies once again are, in many cases, becoming the norm as opposed to the exception. Even with big servers like Sampras, Roddick, Safin, and Ivanisevic, the rallies at Wimbledon and other Grand Slam events have become longer and more exciting over the last couple years.

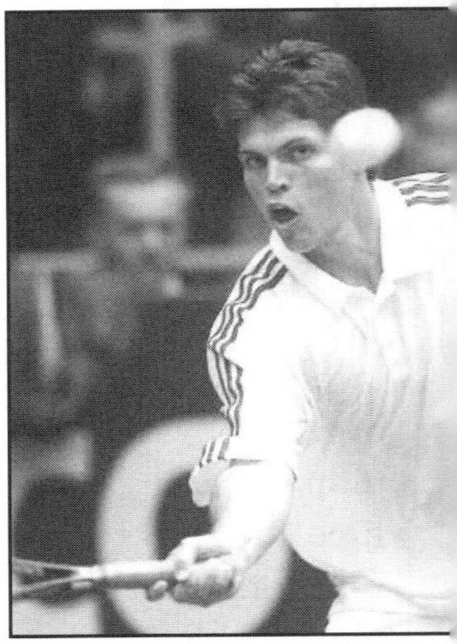

Figures 6 & 7
Players like Taylor Dent (above) and Pete Sampra (below) are net attacking strategists, always looking come to the net.

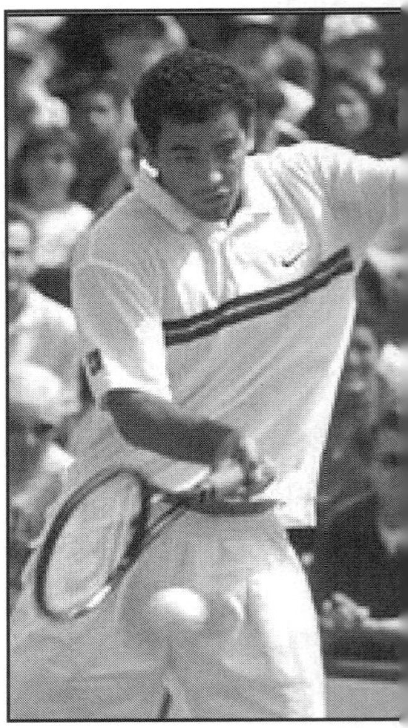

However, the game today is played decidedly differently than that of the days of old. Today's longer rallies, just described, include a barrage of incredibly powerful groundstrokes and-serves,spectacular topspin angles, and displays of incredible athleticism and conditioning by current performers. Subsequently, the strategy of the game has changed from the days of old 'chip and charge' preference to a more resolute game of cat and mouse played between players who possess weapons of mass destruction!

It can be argued that the development of topspin on groundstrokes is the root of tennis evolution. Players who wanted more power needed a technique that helped to keep more powerful shots in play. Of course, the answer to that problem was topspin. Understanding the physics of spin can help us understand the how and why of changes in tennis strategies.

The advent and propagation of greater topspin on groundstrokes has had a significant impact on how the game is played, especially by highly skilled performers. While topspin groundstrokes have continued to be more effective weapons among most skilled players over the course of the last couple decades, the "traditional" shot-of-choice, the slice, has seen virtually no change in its presentation for perhaps one hundred years. As I have mentioned, the simple physics of the slice makes it almost impervious to the kind of changes we have seen associated with topspin shots.

Specifically, how has this consequential shift in groundstroke preference led to the changes in tennis strategy? Before we can address this question, we must clearly identify what those strategies are.

STRATEGIES OF TENNIS

We must identify the various basic playing strategies of tennis before we can correctly identify the how and why of strategic evolution. There are really two basic strategies: Attacking and retrieving.

Attacking strategies include two distinct tactics:

•*Serve and volley*
•*Chip and charge*

Many players of the past executed game plans that revolved around these two strategies. Male players of historical significance who have favored these strategies include Fred Perry, Jack Kramer, Pancho Gonzalez, Don Budge, Ken Rosewall, and Rod Laver. Traditionally, women did not attack the net as often nor with as much aggression as the men. It really wasn't until the late 1960's and early 70's that Billie Jean King and compatriot Rosie Casals demonstrated that women, too, could be aggressive net players. King, Casals, the Brit Virgina Wade, Australian Evonne Goolagong and especially Martina Navratilova were some of the women who set the stage for others to play a more aggressive, all-court style of play.

Certainly, a host of champions have utilized this attacking strategy within the past three decades. Perhaps beginning with Stan Smith, players like John McEnroe, Ivan Lendl, Arthur Ashe and Stefan Edberg led the way for the likes of Pete Sampras, Boris Becker, Patrick Rafter and Tim Henman to make their marks as aggressive net-seeking attackers.

Players camping out at the baseline generally characterize the more defensive or "retrieving" style of play. While playing this "waiting game", these defensive players typically wait for their opponents to make a mistake. Notable players who have successfully utilized this game plan include Bjorn Borg, Michael Chang, Chris Evert, and Tracy Austin. Even a young Andre Agassi played a decisively baseline game.

STRATEGIES TODAY

It is important to recognize that today, top players possess such massive topspin groundstrokes that they often make playing the baseline an aggressive "attacking" game in itself! Never has there been so much power addressed to balls from behind the baseline. In my opinion, this power from the backcourt has brought about the greatest change in player strategies.

Tactics: Topspin versus Slice

As I have mentioned, topspin mechanics have taken on new levels of offensiveness. Conversely, the slice has remained essentially unchanged over time. Thus, a new respect has emerged for a baseline opponent anytime a player decides to come to the net. It becomes ever so clear that the evolution of tennis has moved away from the dominant net-attacking strategies of the past into a methodical dissection of opponents through the weaponry of imposing groundstrokes. Certainly, when players get their opponents in trouble through a course of such spin-related power mixed with geometric placements, they will quite often take the net for the anticipated volley winner they so richly deserve. Today we see far less often the use of the slice being utilized strictly as an approach shot. The slice is still used among most all players—including two-handed backhanders who use one hand in most cases—as both a defensive stroke as well as a change-of-pace ploy. However, as the power and accuracy of groundstrokes and passing shots continue to intensify, the specific net-attacking-only strategies of the past are becoming a liability for those who use attempt them.

Today's "All-Court" Game

Simply playing a retrieving singles strategy, where players hang out at the baseline and engage in a slugfest of groundstrokes, has proven to be somewhat limiting among many players. Much like playing a strategy that consists predominately of serve-and-volley or chip-and-charge points, hanging back, hitting groundstrokes almost exclusively has become less successful in today's professional arena. I remember watching how uncomfortable past baseline players became anytime they approached the net. Not so long ago, Michael Chang looked like a fish out of water when forced to come up and volley. Ivan Lendl liked to stay back with patience and topspin as his main issue of weaponry. He, too, did not look comfortable during times he would approach the net until a little later in his career. Ironically, even as Chang developed a respectable net game as his career proceeded, he never gained the kind of success he enjoyed when he was strictly a baseline retriever.

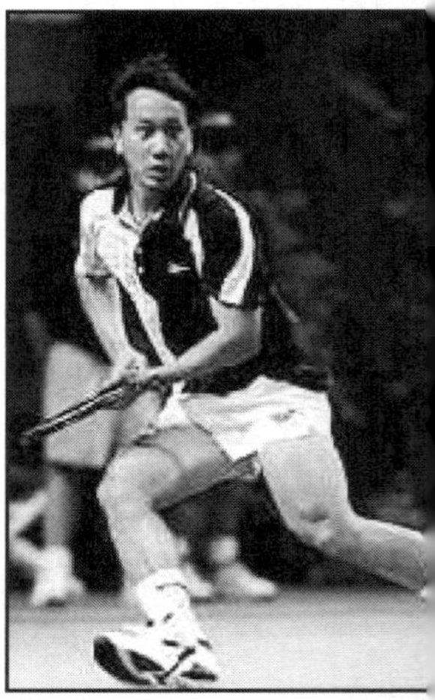

Notwithstanding, the vast majority of men and women tour professionals today play a more identifiable "all-court" game as demonstrated by superior groundstrokes opening up the court for an, oftentimes, formidable volley winner. These volley winners often occur after a chess-like series of precision-guided groundstrokes between players. Few champions of today's modern game have been able to conquer without some mastery of all the weapons available.

In many cases, these heavy-handed topspin groundstrokes force a point to end even before a weak shot is parlayed into a winning volley. Thus, many people might consider these strategies as a "baseline-only" contest when in fact it is a constant battle of respect and confidence between very skilled performers, most of which can play the whole court with expertise.

Figures 8 & 9
Michael Chang (above
and Bjorn Borg (below
are considered to be
"retrievers." Both playe
rely on steely concentr
tion in patience.

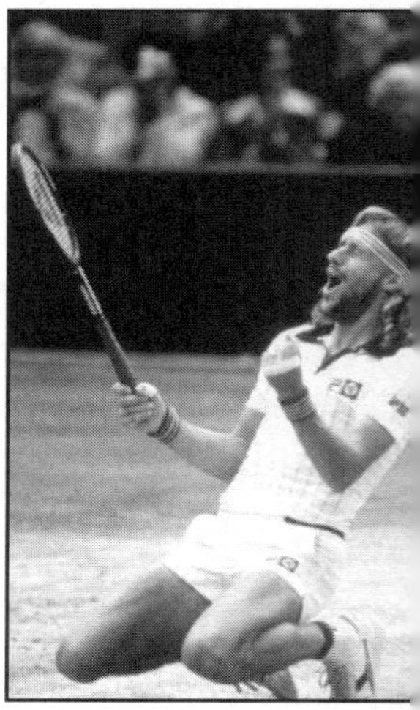

Opening the Door

Skilled tennis players exist in many arenas. Most observers can recognize them easily. A 5.5 club player plays with similar style and mechanics of a 7.0 pro. A top-ranked 12 year-old will often resemble a world-class adult in terms of strokes. While there are a few exceptions, most high-level players play within strategies and stroke mechanics that closely resemble each other. Even among the diversity of stroke idiosyncrasies seen among pros, the "foundation" that ALL pros and skilled players possess are virtually identical. Regardless of whether you are using a one-handed backhand or two, an Eastern forehand grip or western, the foundation of all strokes is essentially the same. At the same time, within this foundation there are specific patterns of play and of stroke methodology that can be clearly recognized as skilled or proficient. Even more obvious are strokes and form clearly associated as mediocre, novice and just plain ugly!

Tennis Mastery is designed to teach you, train you, and prepare you for playing at the highest level possible within your own particular goals and desires. Think of this book as a key, one that opens a door not to incessant tennis mediocrity, but to successful and continual tennis achievements. Imagine a lifetime of tennis enjoyment at the highest possible *personal* level. Not only is this possible, it is attainable by virtually all that seek it.

Section One

The Strategies of Learning

A person's ability to play tennis skillfully is greatly determined by the player's understanding of the processes related to learning and developing what I call the "Advanced Foundation". In this chapter and the following five chapters in this first section you will learn the secrets of skilled player-development based on this concept. From the clear understanding of the Advanced Foundation and its subsequent philosophy of learning to off-court preparation and on-court practice concepts, you will learn how the finest players in the world approach, study, and develop advanced tennis skills. In addition, you will learn why so many players fail to reach their potential while a seemingly select few reach accomplished levels of play. I will show you that highly skilled tennis is a most achievable goal for virtually all that seek to play it at such a level.

Take the time to open your eyes to some very compelling revelations and learn what steps you will want to take in your quest for TENNIS MASTERY!

CHAPTER 1

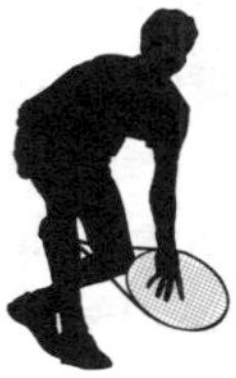

The Advanced Foundation – A NEW Philosophy of Learning

Two Classes of Tennis Players (Which are you? Or, which will you become?)

Tennis, perhaps more than any other sport, has two distinct "classes" of players: in one court there are those who progressively improve and reach what is generally recognized as "accomplished" or "skilled" levels of play. On the other side of our proverbial net are those who learn basic skills, then promptly stagnate at a particular ability level, usually at the 3.0 or 3.5 NTRP levels. (To those just starting out, the NTRP—National Tennis Rating Program—levels go from a 1.0 beginner to a 7.0 professional.) To the untrained eye or to an inexperienced individual this distinction or realization of specifically two classes may be difficult to recognize. However, it can't be argued that there are countless tennis players who have played for years, if not decades, who have *not improved* past the 3.0 or 3.5 level! Of the 12 million tennis players in the United States more than three-quarters of them reside perpetually at the 3.0 or 3.5 levels or below. This statement is not meant to offend anyone or insinuate that players at these levels are incapable of playing high-level tennis. On the contrary, it is my intention to prove that virtually all players, including those who currently reside at the 3.0 or 3.5 levels, are indeed perfectly capable of playing higher levels of tennis... much higher!

This distinction of two classes of players has created an identifiable vernacular within tennis circles. Players refer to "The Big Four-O (4.0 NTRP level)" as being a major stepping stone, a hurdle one needs to vault in order to be recognized as a skilled player. Countless 3.5 level players spend millions of dollars each year in search of ways in which they can "break through" this 3.5 barricade. The question is why do some break through while others have to resign themselves as "mediocre" for life? (With the NTRP levels starting at 1.0 and topping out at 7.0, the levels 3.0 and 3.5 are technically considered below average on this scale. Because so many players are stuck at these levels, many consider these levels to be "average"!)

Many variables can account for such stagnation including lack of desire, lack of natural athleticism, limited playing opportunities, or a lack of available tennis information. However, it is interesting to recognize that the majority of these players who stopped

The Question is: Why to some break through while others resign themselves as "mediocre" for life ?

improving did indeed have similar desires, adequate athleticism, an access to tennis information, and similar playing opportunities of those who continued to improve. If these things are indeed similar between our two classes of players, what factor can be identified as the decisive divergent mechanism? If all things are considered equal, then the answer becomes quite evident. The only recognizable variable, which in this case is indeed a variable, is INFORMATION!

To date, most books, videos, and tennis instructors, for that matter, have never approached nor identified this phenomenon in which some players top out at such levels while others are seen continuously improving through much of their career. A simple explanation proposed by such authors and instructors would be that players in general simply have a varying propensity for the sport. However, this explanation falls short when we consider that even tremendous athletes and players dedicated to learning the game often are seen permanently stuck at our pivotal 3.0 and 3.5 levels.

The existence of such a phenomenon again poses the serious question of "Why?" Anyone who is attempting to play this game and those who professionally teach the sport must recognize that this discrepancy between these two classes exists. Once it is recognized, then one must address this issue in terms of deciding what processes are inherent to continued improvement. If certain techniques, strategies, and/or form contribute to this division of performance, (whether it comes from a self-help book, a video, an instructor, or a helpful friend), then it stands to reason that players will want to avoid those methods which are a deterrent in terms of progress. Obviously, players who want to reach those levels deemed "accomplished or skilled" would want to work within the bounds of those methods that are considered conducive to sustained improvement.

The second big question is of course, WHAT are those methods that will lead players to the world of high-level competitive tennis? That is what this book is all about!

Why Have 22 MILLION Tennis Players Quit Playing Tennis?

This is a most amazing statistic. In the mid seventies, there were around 34 million tennis players in the U.S., according to surveys conducted then by the A. C. Nielsen Company. In 2002, the United States Tennis Association, (USTA) estimates that there were only 12 million tennis players. How can a sport lose over half its player base in only thirty years? In addition, this year (2003) it was estimated by the USTA that 5 million players picked up the game while during the same period another 5 million players quit. These figures demonstrate an obvious problem with player retention.

According to several surveys done recently by such organizations as the United States Professional Tennis Association (USPTA) and the USTA, one of the responses by those who quit playing tennis regularly was the lack of personal progression. Players simply found themselves not being able to move past those levels associated with mediocre play. Thus many found themselves playing a sport that seemed "too hard to improve at". If my perceptions have any validity, then it would become quite obvious that some of the methods in which tennis is being taught (or the processes which players are learning the game) are some of the leading causes of this significant shift in the sport's popularity. Of course, there are many other issues that one can argue which may play a role in this shift as well. Lack of charismatic professionals, poor programming and support by national and local tennis promoting and governing bodies, other sports' rise in popularity such as golf and soccer, and other factors certainly have contributed to the decline of the sport's attraction. I happen to agree that these factors or situations have contributed a significant degree as well to the sport's poor participation levels in recent years.

However, the underlying concept to player participation (or lack thereof) on a personal level include two defining idioms: 1. Player self-perception, and 2. Player progression. These two issues, connected as they are, have a far greater impact on continued player participation then all the other faults in any other tennis entity or stratagem.

How can a sport lose over half its active player base in only thirty years

?

Tennis has lost approximately 22,000,000 tennis players in the past 30 years

!

PLAYER SELF-PERCEPTION

How we see ourselves as individuals is revealed within the perceived performance of the things we do. Our jobs, our relationships, our hobbies, our recreations, all help mold our self-perceptions. Regardless of what others may think of us, how we ourselves perceive our performance in these daily procedures helps develop our personal impression of ourselves. In sports, especially, we usually compare ourselves in two ways: Perceived Performance and Performance Outcome. If we know we have really ugly strokes in tennis but can beat our regular playing buddy, we can have a pretty good—but subjective—self-perception due to a successful Performance Outcome. We may or may not recognize that our actual Performance is appalling! However, if we start playing against others more skilled than ourselves, not only do we recognize just how dreadful our strokes might be, but such players might just thump us in the process! Not only is our "Perceived Performance" dreadful, our "Performance Outcome" is certainly not that which we would prefer as well!

It is amazing for me to watch two beginners' progress within this concept. One player is really working hard to develop skilled strokes, the other simply hacks and dinks balls with unrefined and unspecific form and technique. Usually, the dinker wins hands down during early competitive matches against such disciplined students. But in time, the player developing skilled strokes starts winning…and winning big. And soon, the dinker doesn't like to call the skilled player up to play anymore. (And for that matter, the skilled player could care less about playing the dinker anyway!) I have seen this occur many times in

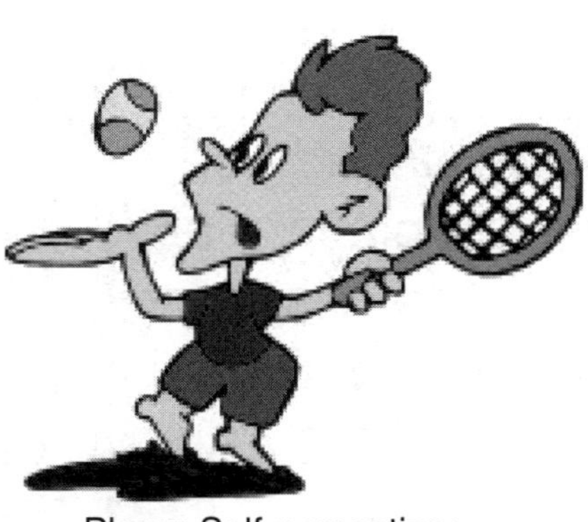

Player Self-perception:
How we perceive our abilities can be far different than what is actually achieved.

the course of my years of teaching tennis. The conclusion: The dinker eventually quits the game while the skilled player not only continues to improve, but he or she finds the sport continuously more exciting, challenging, and thus, rewarding!

PLAYER PROGRESSION

Our second evaluation of personal player participation is the recognition of player progression. Many players will play for years and even take lessons regularly in hopes to see some essence of improvement. If the perception of individual progression is not satisfied, players will eventually lose interest. Just like any endeavor, if the participant sees no real value, results, or chance for improvement, they will likely withdraw completely and find something else to take up their time.

Through these two concepts we can see why millions of active tennis players have indeed quit the game in the past 30 years!

Foundation Building

If we learn to type on a keyboard with just our two index fingers, and proceed to type in this fashion for years, it will be very difficult to learn to type fast with any semblance of accuracy. When we do decide to improve our typing skills through training and the use of proper technique, overcoming the urge to type with our two index fingers will be difficult. Consider a piano student who is learning to play the piano. Would any qualified instructor consider teaching the beginning student by finger-pecking with only his or her index fingers? Perhaps, if the student only had two fingers!

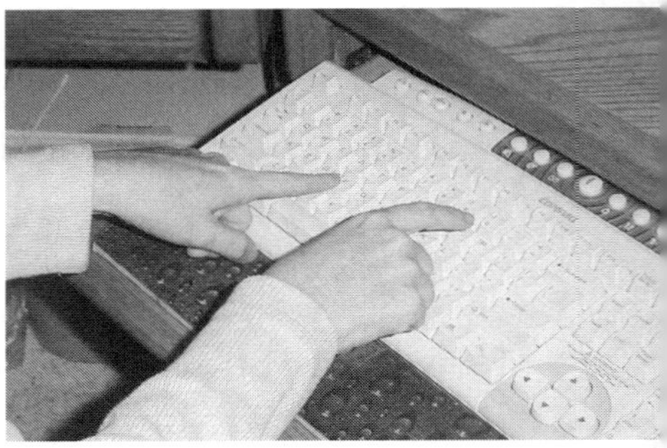

Figure 1
"Hunt and peck." A slow way to type.
This method of typing won't produce
a skilled typist.

Generally, people who have not had any training in playing the piano or typing on a keyboard will try to peck out the keys on both instruments with only their index fingers. Even as they know that this will not lead to mastering either device, they will not have the understanding or the training in using all their fingers in a well-coordinated or skilled fashion. Thus, people who wish to learn these instruments in the manner they were intended, (or in a manner deemed skillful) will need to learn how to coordinate their fingers in a well-defined technique.

Thousands of tennis players are taught tennis using a "Hunt & Peck" method of learning !

The pattern in which a person learns this technique is created in what we call a proper learning foundation. It would not serve the student well in either of these two examples to begin the learning process by pecking out the keys with only their two index fingers! The first thing taught in any piano lesson or typing class is "home" position for all the fingers. This is obviously the first step in building a proper foundation to playing the piano or typing on a keyboard...a proper foundation that incorporates all the fingers. This type of methodology—that which will lead to skillful development in any technical endeavor—is what I refer to as the "Advanced Foundation."

Like learning to play the piano or learning to type successfully, the concept of learning to play tennis within the field of a well-defined foundation for ANY accomplished player parallels the same patterns of skill development found in most activities. Consider other sports. Beginning basketball players are taught the same shooting techniques that the pros utilize; baseball players are taught to swing the bat and throw a ball the way accomplished baseball players do. Tiger Woods swings a 3-wood today, not much differently—in terms of technique—then he did when he was eight or ten years old. Yet, most tennis books, videos and many teaching professionals teach tennis to beginners by offering techniques that the players will need to change if they want to become advanced. Why? Is it that these teaching mediums assume that those seeking to play tennis are so inept that they need to be taught simple methods before moving on to advanced? Sadly, intentionally or otherwise, this is exactly why so many books and instructors employ this philosophy!

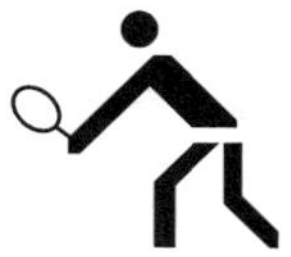

I don't know too many aspiring tennis players who are going to say, *"Gee, I would love to play tennis, but I really don't want to be very good!"*

The underlying argument, which I addressed briefly in the Foreword and will address again in more detail in Chapter Two, is the fact that players who start with one method have a difficult time making the change when it is recognized that a change is needed. Thus, if a person's goal is to play skilled tennis, learning such so-called entry level skills that need to change as the desire to improve changes is an inferior—if not completely foolish—learning approach. It is this type of learning that I directly attribute to the incredible number of players, millions really, who stop improving at the 3.0 or 3.5 levels even though they keep playing and even practicing for years and years! This same philosophy has lead to millions of tennis players quitting the game. Imagine playing the piano and only learning skills that allowed you to play "Chop Sticks" or "Twinkle Twinkle Little Star" even though you have been playing the piano for years. How long would such a student find playing the piano fun? Tennis players who learn simple tennis skills, those that specifically make improving difficult or impossible, are seldom going to find tennis very fun either! (At least not for very long!)

I don't know too many aspiring tennis players who are going to say, "Gee, I would love to play tennis, but I really don't want to be very good." I suppose that if players approached learning tennis this way, then indeed we would teach methods that specifically limit player development. And yet, this is exactly how most tennis texts, videos and even some tennis instructors present tennis information!

Author's Assumptions and Their Ramifications

I have concluded that if you purchased this book, (or borrowed it from a friend—you know who you are!), then you certainly are in search of such methods that will help propel you continuously forward in terms of tennis improvement. Throughout this book, I will describe several examples of how some techniques offered in a variety of tennis texts are, in fact, detrimental to sustained tennis improvement. In fact, it is this very issue in which many books, (many quite notable among tennis enthusiasts and tennis

There is nothing more disconcerting for me than to observe players learning methods that sentence them to perpetual mediocrity!

instructors) actually have perpetuated a player's stagnation because of their teaching material! Unfortunately, there are no warning labels or waivers of liability offered by such books or instructors. Players for decades have been led astray, so to speak, believing that the methods they were learning from teaching pros, videos, or books, would propel them—eventually—into the world of highly competitive tennis. Instead, many tennis pupils have been taught a methodology that very specifically prevents them from becoming the best player they can be.

Not only is tennis a complex sport, it must be recognized that the patterns of player development are very complex as well. In fact, assumptions (that don't recognize this complexity) from past teaching methods have produced a vast number of frustrated and dissatisfied tennis players around the world! Visit any number of tennis "camps" across the country and witness the mass of players searching for solutions to their tennis woes! Yet, among these learning environments we still witness many of the teaching techniques that are prohibitive to sustained learning. There is nothing more disconcerting for me than to observe players learning methods that sentence them to perpetual mediocrity!

It can be argued that if a segment of the playing public does, in fact, improve past the 3.5 level, then the information given out can't be all bad. The reality is that a great deal of the information presented in most texts is indeed helpful to most tennis players. The problem lies in one very distinct assumption most books and a number of tennis teaching professionals make: most books and many instructors assume that all players can make major changes in their strokes when more advanced techniques are required for higher development.

It is important to understand this assumption in order to understand the ramification of its action on each individual.

Most books and many instructors assume that all players can make major changes in their strokes when more advanced techniques are required for higher development.

While it is true that some players can struggle through the frustration and difficulty of making specific changes as needed in their mechanics, most players find the transition virtually impossible. This struggle creates tremendous conflict in a player's confidence and leads many players to uncertainty and doubt about what they should be doing on the court. Players making an educated attempt at a specific change tend to react to this frustration with a normal human response: go back to what is comfortable. If "comfortable" is a form or method that is prohibitive to sustained learning, then the student is destine to a vicious cycle of failure…or at best, sustained mediocrity.

When a player is "ready" to make necessary changes, or recognizes a change needs to be made, a player will have difficulty in effectively changing all the necessary components of a stroke because of the number of components that one change affects. For example, a grip change on the serve also requires a change in body position to the court, a change in the relationship of the racket to the arm, a change in the contact point, a change in the swing pattern, and usually a change in the service toss. A player who changes from the generally accepted novice grip, the Eastern forehand, to the advanced Continental grip on the serve—but fails to adjust ALL of these components accordingly—will ineffectually serve the ball nowhere near the intended target! This pattern of failure alone can account for a player's resistance to making a needed change. Not only is there the strange feeling associated with such foreign swing pattern, the resultant outcome of the stroke being unsuccessful creates frustration as well.

> By Simply avoiding those methods that are necessary for advancement, we prohibit any chance of mastering those very methods
>
> !

Many of these authors and tennis-teaching professionals reason that beginning players, usually young children and women in general, will find it difficult to control the racket using certain grips or stroke patterns. Most books recommend NOT requiring any student to hold the racket in such a grip that feels weak. The consensus is to allow the student to hold the racket with whatever grip is comfortable until he or she has acquired the strength to hold the more advanced grip comfortably. However, this strategy creates a conflicting dichotomy: If a player continues to hold the racket with a grip that is going to prevent them from becoming a skilled player, they will never become comfortable with the grip they will need to use to become that skilled player! Certainly, it isn't rocket science to figure out that if a specific grip is required for advanced play, then we will want to work and practice that grip until it does indeed feel comfortable. By simply avoiding those methods that are necessary for advancement, we prohibit any chance of mastering those very methods. I have a saying that I use to describe this methodology: Elementary methods of practice will produce elementary levels of play.

> Not once, in any tennis book, do the authors mention the fact that such changes will incur frustration or discomfort. Nor do they mention that such changes might even be impossible for some students
>
> !

While we are talking about "required strength," I must add that most shots in tennis, when done correctly and within the bounds of accepted advanced technique, require very little actual strength to produce the shot. I demonstrate the serve, the volley, and the groundstrokes using just my index finger and thumb holding the racket, as an example, to show my students that strength is not the issue in hitting a tennis ball correctly. The reason so many players feel "weak" when executing certain shots or in holding various grips is either because of their unfamiliarity with the grip or stroke or because of improper techniques being utilized. Again, it would be most unproductive if we avoided proper grips or form only to accommodate this feeling of weakness if the feeling is due to one or both of these reasons.

It is amazing to me that so many authors and instructors

continue to teach tennis using a methodology that requires such an obvious need for changes. Almost without exception authors seem to mention that there is a need for such changes under their breath! In just a moment I will provide several examples of authors making this point. Yet, not once in any of these books do the authors mention the fact that such changes will incur frustration or discomfort. Nor do they mention that such changes might even be impossible for some students! Consider too, that each of these authors use complete ambiguity in describing when such changes need to take place. Examples of this vagueness are: "Change when you acquire experience," "Change when skill develops," "As your play improves…we recommend changing." It is no wonder that players who have learned from such means have tremendous difficulty in not only making needed changes, but also knowing when to begin implementation of such changes!

Yet, if we look at any beginning player and compare them to an advanced rendition of themselves later in their playing career, change is going to be inevitable…even if an advanced foundation is taught from the very beginning. I know what many of you are saying: "but if we are going to change from a beginning advanced foundation to a noticeably different "final version" as skilled players, why can't an elementary method be taught from the start and changed later?"

This question is answered within how these changes take place. By offering an advanced foundation, players change ON THEIR OWN through experimentation, through personal preferences, through personality, and/or through natural evolution of swing mechanics—ALL WITHIN AN ADVANCED FOUNDATION. When offered elementary concepts that MUST BE CHANGED to become skilled, the player is not in control of the change process. I have taught over 3000 players, all of whom, with very few exceptions, became clearly accomplished players through the same processes that I teach within these pages. Ironically, almost every player plays this advanced level of tennis differently than most everyone else. And, certainly there exists some variance from the advanced foundation they first were presented as beginners. Yet all these changes among individuals were done within that very foundation that they were first introduced to. (Please see "Tennis Clones" in Chapter 2.) They all have quite accomplished serves, groundstrokes and volleys. However, many of my players use open stances and full Western grips on their forehand groundstrokes, where others will use closed stances and the more conventional Eastern forehand grips. Some use a "pin-point" stance on their serves; others use a "platform" stance. Some are baseliners while others are serve-and volley strategists. The point here is that each player adopted very acceptable stroke patterns—as they apply to advanced play—following very distinct personality traits and development of individual idiosyncrasies. It is easy to distinguish player personalities as they follow individual play. Most of my aggressive, outgoing players play very aggressive tennis—usually serve and volley or an attacking baseline game. More reserved players play more of a patient game of cat and mouse from the baseline or simply play a waiting game. One of the joys of teaching a great number of junior players is to see their personalities emerge BECAUSE of tennis! Many have "found" themselves through tennis, discovering their strengths and weaknesses as they learn the game. You will discover your own patterns of play that suit your needs, your comfort levels, and your personality. But, as long as you learn proper techniques from the start, this foundation will provide you with a base to develop these personal tennis strokes in a way that will seldom, if ever, need major overhauls to accomplish.

Examples

Two of the most glaring examples in this practice of offering tennis advice that requires the student to change their methodology are in the teachings of the serve and the volley. Here are a few examples of the many books that recommend this conflicting methodology and their submission that players will need to make such changes.

THE SERVE:

"The grip for the serve taught to many beginners is the Eastern forehand grip. However, it is advisable to proceed to the conventional Continental grip as soon as possible." *Tennis, A Professional Guide*, the Official Handbook of the USPTA

"Despite the strong preference for the Continental grip, many professionals teach beginners to use an Eastern forehand grip for serving. [However], there is general agreement that the Eastern grip precludes the development of a strong serve, and for this reason, players are urged to change to the Continental when they acquire experience."

Tennis for the Player, Teacher, and Coach by Chet Murphy and Bill Murphy

"I let them use the forehand grip, [Eastern]—but always with the understanding that if they start playing well they must change to the Continental if they want to remain competitive on their serve." *Tennis 2000* by Vic Braden and Bill Bruns

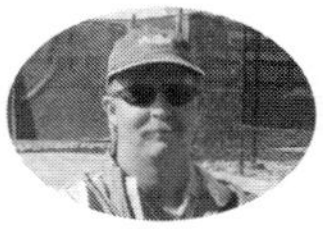

Author's Note

While I have included ten of these examples, I could have included twenty or thirty more from dozens of additional books! Notwithstanding, ten examples might be construed as "over kill" in terms of making my point. However, that is exactly my point! Not only is the subject matter of each of these examples a contradiction of sorts, but the fact that there are literally hundreds of books, most by authoritative authors, that teach such a conflict of learning within this concept. It is important that you, the reader, are very clear on how prolific and glaring this methodology is within the teaching field.

"If you are a beginner, it is probably best to begin with a punch or half-swing serve. Hold the racket with an Eastern forehand grip. As your serving motion becomes more fluid, you can change your grip to accommodate the swing. Players with advanced serves usually hold the Continental grip." *Tennis...Steps to Success* by Jim Brown

THE VOLLEY:

"After you develop solid basic mechanics of the volley, [using the Eastern grips], you can experiment with the Continental grip." *Visual Tennis* by John Yandell

"If you must, and you're quick enough, it's all right to switch grips [between the Eastern backhand and Eastern forehand grips], but not at the "A" or "Open" levels of play. It is best to volley with a Continental grip." *The Real Spin On Tennis* by Jack Broudy.

"The grips for the volley may be the same as those used for the groundstrokes, the Eastern forehand and backhand. They are preferred for most beginners. The Continental grip is used by most advanced players."

Tennis, A Professional Guide, the Official Handbook of the USPTA

"The Eastern grip method is best used to teach the novice player, but the player should change to the Continental grip as skill develops."

High Tech Tennis by Jack L. Groppel, PhD.

"When you first begin to play the net, use your usual Eastern forehand and backhand grips for volleying. But as your play improves, you'll find you won't have time to switch grips...we recommend the Continental grip."

Tennis: How to Play, How to Win. By Tennis Magazine.

"The main difference between the advanced volley and the beginner's volley is that most intermediate and advanced players use the Continental grip."

Tennis...Steps to Success by Jim Brown

These statements and others like them pose two rather perplexing questions for anyone wanting to learn tennis:

- *Why should I learn one technique when another technique is actually desired for advanced play?*
- *If I do learn basic strokes first, WHEN do I make the change to the more advanced?*

Even if players were completely capable of making the transition from a basic form to a more advanced form without the frustrating and incapacitating resistance we so often see, the second question becomes even more undefined. At what point does a player say, "Ok, I'm ready to make the change"? One year? Ten years? No matter what level you are, I believe you can see the deeper problem with this teaching philosophy.

This question also creates a problematic dichotomy: If a player develops basic skills using the beginning form BEFORE attempting the more advanced form, he or she will usually be so ingrained in the programmed response of the beginning form that change will be frustratingly difficult. At this point, any changes from this form will be uncomfortable, exasperating, and, as we often see for a large number of players, almost impossible.

Why is Change so Difficult?

Players ask me all the time, "Why is it so hard to change?" There are many contributing elements to this complexity. These elements can, and usually do, include physical discomfort, psychological blocks, emotional hurdles, and established or ingrained physiological patterns that limit or prohibit change. Let me offer an illustration that might summarize this difficulty more succinctly.

Let's analyze Vic Braden's statement from his book *Tennis 2000.*

"I let them use the forehand grip, [Eastern]—but always with the understanding that if they start playing well they must change to the Continental if they want to remain competitive on their serve."

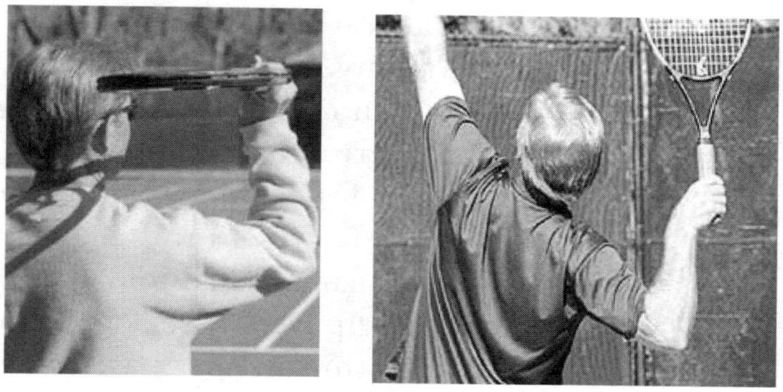

Figures 2 & 3
At Left: The classic "beginner" serve grip and body position.
Right: The "Skilled" grip, body position and swing pattern.

We can easily see where the problem begins: If we start playing "WELL" using an inferior grip, WHEN would we change to the more advanced or progressive grip? Perhaps a bigger question could be posed: "If I start playing "WELL", WHY would I make any changes?" You can probably relate to this enigma. How hard would it be to change grips just when we start playing "well"? IT IS REALLY, REALLY HARD! In this example we see how psychological issues, (the fear of changing or losing what we perceive as improvement) could prevent us from wanting to make a change in our stroke. Yet "well" in this example is only in comparison to the beginning abilities the player first experienced when attempting to play tennis. In reality—and this is true for most players—this example of "well" can be interchanged with words like "below average" and "mediocre" since these terms better describe the typical player who is using inferior grips. Be assured that few players incorporating such grips or technique, or maintaining their use throughout their development, seldom develop into progressively skilled or advanced players, especially on these two strokes: the volley and the serve. (This is why 95% of tennis books recommend the need to change to the more advanced grips or techniques as "skill develops"!)

It is to this end that *Tennis Mastery* recognizes this futile teaching methodology and offers proven and logical techniques that bypass the need for learning rudimentary techniques in such a transitory sequence.

THE SERVE AND THE VOLLEY – REVELATION OF PERPETUAL MEDIOCRITY

It is interesting, too, that these two strokes to which I have just alluded—the serve and the volley—are the two stroke patterns which seem to clearly separate those stuck at the 3.0 and 3.5 levels from those who advance. For the most part those players who are perpetually trapped at lower levels tend to have their limited abilities exposed during serves and when attempting the volley. Typically, these players can have adequate groundstrokes and even fairly good understandings of singles and/or doubles strategies. However, their inability to volley or even fear of the net, (due to inferior volley technique) and of their serve, (usually more specifically their second serve), is the revealing evidence of their fallibility. Ironically, as I have pointed out, these are the two areas that have been clearly taught as transitory by most authors and tennis-teaching professionals.

Are there exceptions to this rule? Sure. There are undoubtedly a few people who, no matter what, will simply do better with the more elementary stroke methods as prescribed by many books and their authors. However, I know for a fact that it is far better to offer players techniques that will prompt continued learning with minimal changes over those methods that presumably offer relatively quick success...however mediocre that success may be. Over the course of my teaching career I believe I only had one player who did indeed meet the exception to my rule. She was an older woman of nearly 70 years who had never played sports nor was she very strong. After a couple of lessons, I found that the Continental grip on the serve was just not going to work for her. A grip closer to the Eastern forehand grip suited her and she was able to get a decent spin serve in (for her age). Even as this change in serving methods worked better for her, it was the only change I had to make. Her forehand and backhand volleys using the Continental grip were excellent, (supporting my assertion that strength has little to do with hitting an advanced volley!)

Band-aid Repairs

I have found that players who learn methods that require some change as advancement is desired begin to look for "band-aid" repairs for their ineffective strokes, especially once they realize they are not improving. These short-term fixes tend to complicate the overall understandings of tennis mechanics and corrupt the player's ability to execute anything close to what is considered skilled form. Many times these band-aid repairs don't address the root cause of the player's mediocrity or frustration. Instead of identifying, incorporating, and practicing the specific changes required to improve one's stroke, band-aid repairs tend to produce "instant gratification" through questionable technique only utilized to satisfy that specific shot for a player in that instance. This methodology seldom, if ever, produces long-term improvement. Such band-aid fixes rarely provide for better results against more effective shots by our opponent. Finally, this teaching philosophy fails to provide for long-term adoption of any reliable stroke pattern. True change from such inferior technique usually requires much more discipline by the student than simple quick-fixes that are often offered in the place of proper technical instruction.

OUT WITH THE NEW, IN WITH THE OLD THE "COMFORT ZONE" SYNDROME

When a player has learned inferior strokes at first then makes a dedicated effort to change, we observe these students often falling back on their mediocre strokes in the heat of any competition. Even when players know what form they SHOULD be using, these players almost always and immediately go back to their inferior—but *comfortable* stroke patterns in various playing situations. (Comfortable because they learned these mediocre strokes first!) I call this tendency to revert back to this inferior—but comfortable—pattern of play the "Comfort Zone Syndrome". (I probably should call it the comfort zone "plague" since it affects so many players who are attempting this pattern of change!)

What is the point of using such inadequate methods if they are still fallible even in their simple use ?

A player, who continues to only use rudimentary form on strokes such as serves and volleys (as described earlier) or any other inferior form in match play, will *never* move out of such simple form. I think it is obvious to any reader or student of the game, regardless of experience, that repeating strokes/form/technique, which are prohibitive to improvement, will prohibit any substantial improvement in their game!

For example, if we all can agree that a spin serve is needed to increase pace, error room, and effect on our second serve, would it help us in any way to hit paddy-cake after paddy-cake second serves in competition? Obviously not. Yet, even students who are quite familiar with the grip needed and the form necessary to hit a spin serve sadly revert right back to that which is perceived as safe or comfortable. I use the word "sadly" because these players who paddy-cake their serves are often seen still double faulting! What is the point of using such inadequate methods if they are still fallible even in their simple use?

If it is your desire to become a skilled tennis player then it is critical to use correct form, that which you know to be within the context of skilled play. To play better competitively as well as produce the greatest development and overall improvement of which you are capable, this concept is absolutely critical.

> *It is almost without exception that players stuck at the 3.0 & 3.5 levels all play tennis incorporating unsophisticated stroke mechanics that are commonly taught to beginners.*

LINEAR PROGRESSIVE LEARNING VERSUS TRANSITIONAL LEARNING

As mentioned, the assumption that players must learn stroke mechanics that are considered basic or rudimentary before they can transition to more advanced techniques is unique to tennis. It is assumed that advanced methods are too difficult and will result in player frustration if attempted prior to more basic techniques. While certain highly advanced methodologies, (or more specifically, advanced *idiosyncrasies*), are not recommended for the beginner without first establishing a proper foundation, what is important is that the player be taught methods that allow for the Advanced Foundation to be established. I call this foundation a "Progressive Player Foundation" since it describes and provides for the concept of constant player improvement.

In observing those 3.0 and 3.5 players who are exhibiting frustration and difficulty in moving past such levels, I have found almost without exception these players all play tennis still incorporating the unsophisticated stroke mechanics which are commonly taught to and associated with beginners. It is interesting to examine many of these same players who express an intense desire to improve while they attend clinics, lessons, workshops and camps. Almost unanimously these players all acknowledge some understanding that they need to make changes in their game in order for them to improve. Yet, (and this is perhaps one of the most frustrating aspects of being a tennis teaching professional), when such players are introduced to new and necessary mechanics they will need to employ in their game, there is an immediate and glaring resistance to these changes. Sometimes this resistance is due to the knowledge that a change is going to be difficult. Sometimes the resistance is due to incorrect psychological perceptions of what the player interprets as correct mechanics in their mind. Sometimes the resistance is simply because the discomfort of making the change

> *Sometimes...the discomfort of making a change (in one's game) is greater than the discomfort of losing to opponents*
>
> *!*

is greater than the discomfort of losing to opponents!

Consider a player who is beginning to meet with some element of success using simple form. Regardless how mediocre that success may be, asking him or her to now change his or her technique in competition—and thus digress in perceived skill level until comfort and confidence in the new technique is gained is one of the hardest things for any student to do! The natural human condition of wanting to win usually supercedes and overrides the desire, and even the awareness, of using proper form in competitive play. And the sad part is that all those players who refuse or resist those changes toward better strokes and technique during competition still can lose! Not only do they lose, they fail to get much better in the process.

Obviously, players who are just starting out don't have faulty stroke patterns that are as deeply ingrained as those who have been playing tennis inaccurately for years! This is one of the reasons why knowledgeable pros have such great success with little kids! Even beginning adults are easier to work with than those who have been playing for decades at the 3.5 level are! It is sad for me to watch some of these long-time 3.0 and 3.5 adults who become so complacent with their mediocrity that they actually give up hoping to become a better player. This personal grief stems from two reasons: One, the player was cheated when they learned the game in the first place; and two, the player has lost the sense of goals and personal values that come with the desire for improvement and its consequent acquisition.

This concept, the resistance to change by those who have previously learned such transitory methods, has a similar relationship within the Martial Arts. In his excellent book *Zen in the Martial Arts*, author (and tennis player!) Joe Hyams relates the analogy of a full cup of water when confronted with recognizing a need for change or growth:

> *"Like this cup, you are full of your own opinion*
> *and speculations.*
> *How can I show you Zen unless you*
> *first empty your cup?"*

Any player who has ingrained strokes that are recognizably a hindrance to progressive improvement must let go of those patterns before new patterns of play can take root. This is not an easy task! Oftentimes, correct stroke patterns have component parts that are closely related to the undesirable stroke pattern. Thus, even as there might be significant changes in a new stroke, such as a grip change or stance change or the like, there are still going to be similar movements between the old and the new. This ingrained stroke pattern is sometimes called "muscle memory" since the body tends to repeat that which it is most used to, even if the movement is not a desired one. Players must physically and mentally "empty their cup" to allow the complete conversion to occur.

Incongruously, some 3.0 and 3.5 players—especially those who have been playing for decades—will take a lesson but will caution the pro at the start, "I don't want to learn something that will ruin my old, reliable stroke." If their "old" stroke was so reliable, why, after twenty years are they still playing at the 3.5 level? This is like a server who still double faults while serving a 20-mph puffball second serve. Notoriously, when such a player learns a more effective and progressive slice or topspin serve, they double fault once or twice and immediately complain, "this serve isn't working!" They proceed to return back to their feeble dink serves, guaranteeing themselves a life of serving mediocrity!

Notoriously, after learning a more effective serve, players double fault once or twice and immediately complain, "this serve isn't working!" They proceed to return back to their feeble dink serves, guaranteeing themselves a life of serving mediocrity!

Players must understand that using proper form does not guarantee against failure! Heck, even the pros double fault, miss overheads, hit groundstrokes into the net, as well as a slew of other errors, although they have refined and skilled stroke patterns. Using proper strokes will still require the refinement of aim, the understanding of limitations, and the recognition of human frailties. It is the continued application of proper strokes in competition that will not only eventually create comfort, but also will reduce errors over time. All the while, this effort will put into motion a course of action for the player to eventually hit more effective strokes while reducing those errors in the process. That is technically what skilled play encompasses: Hit more effective strokes consistently.

Is it TOO LATE for ME?

Naturally, the longer you have ingrained inaccurate stroke patterns, you generally will meet with greater resistance and increased difficulty in making the necessary changes. For those of you with established, yet flawed stroke patterns, your propensity in making necessary changes is going to be dependent on your aggressiveness in creating desire for the needed change.

The teaching tools in this book will help you overcome this resistance in several ways. The same tools that a beginner will use to establish a proper foundation and methodology will be the same tools which our proverbial long-standing 3.5 player will use to overcome stroke flaws and master new techniques. I have had players who have played for decades using these ineffective strokes patterns discover and achieve stroke mechanics that allowed them for the first time to reach 4.0 levels and above!

If you really want to make the necessary changes in becoming an accomplished player, follow the lessons presented within this book and you will be well on your way to not only "playing a better game of tennis," but you will also be a much more "knowledgeable" player as well!

How will this book help YOU?

Because this book is written to help every level of player, it is important to identify specifically HOW it will help YOU at your present playing or learning level. The vast number of students reading this book will have had some background in tennis. However, some of you will have never played the sport before. Likewise, there are those of you who are already reaching higher levels of skilled play and want to gain an edge on your opponents who are also playing at higher levels of play. Here are specific advantages that each level of player will gain from reading *TENNIS MASTERY*:

The "Beginner" Player

You are in good hands! The tennis "foundations" taught in this book will provide you with a "linear learning progression". This means that from the first page of instruction to the last, the learning will build upon each concept. It isn't important for you to have the goal of becoming a "world-class" player, (unless you do indeed want to be a world-class player!) However, one of the mistakes most books make is to assume that players who want to achieve tennis greatness should be taught differently than those who just want to play casually or socially. On the contrary! Anyone who wants to learn tennis, should be taught methods which will not only allow them to play tennis for fun, but the methods taught should offer them the opportunity for continued improvement and success AT ANY LEVEL THEY HOPE TO ACHIEVE! Thus, if you are a true beginner understand that you need not pursue tennis as a career or livelihood! Likewise, if you have an earnest desire to pursue tennis to your greatest potential, the methods here will give you the tools and knowledge needed to reach those goals as well!

The "Intermediate" Player

The "intermediate" player is perhaps the largest segment of those who are reading this book. The vast majority of players who indeed purchase instructional books or videos are those who have been playing tennis at least a little while.

If you have recognized that you are not improving or you know that you are doing things wrong in hitting a tennis ball, then you must first understand WHAT you are doing wrong. A lot of players know that they don't hit the ball correctly. The problem is that they don't know what exactly is wrong with their stroke or form. Tennis is certainly complex enough that many players may be doing several things wrong on just one stroke! This concept alone tends to make the intermediate player more resistant to change. Knowing that several things need to be changed make some players very nervous about beginning a course of action that they hope will correct the incorrect methods they possess! The human ego is a very delicate device! Nothing is more humiliating to an individual than the recognition that not only have they been doing something wrong…but that they may have been doing it wrong for a LONG TIME!

Nothing is more humiliating to an individual than the recognition that, not only have they been doing something wrong....but that they may have been doing it wrong for a LONG TIME

!

After reading this book you will come away not only knowing WHAT you have been doing wrong, but you will also head to the courts with the knowledge of HOW to correct that which is indeed wrong! The strength of this book lies in the teaching tools and "Key Position Points" teaching methods which provide ample strategies for you to quickly gain the stroke foundations needed for continued growth and improvement.

The "Advanced" Player

Perhaps the smallest group of readers is the advanced group. There are several reasons for this. First, advanced players generally feel they have mastered most of the proper strokes and strategies in tennis. That is, they believe they have already learned many of the concepts presented in a book such as this. Second, advanced players believe they should spend most of their time "fine-tuning" their game on the court. They seldom feel the need to spend additional time reading about things they think they already know!

Advanced players are sadly mistaken on both of these counts. It is even more important for the advanced players to learn everything they can about tennis. The one item that separates one advanced player from another might just be a subtle piece of knowledge or strategy that can only be picked up from such processes. Jimmy Connors once said, "The day you say you know it all about tennis is the day you do indeed stop learning!" If you are an advanced player, explore every opportunity to learn more.

New Teaching Techniques

In addition to recognizing that certain methods are detrimental to advanced learning, I have discovered specific patterns of learning that increase the likelihood of players developing their Advanced Foundation as early as possible. One example of these *patterns of learning* has been my fifteen-year study of the two-handed forehand topspin groundstroke—both as a learning tool and as a weapon for many advanced players. *Tennis Mastery* is one of the first publications that not only instructs the two-handed forehand, but also identifies it as a solid stroke option for many players who want similar results as produced by a two-handed backhand.

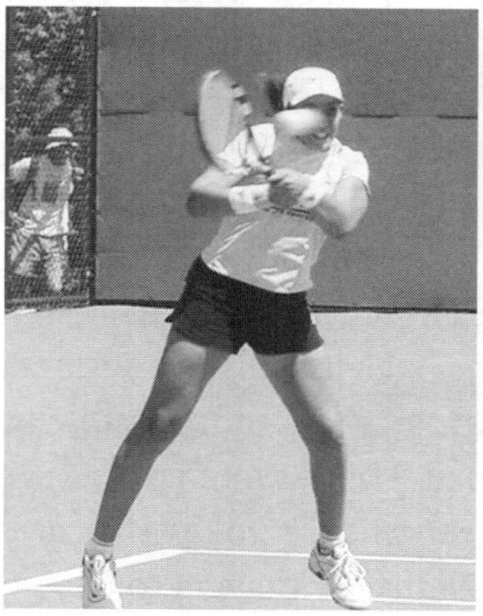

Figure 4
The two-handed forehand is making its mark in tennis, becoming both a learning tool and weapon! Here, Marion Bartoli of France hits her two-handed forehand. *(Photo by Dave Smith)*

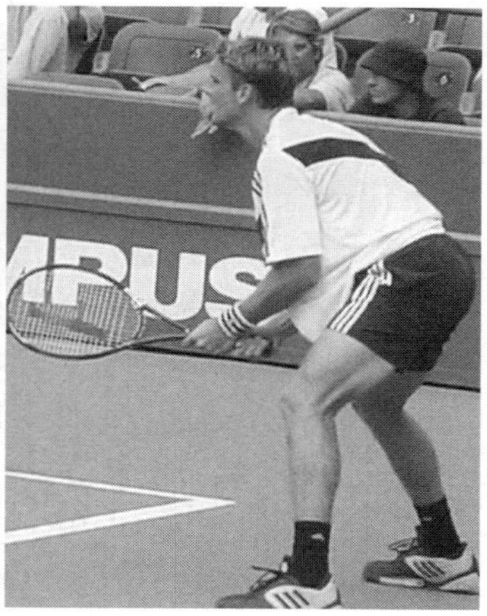

Figure 5
American Jan-Michael Gambil uses two hands to hit groundstrokes on both sides of his body.
(Photo by Dave Smith)

This stroke is nothing new to tennis as witnessed by its use by Marion Bartoli of France (Figure 4) and Jan Michael Gambil (Figure 5) on the men and women's professional tour. As early as the 1930's Pancho Segura demonstrated that the two-handed forehand could be used in world-class tennis of that era. In addition, it has quietly become a weapon of choice by many top junior players in sections of the country. I hope, that through this publication, the stroke will be viewed as a new tool for teaching pros and a new weapon for many players who may be struggling with their one-handed forehand. In its description you will find the many benefits of its implementation for players of all abilities. Having taught the stroke for over 15 years, I have seen the rapid speed of achievement among players who institute the shot, producing both greater effectiveness of the forehand itself as well as the speed in which players master the forehand.

Even as the sheer numbers of one-handed forehands overshadows it, the two-hander is making a significant emergence among many players around the world. However, the two-handed forehand, as it will be taught within this text, is also a strategic learning tool for all ages of beginners. From almost a self-working topspin *advanced* swing pattern to the early development of proper shoulder turn and footwork, the two-handed stroke is a remarkable learning tool. Unlike the one-handed forehand, (which features an array of calamities and stroke faults among a great percentage of current beginner, intermediate, and even some advanced players), the two-handed stroke provides a stability that results in far greater mastery of the forehand stroke.

For those who want to develop an Advanced Foundation on the one-handed forehand, I have included the most modern and up-to-date methodology being taught by the world's top instructors as well.

As for all the shots—from the one and two-handed backhands, the various advanced serves, slice ground strokes and drop shots, overheads and half-volleys—you will indeed learn what is recognized as the Advanced Foundation for each shot. And you will be given the tools necessary to learn, practice and master each shot within this book.

Research-Based Common Sense

One issue I have had with many books on "technical tennis" is their insistence that because something is biomechanically correct, players should adopt only stroke patterns that arguably produce the greatest efficiency. While I don't dismiss any research done in the name of improving the game, many authors sit themselves on a pedestal claiming their research proves their methods are infallible. My contention with any of the methods produced by such a procedure is in the following comparison. If a technical method produces 100% efficiency yet is difficult or impossible to attain by individuals, would we be better off teaching a stroke that is perhaps 95% biomechanically efficient yet easy for the player with which to advance their play? My answer is yes. Consider, too, that virtually no shot is ever hit at 100% maximum capacity of any player, even the pros (with the possible exception of first serves.) So, if we almost never attempt to hit at 100% maximum speed (swinging as hard as we can), why is it critical to learn biomechanical strokes that are assumed to be 100% efficient? I have found it is far more important for players to develop sound strokes that lend themselves to advanced play instead of attempting strokes that provide debatable efficiency.

A classic example of this comparison was clearly illustrated to me when I discussed serving methods with a well-known tennis researcher who claims he teaches the most efficient service motion. My question to him was "How many pros serve the way you profess in attaining an efficient serve?" His honest reply was "only about 5 percent." Now if *ONLY* the top 5 percent of the men and women professionals were the ones utilizing his technique, I would say his method indeed has merit. However, in researching all the current players on tour, I could not find one player in the top 50 players on either the men's tour or the women's tour who served using his prescribed method.

If the vast majority of the world's top players can't (or won't) master this so-called efficient service motion, then can we expect the rest of us to create an effective serve this way? Ironically, this service model is based on that of Roscoe Tanner, a player who played over 20 years ago and had minimal success and even less longevity on the pro tour. Even as Tanner had, at one time, the fastest serve in the world, his motion was quite exclusive and unique. In addition, even if this "research" of such a serve might produce arguably more efficient racket head speed, the swing pattern for the vast majority of players of all ages and abilities is very difficult to master! On top of that, it has been shown through high-speed video research that such a service technique prevents more critical aspects of the serve required for maximum power and higher levels of skilled play. If the best players in the world (those who make their living on winning tennis matches) DON'T prescribe to such a method, there is probably a reason for it! Finally, it should also be noted that a fast serve does not always equate into an effective serve. As we talk about the techniques used to deliver a skilled serve in Chapter 11, we will discuss all the concepts that not only produce a fast serve, but one that is effective, consistent, and, most importantly, achievable!

DEPTH OF COMMON SENSE

Another concept on this issue of methodology revolves around a method's depth of common sense. Let me explain.

There are a few pros who teach that the toss of the ball on the serve should only be to the apex of the contact point. That is, the ball should only be tossed as high as the player can reach with his or her racket. Their explanation for this is that the ball is momentarily suspended in air at that point. This is true. These pros further assert that players who toss the ball higher than the apex of contact have to negotiate the timing of hitting the ball as it is falling—which is arguably more difficult. Again they are correct. Up to this point, students can be seen shaking their heads saying, "yes, this all makes sense". Their conclusion is you shouldn't toss the ball higher than contact point. However, there are some other issues that these pros fail to identify. Intentionally or otherwise, this information is only correct within the issue of relativity. The first relative point is found within the difficulty of creating correct coil and rhythm by having to rush to hit such a low toss. As players develop an advanced serve, such a low toss generally prohibits the required rhythm necessary to achieve desirable racket head acceleration for most players. The second issue is, while it is true the ball is falling faster at contact if tossed higher than the contact point, the ball is falling exceedingly slow, even if tossed fairly high. (Tossed 10 inches above contact, the ball will only reach about 5 miles per hour at contact. Even a toss a full two feet above contact will only be traveling approximately 10 miles per hour at contact.) Intermediate players hit volleys and groundstrokes at speeds of upwards of 40 to 50 miles per hour. How hard would it possibly be to hit a ball that is barely moving at 8 or 10 miles per hour? Even beginning players have minimal trouble hitting such a toss.

John Yandell of Advanced Tennis Research has found through extensive high-speed video tape research: "When it comes to tossing height, the fact is that virtually every player on tour hits the toss when the ball is on the way down. In most cases the ball has fallen substantially from the top of the toss, up to two feet or more at contact. Without enough time, there is no way to develop a relaxed, comfortable rhythm. To get the time they need, skilled players toss the ball substantially above their contact points."

As you can see, one common sense idea might be sensible only within a relative aspect. If we are going to explore the best methods to play tennis, we must look beyond that first sensible thought and see if there is something more beyond it.

LOOKING FOR BETTER WAYS

Certainly, many of the advances in tennis research have helped players attain higher degrees of speed and spin on tennis shots. Compare the speed of the ball by the pros today to what it was thirty or forty years ago. I am in deep appreciation of those who have spent years in search of better ways to play tennis. My father, nationally recognized tennis coach, Bruce Smith, always said to look for ways to do things better. That combination of philosophy and research has made this book a reality. My goal is to take that which has been studied and couple this research with decades of application and observations. This process has resulted in methods that will provide the most productive and progressive learning opportunity for every individual. The result from this process is what you are reading: a fusion of the absolute best tennis methods and techniques to date. These findings will provide dedicated tennis players of every level and ability with a clear path in which to take on their road to tennis success. If prescribed tools and methods of practice to better master those techniques are added, then the student has that much more opportunity to meet their desired level of ability within their realm of potential.

That is exactly what I have done in this book.

Tennis is a great game. No one should be neglected the opportunity to explore, experience, and attain the highest degree of accomplishment possible in playing the game. I have seen, all too often, players who have had the ability and desire to excel at tennis, who are thwarted time and time again by an inadequate methodology. I have also seen too many players give up the game because of this very issue. In addition, I have witnessed players who seemed to lack any natural tennis athleticism, become highly recognized skilled players through learning the techniques in this book. Tennis is one of the rare sports that can be played competitively for an entire lifetime. It can be played enjoyably and competitively between the sexes and across all age groups. It is a pity that so many players don't achieve their maximum potential because of a flawed learning philosophy perpetuated through many decades of tennis misinformation. Regardless of nationality sex, age, and socioeconomic background, if you establish an Advanced Foundation, you will continue to increase your skill level as well as your potential.

CHAPTER 2

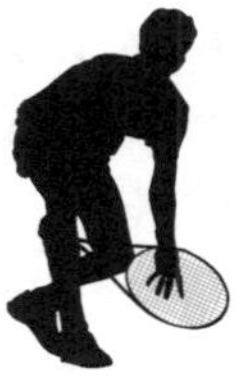

Discovering the "Advanced Foundation"

One of the most debated subjects in tennis is the concept that there is more than one way to hit a tennis ball. No one should dispute this statement as it can be witnessed on tennis courts all across the country. There are, indeed, multitudes of techniques that allow a person to hit a tennis ball over the net. However, if we are discussing how many different ways skilled players hit the ball over the net, we narrow down the options considerably. Just as in any sport there are fundamental tennis methods that are recognized as skilled, advanced, and/or expert. Likewise, there are other techniques that can be clearly recognized as beginner, rudimentary, and/or underdeveloped. In tennis vernacular, terms like "dinker" and "hacker" are sometimes used to describe those who don't play tennis skillfully!

There is a common saying in tennis: "Dinkers have tons of trophies." While this statement is usually more true than not, it is very misleading. The reason for this is that most dinkers only play tournaments at the 3.0 or 3.5 levels and they seldom, if ever, progress past these levels. Through years of experience in such levels, dinkers will initially beat developing players, those who are working on developing strokes associated with skilled play. Yet, as I mentioned briefly in Chapter One, players who are dedicated to learning and practicing within the Advanced Foundation eventually pass such dinkers and move on to higher levels of skilled play.

Those players who do advance in tennis recognize a progressive need to address several key issues associated with more highly developed play. These can include:

- Hit more accurately
- Hit with more pace and depth
- Hit with more spin
- Hit with greater angles
- Hit with greater consistency
- Hit with more touch
- Hit with disguise
- Hit with greater variety
- Hit from a variety of position
- Hit off a variety of opponent's shots.

As players develop, certainly many of the possible ways to simply hit a tennis ball over the net will not meet the criteria that these higher levels of play demand. These elevated levels of play require a specific foundation within the area of each shot. This foundation is what makes up the Advanced Foundation. Players who practice or play using stroke mechanics that are not included in this foundation seldom, if ever, reach recognized levels of skilled play.

Advanced Players: Different Play, Similar Foundations

In observing the pros and players recognized as skilled we see an assortment of strokes executed by a variety of these accomplished players. It isn't difficult to identify these differences: one and two-handed topspin backhands, slice backhands, open and closed-stance forehands, two-handed forehands, swinging topspin volleys and abbreviated slice volleys, pinpoint service stances and platform stances, forehand groundstrokes with Eastern grips and full Western grips. Depending on what you are looking for, there is diversity even among the pros. Idiosyncrasies that top players exhibit widen the apparent disparity in stroke diversity. It is easy for many observers to come to the conclusion that there are indeed many ways in which a tennis ball can be hit correctly. This conclusion is what contributes to the perpetual insistence that there are not only many ways to hit a ball over the net successfully, but also there are many ways in which players can learn to hit the ball skillfully. Within the field of advanced play this simply is not true. While there are, indeed, a multitude of successful teaching STYLES, the truth is for each shot hit, there are only a select number of foundations which will lead to the production of skilled tennis shots. While there are a few identifiable exceptions to this rule, the vast number of players who follow foundations identifiable as "skilled" increase the likelihood of sustaining improvement and, thus, reaching skilled levels of play (and reach their considered potential).

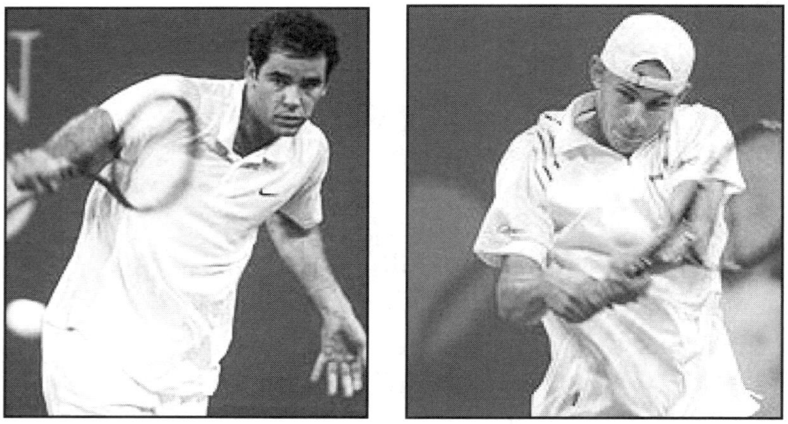

Figures 1 & 2
While professionals can be observed playing the game using a variety of methods, (such as Pete Sampras' one-handed backhand and Andy Roddick's two-handed backhand), the vast majority of pros and skilled players alike play within a specific foundation.

For decades the perceived theme of most tennis books has been to provide several "accepted" forms of tennis methodology. This concept, upon initial review, seems to offer the student many choices in deciphering which method is right for them. In reality, most books introduce a beginning method followed by the recommendation of changing from the beginning method at some point to a more advanced method. (As witnessed by the examples I listed in Chapter 1.) However, if we analyze how top players learn the game of tennis, we find they don't follow this pattern of learning. From top juniors to top touring pros, from top college players to top club players of all ages, we seldom, if ever, see these proficient players incorporating these beginning methods at any point of their development. (There are exceptions to this where players may briefly engage in some aspect of a beginner form yet quickly adopt form that will propel them to higher levels of play.) Furthermore, it is interesting to note that millions of players, specifically 3.0 and

3.5 players, who indeed have been playing for years, if not decades, still play tennis using the same basic or rudimentary strokes to which they were first introduced as beginners! Somehow, millions upon millions of players who were introduced to "transitory" methods literally failed to make the transition from beginner to skilled.

TWO TEACHING ASSUMPTIONS:

There are two distinct assumptions made by many teachers and authors alike that often prohibit or stifle a player's improvement.

Assumption #1

It is assumed that all players will interpret the information correctly when they take it to the court.

There is considerable misinterpretation and misunderstanding of what exactly some authors and teachers are trying to communicate. A simple phrase such as, "power comes from the ground up with most all shots" can be misconstrued in a wide variety of interpretations. Does this mean the player should jump from the ground on all shots? Should the emphasis be on the legs, knees, and/or feet? Obviously, there needs to be much more specific information that the player can use when attempting to take what they have learned onto the courts. Under this same assumption many books or instructors overemphasize some concepts or minimize others, all the while creating uncertainty in the mind of the player when it comes time to apply what is presumed!

An excellent example of this misinterpretation was demonstrated to me when I heard Luis Mediero, one of the most recognized tennis coaches in Spain speak at the World USPTA Convention in Phoenix, Arizona. Mr. Mediero stated, "Eighty percent of the power on the serve is generated by the legs." According to this statement one would conclude that the arms and upper body generate only 20 percent of the speed of a serve. I found this to be quite amusing, if not confusing because I can serve from my knees using absolutely no legs, and serve at 90 miles per hour in the service box! (This isn't anything special since many pros demonstrate the serve from this position to emphasize that a short player can still serve effectively.) If this serve was generated only by the so-called 20 percent of power from my arm and upper body, (as Mediero would lead us to believe), then it would stand to reason I should be able to serve at over 700 miles per hour standing and using my legs! Since the fastest I can actually serve is about 120 miles per hour, it would be far more accurate to conclude from this scenario that the legs—when used correctly—can add approximately 20 percent more power to my serve! NOT eighty percent!

A related problem to this assumption is the lack of comprehension of what is actually being done by top players when observed by those who wish to learn from them. When students watch the pros play, they oftentimes miss the core elements that these professionals execute while hitting specific shots. Oftentimes, the pros hit with such speed and force that students will miss a key position that was actually accomplished, seemingly invisible to the naked eye. And, quite frankly, sometimes the pros, through tremendous training and skill, can use a technique that would not be advantageous to lower level players. (Although, even in these situational shots we can still identify key position points within the stroke or shot that follow our Advanced Foundation.)

And speaking of "key position points," most books fail to provide this very concept which allows players to accurately assimilate that which is being taught. As mentioned, the complexity and diversity of the game of tennis can't be conceptualized by most players without some points of reference. When a player has specific key position points that they can feel, see, and associate, they can then be assured they are working towards a proper foundation. When offered only generic phrasing, the student won't necessarily have a starting block from which to work.

Assumption #2

> *It is assumed that social players, those who are not trying to make it to the professional level or expect to play in high-caliber competitive events, should be taught differently from those who seek such high levels of play.*

In this second assumption it is beyond reason why some tennis players should be taught specifically different tennis strokes than others! (There are some rare exceptions to this statement that I will cover in a moment.) Players who want to achieve relative tennis greatness should not be taught a foundation any differently than that of social players who want to improve within the bounds of their effort! Tennis progression should not be dependent solely on player-expected outcomes. As I have mentioned, tennis is perhaps the only sport that considers this transitional method of learning. From my extensive experience, any player, who is provided the learning tools in which proper progressive tennis foundations can be developed, can learn "advanced" methods just as easily and quickly as methods which are deemed basic.

Players who want to achieve relative tennis greatness should not be taught a foundation any differently than that of social players who want to improve within the bounds of their effort.

The one exception to this statement is that when a student is determined not to learn more advance methods. The psychological power of the mind oftentimes won't let a player even attempt certain strokes or form if they believe they won't be able to master them. In this case these players will stay very close to what is only comfortable and they won't waiver from this stance. In this situation a player will need to be taught methods that will allow them to be as successful as possible within the limitations set forth by the individual. And since there are literally hundreds of books that already provide many of these basic instructional methods that are for a beginner in nature and dependent on change for advancement, I will leave those methods to those books and authors.

In my opinion, the only time a player should adopt such elementary methods is if they were only going to play tennis for a few days and never attempt to play it again. It would be in this scenario that a player might want to learn a perceived quick method of simply hitting the ball over the net in the general direction of another player's court. Such a method would indeed be whatever worked for that individual in the shortest time possible. And such a method would surely include as rudimentary a technique as possible. I call this the "backyard badminton" method of playing tennis.

Advanced Foundation = Sustained Progression

The development of the Advanced Foundation—or more specifically, "a system of learning that reduces the need for change as players develop"—creates a logical need for more dynamic learning tools. Every specific movement understanding, from weight transfer to angular momentum, from racket collapse to wrap follow-throughs, will fall in a natural progression within the Advanced Foundation. High-level physical properties dealing with sophisticated motion, physics, and human motor learning—as they deal with tennis—are conceptualized by the student easier through the processes inherent to the Advanced Foundation. It makes sense that if certain advanced strokes involve complex motor learning, overall simple movements would not be part of the more advanced and desired patterns of skilled play. Consider players who are taught simple methods of playing tennis. If they remain playing within these simple strokes and strategies for the duration of their playing career, not only will it be more difficult to comprehend more advanced patterns of play, but it will be extremely difficult (if not impossible) for the players to execute these advance patterns. Thus all players, from those new to the game to those who are stuck within our proverbial levels of mediocrity, will need to be exposed to new teaching techniques that can increase the probability of every player reaching their potential within this Advanced Foundation.

INDIVIDUALITY WITHIN THE ADVANCED FOUNDATION

One thing that has impressed me in developing this methodology over the years is the resounding profusion of individuality within the Advanced Foundation. As I have mentioned, even as I taught the same foundation strokes and mechanics to thousands of players, each and every student has developed their own idiosyncrasies that favor their personalities, physical strengths and weaknesses, as well as their own sense of need. However, the foundation is seldom lost during this natural "customizing" process. Such idiosyncrasies include the integration of more topspin-oriented grips on groundstrokes, incorporating open stance positions, exaggerating backswing components and follow-through effects on forehand and backhand groundstrokes, and the many preparatory positions on which servers settle. Yet, most of these idiosyncrasies do not compromise the foundations that are necessary for players to develop high-level skills. In fact, such peculiarities are usually a result of experimentation within the Advanced Foundation. Oftentimes, students will develop situational shots that can either hinder or assist the advancing process. Students must evaluate objectively if certain stroke patterns are contributing to successful development. In other words, did a specific swing pattern produce a "lucky" winner, or could that same swing pattern be developed into a consistent, high-percentage stroke? Certainly, this is where experienced teaching pros are employed to evaluate a player's mechanics and help guide the individual towards what is recognized as proper development if the player themselves can't make their own evaluation.

IMMEDIATE GRATIFICATION VERSUS LONG-TERM SUCCESS

In tennis, there are what we call "proper" strokes and then there are what we would call rudimentary stroke patterns or mechanics. The word "proper" would insinuate that there are indeed "improper" strokes available as well. I think we would all agree that in every sport there are far more ways to improperly attempt sporting mechanics than ways that are deemed proper. Just like throwing a baseball or swinging a golf club, there are mechanics that anyone familiar with the sport would recognize as just plain inferior. For example, I can throw a basketball over my head like throwing a soccer ball into play and make a basket. Just because I made a basket with such form, would I justify this method as one I should teach to everyone wanting to learn to shoot a basketball? Obviously not. It might even be easier for a player to initially get the basketball closer to the hoop with this method. Yet, this would still not justify my teaching of this particular shooting method to would-be basketball players just because it produced a desired outcome. Ironically, this is the same concept of teaching that most tennis books and many tennis pros adopt.

Understanding this concept I have come to the conclusion that many tennis pros and authors are embracing a teaching methodology that I call "immediate gratification" in their process of helping players experience a certain level of success. This temporary fulfillment comes at the significant price of substandard long-term player development. This practice must end if we hope to provide all players with continued improvement and enjoyment within their bounds of desire and ability.

ADVANCED FOUNDATION "TENNIS CLONES"

One of the remarks that some pros say is that they don't want to be accused of producing the "Tennis Clones". Have you ever watched skilled basketball players shoot? Professional baseball players bat or throw? PGA golfers swing a golf club? PBA bowlers bowl? Tennis professionals serve? These advanced players all accomplish their expertise in their professions within specific parameters of nearly exact mechanics. Certainly, there are player idiosyncrasies that give each player unique human qualities or characteristics.

Yet, when you put these players side-by-side or even overlay their image over another professional's image, you find that the foundation of their mechanics in each and every

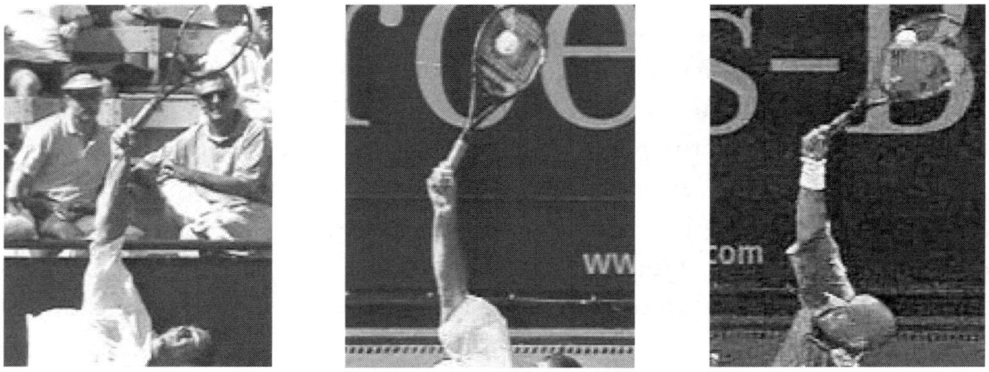

Skilled players usually resemble other skilled players within the context of the Advanced Foundation. Note here that each of these professionals all have essentially the exact same grip, same shoulder position, similar upper body configuration and essentially the same arm position.

sport is nearly identical. Can you say that about the vast majority of tennis players who occupy tennis courts across our country? Of course not.

So, is this attempt to TEACH methods that perhaps resemble "proper" mechanics to all that wish to play quality tennis such a bad thing? Absolutely not. The reality is this: Players who are taught tennis essentially the same way will NOT all play tennis the same way. This is a fact. Amazingly, of the 3000 players I have taught using the same meth-

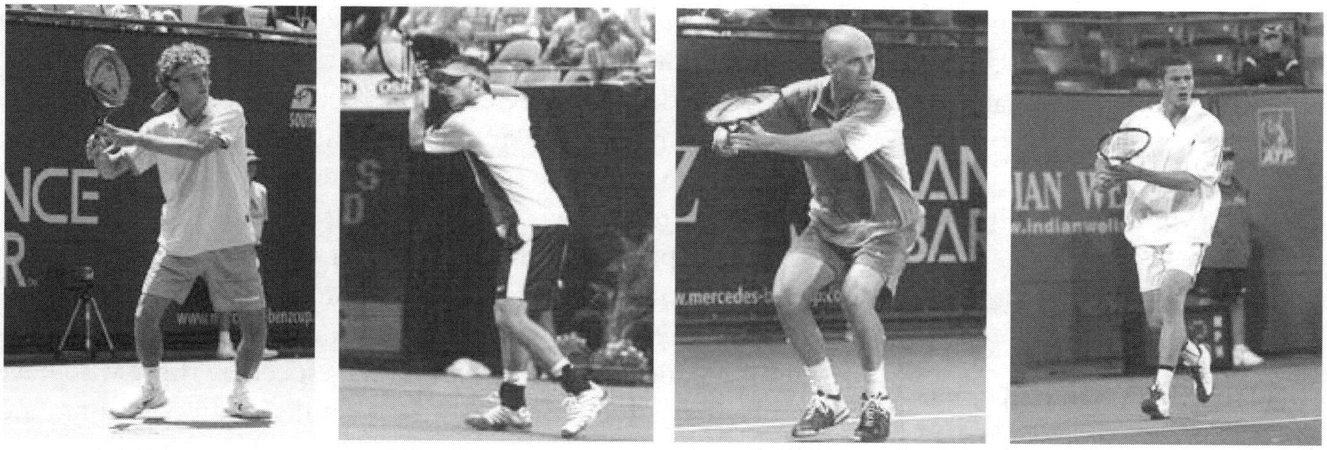

Top-level players create strokes that are similar within the Advanced Foundation. Note that while each player has subtle differences, (differences that can be attributed to variables in ball location as well as player idiocracies), there are comparable characteristics between Gustavo Kuertin, Andy Roddick, Andre Agassi and Marat Safin in their racket preparation on the forehand.

ods, technique and progression, no two players play exactly alike! Yet, all of those students who have given the game the proper time and dedication became exceedingly exceptional players, far surpassing the national majority of 3.0 - 3.5 NTRP levels.

Here is an analogy that might help you to understand this concept more clearly. With few exceptions, learning the piano (or any other musical instrument) is a process that is quite straightforward. Piano players must first learn to coordinate the movements of their fingers so they can consciously play specific notes and/or chords in a specific order or rhythm. Once a piano player masters this ability, their preference as to what style of music they are going to play begins to develop. Even as a mass of piano students can take

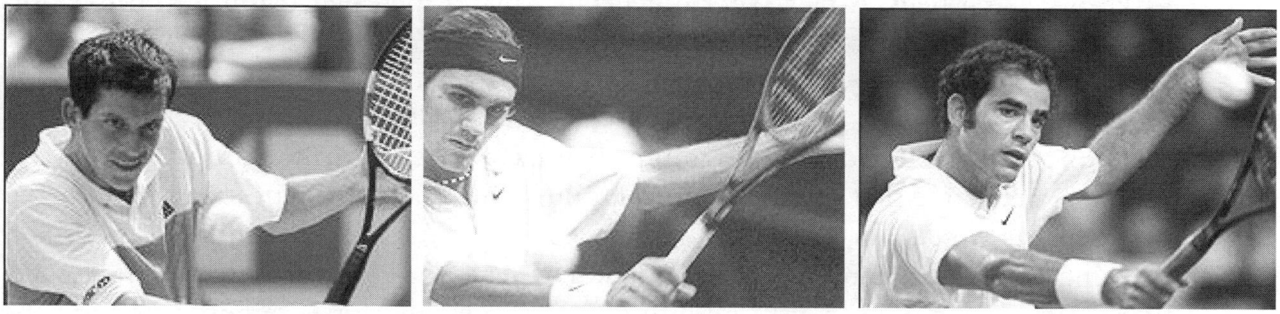

Even as these top-level players hit backhand volleys using almost identical form, they all play distinctively different. Like playing a musical instrument, all top players will play tennis with a distinct rhythm, pace, and feel.

from a single individual teacher, most of these students will develop their own style, feel, rhythm, and idiosyncrasies. At the same time, these same piano students will each end up playing types of music they enjoy the most. Even the same song played by each individual will have a different feel, pace, or accent.

This same effect can be seen on the tennis courts among those learning the game: Developing methods that are recognized as skilled will ALLOW a player to progress, improvise, evolve, and ultimately enjoy the game at much higher levels. Yet, those levels will retain personal individuality for each player.

One final analogy: Allowing a player to adopt a method that might be comfortable or initially somewhat successful—yet is clearly not what is accepted as advanced form—

is like building a house with an incomplete blueprint. Of course we can hammer nails in wood, pour concrete slabs and dig holes. We can get through a portion of building our house, then all of a sudden we can't seem to make any more headway in completing the house. Doors might not fit; walls might be in the wrong place, etc. In order to build the house correctly the builder would probably have to tear down some parts of the structure and start again. Tennis players who adopt inferior tennis strokes, regardless of rationale, will not reach their true potential and will meet similar results as our analogical flawed homebuilder! This process certainly explains why so many players, especially those who have been playing a long time, head to tennis clinics, lessons and camps to "rebuild" their game! This analogy is yet another explanation of why millions of tennis players who embrace inferior mechanics literally stop improving at such low levels.

There has been a great deal of study on what methods are clearly being executed by skilled players. We have a tangible blueprint of what our "proper" form should resemble. And like decorating a properly finished house with personal touches, we can embellish upon our proper tennis foundation; employing personal characteristics that help refine our proper tennis strokes into something more. By embellishing on rudimentary or improper strokes, you simple make your already flawed "tennis blueprint" (if one exists at all!) that much more chaotic.

By embellishing on rudimentary or improper strokes, you simple make your already flawed "tennis blueprint" (if one exists at all!) that much more chaotic.

I think you can now easily recognize why so many thousands of tennis players seek tennis instruction, and you might also recognize why so many of these thousands of players keep seeking help. A flawed form generally invites increased confusion, frustration and minimal progression even as the player continues to search for a cure.

Human Tennis Machines

I don't think God had tennis in mind when He decided to make a human. If we were to design a machine that produced efficient, powerful, and consistent tennis strokes, the moving parts would not resemble a human body per se. Look at tennis ball machines! Spinning wheels, air compression tubes, and ratchet-torque machines don't quite resemble normal human movement! And in most cases, these machines certainly are not constructed simulating the human swing! The point is that when players first pick up a racket with no preconceived or instructional input, their swing almost never resembles what we would recognize as one that is sophisticated or highly developed. Why? In addition to the fact that, for most of us, advanced tennis mechanics are not natural human characteristics, there are several factors that limit a natural understanding and production of advanced tennis strokes by would-be tennis players. These would include:

- *Most players don't know what accomplished swings look like beforehand*
- *Everyday human movements don't resemble sophisticated tennis strokes*
- *Advanced strokes are thought to be so complex that players may not think they know or understand them.*

- *Psychological fears of making a mistake influence players to simplify mechanics*
- *Most simplistic approaches to hitting a ball do not tend to be inherently efficient or productive.*

Most people recognize some or all of these factors and turn to books, videos, tennis camps, and instructors to learn and then master the strokes that they hope will resemble advanced play. Unfortunately, for decades there have only been a handful of pros who understand the complexities as well as the "cause and effect" of certain teaching methods. Unknowingly, many a pro, book, or video has caused what I call "Long-Term Negative Progression." This is the ramification of certain teaching methods and strategies that don't allow a player to reach their full tennis potential. Inferior methodology can actually cause players to become paralyzed, in a sense. When attempting to move away from rudimentary strokes—when advanced strokes are deemed necessary—most players simply can't make the change. Unfortunately, many players and numerous instructors are completely unaware that certain methods will lead players to tennis prosperity while other methods will essentially doom them for life!

Overcoming Human "Deficiencies"

When we come up with ways we hope will generate more power, spin and placement using our human body, we have to change our customary way of thinking. "Natural" positions of the body, (whether they be natural because of condition or natural because of cognitive limitations), are not usually the methods we associate with championship form. If they were, most every newcomer to tennis would be burgeoning in rhythmic and prolific tennis form!

In determining those factors that clearly separate the static 3.5 players from those players who successfully move on, I see an amazingly clear picture. For decades tennis "authorities" have lamented on learning processes that center on comfort, on simple, and on what will "get players on the court playing tennis the fastest." However, when we observe these general teaching strategies in action, we find a chasm of difference between the 3.0 – 3.5 players and those who are far up in the echelons of tennis! We find most instructors and books chalk these "pre-transitional" strategies up as the "initial steps towards advanced tennis." However, if millions of players end up stopping this advancement at some stage of their development, and it is not by choice, then we must stop and say, "There is something wrong here."

Indeed, there is something very wrong in the way tennis has been taught over the course of time. However, it is obvious that not everyone is wrong in how they learn to play tennis. Otherwise, we would have the pros hitting balls much like we see players doing at the public parks!

Many of us have observed youngsters cranking out strokes that are obviously associated with high-level play. I have 7 and 8 year-olds hitting strokes that more closely resemble pros than many adults who have been playing for decades! What is more amazing is that these adults are still using strokes similar to those many books and instructors are using to first introduce players to the game! If such basic strokes are considered "steps towards advanced tennis" why are many players still using them after dozens of years of

If such basic strokes are considered "steps towards advanced tennis" why are so many players still using them after dozens of years of playing? Why have they not made another "step" forward ?

playing? Why have they not made another "step" forward?

The obvious answer is that advanced players, for the most part, didn't try to learn those "initial learning steps" when beginning. They were taught methods that didn't require them to "relearn" or abandon initial methods as they progressed further. They were taught methods that would allow them to move on in a linear progression…as opposed to a transitional one as I mentioned earlier. No matter what age a player starts learning tennis, if he is taught the right strokes and mechanics, gives the game the necessary attention, he or she will continue to improve over time.

Your advancement will also be dependent on several other issues that are not necessarily related to how you learn the game. The most important variable will be your ***desire*** to learn. Everything else takes a back seat to the importance of what you want to do. Obviously, the ability to compete, practice, and utilize elements learned will play an important part in your development. In the following chapters, I will delve into many of these "other" aspects essential to your learning and mastering tennis.

How does one prevent becoming a "Dinker"?

Tennis is probably the only sport that has the word "dinker" as part of its jargon. The word itself describes quite accurately the style of play or strategy such a player enlists. Why is it that the sport of tennis is essentially the only sport relegated to such a playing term or tactic? For those of you who might not be familiar with this term, it refers to the act of "dinking" the ball over the net. As opposed to stroking topspin or underspin shots with some essence of authority, dinkers typically push the ball over the net with minimal spin or pace.

If no one starts out by wanting to become a dinker, yet many do become just that, there must be an ensuing force causing this outcome.

I honestly don't think that any tennis player starts out wanting to become a "Tennis Dinker"! If this is true, then how does someone unintentionally become a dinker? This type of thinking made me begin to look at many of the tennis-teaching concepts on not just a progressive level, but also on a level that I would call a "Digressive Level". If no one starts out by wanting to become a dinker, yet many do become just that, there must be an ensuing force causing this outcome. But what situations, teaching or learning methods, and/or tennis experiences are resulting in players becoming dinkers? The answer to this question deals with a very simple concept: Gravity.

GRAVITY-RELIANT PLAYERS

Most beginners play tennis within the context of gravity. That is, they hit balls hard enough and high enough to go over the net, but soft enough for the force of gravity to bring the ball back down into the opponent's court. Consequently, players learn to play within this constant force of nature by attempting to maintain a relative balance between velocity and gravity. As everyone discovers, when the ball is hit harder gravity has less effect on the downward movements of the ball. Those players who are taught methods that provide the use of spin discover how they can increase the downward movements of the ball beyond that of the constant pull of gravity. Topspin, (which will be discussed in detail in Chapter 7 on "Tennis Physics") is critical to increasing this downward movement of the ball.

Even as the opposite of topspin—slice or underspin—which if hit with enough velocity will work against gravity, the rotational action of the ball can actually be used to contribute to a ball's downward movement if used properly in specific situations. Typically, a ball hit hard enough with slice or underspin will actually rise in relation to the opposite downward movement that topspin produces. However, slice used correctly can also help a ball stay low while the stroke is still firm. For example, if a player hits a ball from a very low position near the net, he or she must hit the ball upward at enough of an angle to clear the net. However, if this shot is hit with too much velocity, the ball, of course, will sail long. Now, if the same player hits this low shot with underspin or slice, the ball's velocity is decreased with the force of the shot being changed from velocity to spin. Yet, even as the ball's velocity is decreased, the force of the stroke can still be solid. Thus, this shot will drop because gravity's force can work with greater effect on a ball because of its lower velocity.

Another way the application of slice helps a ball drop is the action of air friction on the spinning ball. A spinning ball will tend to slow earlier than a ball with minimal spin. As you will learn in Chapter 7, air friction acts in both the movements of the ball in relation to its trajectory as well as slowing down a ball's velocity.

Finally, one other principle of physics that applies to a tennis ball in flight is the gyroscopic control spin adds. The action of spin helps a ball maintain a true trajectory. A flat ball tends to act much like a knuckle ball in baseball: wind and other factors diminish the control of a flat ball in flight. A spinning ball will curve a controlled amount based on the amount of spin applied and the ball's velocity and trajectory. This does not count the added need for perfection during contact on flat balls. Hard, flat shots must be hit relatively perfectly to achieve the desired trajectory. Any slight variance in racket angle will adversely effect of the control of any flat shot. As I will point out in later chapters, the mechanics of hitting a ball flat usually will require greater control. Even as good as professionals are, you will seldom see a tennis pro attempt to hit a ball perfectly flat. Typically, spin shots are not only easier to control, they are easier to reproduce mechanically.

How does all this talk about spin and velocity galvanize a player into becoming a dinker or not?

If a player a simply hit most shots relatively flat, the only principles that this player can count on is gravity and the actual trajectory based on the racket's angle at contact. If gravity is the only way a player can make a ball drop down into the court, then the only course of action for this player is to hit either hard shots low across the net, or, hit higher shots softer. Since hard hit balls are very hard to control, the player will resort to hitting progressively softer balls for control and consistency. Thus the dinker is born!

Skilled players create their own "gravity". Through the use of strokes that pro-

It is not uncommon to see "experienced" 3.0 or 3.5 level players still serving essentially the same exact way they did the first time they learned to serve !

duce spin, they can hit the ball harder with greater margins for error through the use of spin.

A good example of this is the myth of the "flat serve". So often, mediocre players are seen belting a flat serve only to get this serve in about once every lunar cycle! This serve is hit with terrific speed; however the ball lands not only outside the service box, but also often outside the entire court as well! In reality, pros like Pete Sampras, Gregg Ruseski or Andy Roddick who often hit serves reaching speeds of 130 miles per hour or more, hit with tremendous spin. In fact, most pros that do average such high-velocity serves hit with ball rotations between 2000 and 4000 rpm's. In other words, even at 120 miles per hour a typical Pete Sampras serve will be spinning somewhere near 30 revolutions per second! This is far from flat! (I will talk about this concept in detail in Chapter 11 on serves.) It is this spin, coupled with a specific axis of rotation, which allows such hard serves to land in the service box. Without this spin, it would be next to impossible for any serve, hit at these velocities and hit from the normal height of these players' reach, to ever land in the service box.

Dinkers, of course, rely only on the forces of gravity to keep balls in play. The result of such a hitting style on the serve is the aforementioned out-of-control flat serve followed by a puffball serve that my four year old daughter could return. And, ironically, even at such slow speeds, these players still double fault with regularity! Most of these players have a fast windup on the second serve followed by a marked deceleration of the racket in order to hit the ball soft. This deceleration of the racket makes a repeatable swing very difficult. Thus serving dinkers often find themselves guessing where the ball will land...even on such soft second serves!

This pattern of learning is why players, even those who have been playing tennis for years, seldom have their serve (or other strokes hit in the same dinking fashion!) improve. In fact, it is not uncommon to see even experienced players, (3.0 and 3.5 levels), serving essentially the same exact way they did from the first time they tried to serve!

So, You Want to Be a 5.0?

Tennis players of all abilities and those seeking higher levels of skill (and thus a higher rating) must understand this very simple but very true statement:

> *"If you don't ever seek to create stroke patterns that are decidedly at higher levels of play, you will never reach those higher levels of play you seek."*

This statement is critical on three points. First, players must be willing to make errors while attempting more advanced form. Second, players must clearly understand what advanced form is. Third, they must know how to attempt it themselves, (especially without falling back to old stroke habits in the process.)

Let me break down these concepts so players can clearly understand how they relate to them personally.

1. PLAYERS MUST BE WILLING TO MAKE ERRORS WHILE ATTEMPTING MORE ADVANCED FORM.

Understand that when a player attempts more advanced stroke patterns, some element of failure is inevitable. Yet, failure should not discourage future attempts! Consider the toddler who is trying to walk for the first time. Failure (in falling) is a given. Yet, we as wobbling infants get up and try again and again...until we are actually walking. Tennis players must keep attempting more advanced stroke patterns regularly in competition and in practice if they ever hope to reach such skilled levels of play. If we as toddlers reverted back to the safety and comfort of crawling the first time we failed at walking, we would probably find ourselves on all fours playing tennis! Tennis is no different! If we sincerely want to achieve high levels of play, we must continue to attempt such advanced stroke patterns. Yet, millions of tennis players, when attempting what they know is the correct serve, volley or groundstroke go right back to that which is comfortable and safe. (And then they wonder why they can never get past the 3.0 levels of play!) As you will read in this book, advanced stroke patterns can include both stroke mechanics that are deemed "advanced" as well as stroke patterns that are more effective through their application (such as greater spin, angle, depth, pace, etc.).

Player personalities can contribute to the likelihood of such higher level attempts. For example, an extrovert (usually a young male!) often goes for more shots or greater difficulty in shots than they are usually ready to do. While this premature effort often leads to disaster, these same players, when working within stroke mechanics deemed proper, eventually master such high level strokes just because they are constantly attempting them. On the other hand, a very conservative individual might never attempt anything out of their comfort zone. Thus, they languish at mediocrity; their level of mediocrity is determined only by the level of comfort they possess within their perceived conservative play.

2. PLAYERS MUST CLEARLY UNDERSTAND WHAT ADVANCED FORM IS.

Simply swinging harder or aiming for severe angles will seldom lead to consistency or success for any individual. (Swinging harder is seldom part of the Advanced Foundation. However, players who develop the Advanced Foundation will indeed begin to naturally swing harder with greater success and consistency.) Without swinging within defined and proper stroke patterns, the likelihood of mastering any shot is practically impossible no matter how many times you attempt it. This is because most wild or extreme strokes are seldom repeatable within the vast diversity and location of our opponent's shots. Thus, it is paramount that players KNOW what advanced form is and how it applies to each shot attempted. This is where lessons, books, videos, and simply watching tennis on television or in person can be of such help. Without having a clear understanding of all tennis strokes, it is highly unlikely a person will spontaneously hit tennis balls with advanced form.

3. PLAYERS MUST KNOW HOW TO ATTEMPT ADVANCED FORM THEMSELVES.

Understanding and knowing what specific strokes and shots look like is one thing. It is another thing to know how to physically reproduce them. Through my years of training players, I can say without a doubt, that every single player has a different baseline level of kinesthetic control of their own bodies. Therefore, some players must be more disciplined and patient in their development of strokes, while others can mimic and replicate exactly what they see and understand almost immediately. And players who have played many years using inferior form will be most pressed into first overcoming prior stroke tendencies before proper and, then, advanced stroke patterns can be instilled and mastered.

Players must understand the desired stroke pattern as well as understanding what their body and appendages are doing. A number of players to whom I have been exposed actually thought they were hitting topspin when in fact they were hitting a slice! Certainly, if a player has not developed the necessary comprehension of personal movements of body parts, then executing strokes deemed proper will be most difficult.

Be assured that the tools and practice methods prescribed throughout this book will help even the least gifted of players! In fact, many players only perceive a limited athleticism. After proper training most players will end up mastering the game far better than they ever imagined!

Adjustment Period

When beginners play, they will play within a performance pattern that is comfortable. Since they have minimal understanding or experience in stroke development, they can only do what they "feel" is correct. Obviously, if skilled form is foreign or uncomfortable, a beginner will seldom explore such form—at least not with conscious effort! This concept alone clearly contradicts those teachers who believe in letting players blindly explore the game through self-discovery or within passive explanatory means. While skilled players play within a methodology that resembles "simple,"(or as many often say, "they make it look so easy!"), the actual methods that lead up to such simple stroke patterns are not natural, comfortable, or simple to most people.

Experienced players in competition will to tend fall back on old strokes and form which is most familiar. As with most intermediate players, the most familiar stroke pattern is the way they FIRST learned the game. If this pattern is based on inferior, mediocre methods, than the player will indeed revert back to inferior and mediocre strokes.

In either case, players must understand three things:

1. *They will never become familiar nor successful with more advanced strokes if they never attempt them, or if they attempt such strokes only when there is no pressure—as in practice only*
2. *If they continue to use inferior—but comfortable—strokes, they will nevertheless still make errors with such form*
3. *While continuing to use mediocre form such players will seldom be competitive with skilled opponents.*

It is far better for players to use the best form they have been taught, and make mistakes with those strokes than it is to continue using simple or inferior strokes and *perceive* some idea of success. (That is IF they indeed want to become skilled tennis players!) I say "perceive" because players can actually make more mistakes with their old, inferior strokes and feel more successful than when making fewer mistakes with new, more advanced strokes. This perceived success (within such failure) is due to familiarity. Typically, when players start trying to use new strokes, the unfamiliarity creates discomfort and uncertainty. For many players it is more comfortable to miss with shots with which a player is familiar than to make successful strokes using something new and unfamiliar! This is why players must understand that an "Adjustment Period" will need to be tolerated while using proper form.

Even when a player applies proper form, mistakes often occur. These can be caused by:

- *Using the correct grip but using improper footwork*
- *Using the proper footwork and grip, but hitting with an improper swing pattern*
- *Using the proper grip, footwork and swing pattern, but swinging with poor timing*
- *Using proper grip, footwork, swing pattern and timing, but miss-hitting the ball*
- *Using proper grip, footwork, swing pattern, timing and hitting the ball in the sweet spot, but aiming wrong.*

As you can see, there can be many incriminating factors that can produce an unsuccessful shot. Thus, a player must understand that while many components of a shot can be correctly executed, one or more other stroke-components might be off or wrong... producing an unsuccessful result. I can't tell you how many times I have heard a student say, "I did what you told me but the ball still went out." Teaching pros around the world can all probably attest to this! And we can easily see from the description above just why a player can actually do almost everything right...yet still not have the desired outcome!

However, there is hope!

With every mistake using proper form comes learning. For example, if a player is trying a new two-handed backhand and hits it into the net or long, a realization of racket control and body movements is initiated. Each succeeding hit will ingrain the understanding of what the racket and body is doing in conjunction with each hit. Each time we revert back to inferior form, we prohibit what we are trying to accomplish in favor of accomplishing what we are trying to eliminate!

The Duality of Mastering Tennis

TENNIS MASTERY (and playing tennis masterfully!) is a two-part continuum. As mentioned earlier, the methods in which a player is taught certainly is the core of a player's mechanical development. If methods that are taught prevent a player from reaching their potential, then those methods are faulty. By providing a "Linear Progression" learning process and using highly effective teaching methods, tennis instructors will develop an "Advanced Foundation" for players on which to build their tennis future. This concept makes up the first part of this duality. The second part is called your "Practice Foundation".

Practice Foundation

Every successful athlete must address, understand, and be willing to adhere to an "Individual Practice Foundation" in order for them to reach their greatest potential. An Individual Practice Foundation coordinates a proper on-court routine based on several factors:

A) What level the player is currently playing?
B) What level the player wants to achieve?
C) How quickly does the player want to achieve the desired level?
D) What limitations or handicaps does the player possess?
E) What is the player's schedule of competitive matches?

In reality, a player's Individual Practice Foundation begins BEFORE they step onto the court…even for the first time! To maximize learning and gain the greatest value from the methods learned in this book, the Individual Practice Foundation begins with THE BRAIN. The following chapters of TENNIS MASTERY deal with concepts that are directed at the player's mind and cognitive understandings surrounding tennis. Back in 1974 W. Timothy Gallwey wrote a revolutionary "psychological" book called Inner Tennis. The entire book dealt with the mental side of tennis. Not a single picture, diagram, or instructional tip that dealt with tennis mechanics was discussed in the book. However, the book consisted of over 160 pages and sold over 700,000 making it one of the greatest selling books in tennis! This should tell you that there is a great deal of information that includes the brain, including psychological, emotional, strategic, and motivational components of the mind.

However, there are even more ways to not only incorporate the mind, but to exercise it as well. This is your starting point, no matter what level of player you currently are!

There is a cliché; "Practice makes perfect." This has long since been revised to say, "Perfect Practice makes perfect." Your on-court practice technique must follow a similar objective. After learning techniques that will allow for proper progression, players must then utilize practice techniques that not only reinforce those learned procedures, but also provide for a multitude of other important learning criteria. These can include:

- *Strength building*
- *Stamina building*
- *Improving reaction time*
- *Targeting*
- *Finesse and touch*
- *Quickness*
- *Concentration* • *Consistency* • *Mental toughness*
- *Strategy understandings And more.*

Each time we revert back to inferior form, we prohibit what we are trying to accomplish in favor of accomplishing what we are trying to eliminate

!

Levels of Competency

It should be understood that, in reality, competency can be discussed within four distinct criteria. When a player understands these four levels, they are better equipped to attack learning—and, eventually move closer to the highest level of Competency in competition. The four levels are:

•**Unconscious Incompetence**: This is basically the lowest level that describes individuals who are terrible but don't know how terrible they really are! Don't laugh; this is actually a very real situation. I've had players actually believe they are either very good, (when they simply were not!), or had no idea what they were doing on the court. A couple examples of this level are as follows:

•In a clinic where the drill was to execute a topspin crosscourt stroke, a woman repeatedly hit a hacking-type slice stroke, hitting severe underspin, with very poor form to boot. As I discussed the results of the drill, I turned to the woman and said as amicably as I could, "And Suzie, those were really nice slices on the forehand side." Suzie turned to me and said, "Oh no, those were topspin forehands." Obviously, Suzie had no concept of either what topspin really was as it pertains to a tennis stroke or had no idea what she was actually doing with each shot. Either way, she would need to recognize this failure and learn from it as quickly as possible if she were to progress.

•The second example I've seen with Unconscious Incompetence was when I was working with a middle-age woman. Prior to our first lesson, her comment to me was, "Dave, I've played a lot of volleyball and other sports, so I think I will take to tennis very quickly." I, of course, looked forward to having such an experienced athlete to work with. However, within only a few shot attempts, I could see very quickly that this woman had absolutely no hand-eye coordination. No matter how easy I made the drill, even going to a dead-ball, drop-fed shot attempt, she simply had no inkling of how to hit the ball. Even after very clear directives, demonstrations, guided movements and even breaking the stroke down to the simplest level I could, she did not respond as 99.9% of my other students did. Yet, all the while this woman felt she was actually quite competent in each attempt.

•Conscious Incompetence: Here a player is very aware that they are doing things wrong. They usually don't know how to correct their problematic stroke element; however they are aware that what they are attempting is not what they know they should be doing. Here, we are now on a path towards improvement. It is a little like going to an Alcoholic's Anonymous class: The first step towards improvement is recognizing one has a problem. In tennis, we must be open to recognition that we are not doing things within acceptable patterns as they pertain to skilled tennis. Obviously, the ability to improve towards skilled play is dependent not just on our recognition that we are not doing what we should, but it is also dependent on our desire to achieve skilled play. For what ever reasons, some people are simply satisfied with where they are at. And, quite frankly, I have no problem with this. Yet, even people who claim to be satisfied often have a deep secret of wishing they could become better tennis players. Some believe they just can't. Others feel that making changes is simply too difficult and they want to avoid the frustration of making changes.

•Conscious Competence: Here we are gaining understanding of what we want to do and how to do it. This is the second step towards reaching Tennis Mastery. While the first one is recognizing we have a problem, this step is recognizing what we SHOULD be doing…and doing it in a conscious effort. We now know how a stroke should look; we are able to emulate the stroke consciously. However, the minute we are pressed into a situation where we don't have time to think, or, we are under pressure to the point that we revert back to something more comfortable—yet a pattern we may know won't make us better—we are not able to execute this new or desired competent pattern. We have not fully "Mastered" the technique.

•Unconscious Competence: The highest degree of achievement…in ANYTHING! Without thinking about any major concept of a stroke, we execute the shot correctly, even under pressure or in situations where we must react quickly without any thought. We often compare this level with terms or phrases like, "Playing in the zone" or "Playing unconscious". While even with unrefined swing patterns, players can play in this so-called zone…hitting shots that they normally don't succeed with, with any regularity. However, truly skilled players are able to execute optimal shots, (and strategies, for that matter!), on any given day, regardless of whether they are playing well or are having an off day. Remember, the pros miss too. They don't go out there after missing a serve or a backhand and say, "Heck, this shot isn't working, I need to change my technique." This type of statement is usually done by players in the first or second phase of competency. They often don't recognize the difference between "aim" and bad form! Good players who have mastered the game seldom look at misses as improper technique. (Although, sometimes a stroke can break down through many causes: stress, tiredness, poor focus on the ball, miss steps, etc.) Most good players know that a miss is usually from some element of their aim being off.

When players begin to accept these stages they may be currently in, they have more clarity in what to work on in practice.

CHAPTER 3

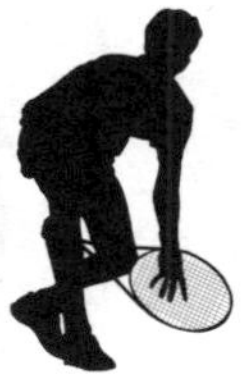

The Advanced Foundation–Defining Tennis Mastery

Tennis Mastery: Two Foundations

Progressive Stroke patterns, those that will provide sustained improvement, makes up what we call the Advanced Foundation as it applies to the actual methods of hitting a tennis ball. It is obvious that players who want to play tennis well will need to be able to replicate desirable strokes under the pressure of competition. There are many people who can hit nearly flawlessly off a ball machine or a wall. However, when they get on the court against another human player, the realization that their stroke patterns are not reliable is exposed.

Thus, it is critical that players learn an equally important foundation: the "Practice Foundation". The Practice Foundation describes how the player will acquire and then incorporate the desired strokes in actual competitive environments.

The "Practice Foundation" describes how the player will acquire and then incorporate the desired strokes in actual competitive environments.

The following information will help you understand how both of these "Foundation" concepts interrelate. The Advanced Foundation is based on cognitive learning and understanding of what strokes a player will want to emulate, practice and, eventually, master. Your Practice Foundation is the "action phase" of this knowledge.

Understand too, that this "action phase" is not relegated to on-court practice alone. There is much a player can and should do off the court as well. This is perhaps one of the big differences between champions and just "good players".

These first few chapters on defining the Strategies of Learning, are the "starting point" of a player's trek to Tennis Mastery. Like trying to get through a maze, players can go many ways in terms of learning how to play the game. Following the correct path takes us to our "finish point" or, more appropriately our goals. More often than not, players who follow other paths, faulty in their direction, can lead to dead ends. (Our "finish point" in reality is never finished! If a player learns methods that provide continued improvement, they will really never be "finished" learning and improving!)

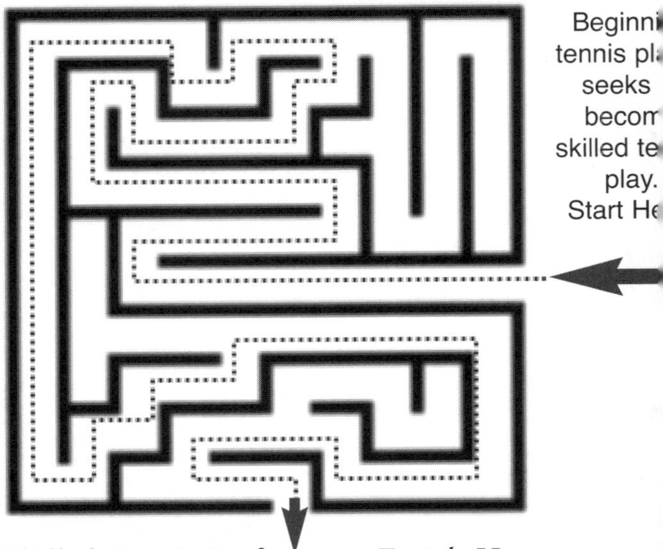

Skilled Tennis Performer - Finish Here.

Figure 1
Learning tennis is like a maze. Going down the wrong path usually meaning having to go back and try another way.

Just as in our proverbial maze, some players who choose the wrong path must go backwards and try another one. Unfortunately, some people get tired of going down the wrong paths and eventually end up quitting the game. Some players continue to play but relegate themselves into believing that they will never reach high levels of skilled play. Either way, players who are introduced to—or continuously taught—inferior tennis methods are doomed if the goal is to play skilled tennis.

Imagine that someone, who knew the correct passageway through our "Tennis Maze", illuminated the correct path for you with a Highlighter pen. Such an advantage would certainly save time, but perhaps more importantly, such help would save us from unnecessary frustration of having to "start over". These chapters will highlight a clear path for you to follow with no dead ends at the very least. A practical practice foundation, one that incorporates the Advanced Foundation as the technical methodology, will provide each player with efficient and productive improvement. If either the practice foundation or the learning methodology is flawed, players will indeed meet dead ends.

WHEN IS "EQUAL" NOT EQUAL?

What separates two tennis players who appear equal in all respects? Observe two players, both hitting solid groundstrokes and/or volleys, both possessing a good serve and both seemingly equal in terms of footwork or speed. If someone asked you who you thought would win before they began the match, would it be possible to predict who would come out on top?

Possibly.

It is a given fact that when these two hypothetical players meet in a tennis match, one will win and the other will lose. There are no ties in tennis.

Now, what *really* separates these two players?

Separating the Winners from the Losers

The fact is that some players win more than their share of matches. An obvious statement was once mentioned: half of all tennis players lose in match-play. If this is true, (and of course it is!), and some players are indeed, ending up winning more matches then they lose, it stands to reason that other players are losing more than 50% of the time!

Just who are these consistent winners and losers? Do the winners possess some kind of magic potion, a secret weapon? Are the losers predestined to meet defeat because of who they are or where they live or what they eat?

Again, what separates our two so-called equal players mentioned above?

Looking solely at match performances, you will not fully understand how the winner won by those observations alone. Sure, you will observe that the victor made fewer errors and, perhaps, hit more winners. But what made it possible for the winner to do just that:

Make fewer errors; hit more winners?

It is this phrase and this phrase alone that separates the winner from the loser *during* a match. It also separates those who possess a greater amount of Tennis Mastery from those who are lacking it.

> Everything we have accomplished in learning to play tennis and in preparing for competition will have a direct impact on what is happening at any given moment of competition.

Take a Closer Look

Those of you who are experienced tennis players can readily identify the mistakes made or the intelligent shots hit by players in competition. It is possible for all of us (beginners to tournament players) to recognize when a player's momentum is on the rise or if it is collapsing like an avalanche! We might wince when witnessing a player in the process of choking, perhaps because we have all experienced some level of the choking syndrome ourselves. Likewise, we might be able to similarly relate to those moments when a player's confidence lifts them to perform at extraordinary levels.

All of these match-play scenarios by the player (or opponent) happen in what we call "Real Time" experience. In other words, everything we have accomplished in learning to play tennis and in preparing for competition will have a direct impact on what is happening at any given moment of competition. Based on this statement, the winner would almost seem *predestined* to come out the victor because of this preliminary preparation. In reality, this is quite true.

Can you tell a Winner from a Loser by watching them *before they compete?*

Sometimes, just by observing players before a match, we can predict who will win with some degree of accuracy. Simply looking at the physical appearances of players can help us form our opinion regarding the predicted outcome of a match. Strong, athletic-looking players with defined muscles and five tennis rackets often creates an image of a potential winner long before that player has stepped onto the court and taken his first swing.

Yet, these images can be deceiving.

In 1974, one of the top junior players in the prolific tennis area of Southern

California was a five-foot, one-inch, 97 pound high school senior named Roger Hillie. Hillie won ninety-two tennis matches and lost none during his senior year. Prior to that, in his junior season he went 83 - 2 when he weighed in at a paltry eighty-eight pounds. His legs were no bigger around than most kids' arms and he could fit into clothes purchased in the children's section of a department store. His mop of sun-bleached blond hair reflected his love for surfing the beaches of Southern California whenever he wasn't on the tennis court playing or practicing.

What made Roger Hillie so darn tough? To look at him standing on the court, you would swear even a sudden breeze would knock him down. Yet, he took on the likes of players standing a foot and a half taller, and in turn, knocked them down as the proverbial David conquering Goliath! I personally saw him diminish such Goliath-like players into whimpering fools. Roger was unbeatable until his untimely death from a car accident in 1980.

Why was he so unbeatable?

Here's why:

Roger Hillie hated to lose. Is this part of Tennis Mastery? You bet it is!

My father, nationally recognized coach Bruce Smith, used to love to tell this story about Roger and his tenacity for not just wanting to play well, but for his persistence for wanting to play competitive tennis:

> *In the finals of the regional playoffs, Roger was playing teammate Mike Chewalek, a strong, athletic boy with extremely fast feet and hands. The score at the end of the finals was 6-2, 6-3 in favor of Roger. As the two boys approached the net to shake hands, Roger punched Mike in the chest in anger. Startled by Roger's outburst, especially since he had won the match, my father ran out to the court and held Roger back from sending another punch in Mike's direction. When asked why in the heck he had hit Mike, especially since he had won the match rather easily, Roger replied in anger, "Coach, Mike didn't try hard enough to beat me."*

While most kids would be overjoyed to have won such an important match, Roger was more concerned that his opponent hadn't tried hard enough, in his opinion. Neither my father nor I ever condone violence of any kind, yet this kind of determination and expectation that Roger displayed was evidence of his desire for truly competitive competition.

Can a player who seems to lack abhorrence for losing develop this determination? Isn't it a little like having a "killer instinct" on the court? Can a nice guy finish first, also?

Yes, yes and yes!

By developing progressive strokes within the Advanced Foundation players will not only achieve sustained improvement, they will develop a "progressive confidence foundation" as well. This combination of proper stroke mechanics and player confidence helps build a player's competitive "character." Certainly, individual player personalities and natural competitive spirit will contribute additional characteristics and responses to competitive situations. However, players can, indeed, train themselves to gain both a "killer instinct" as well as a thirst for competitive success no matter what their predisposition to these characteristics might be.

* * *

I remember a story told to me by my father, a story that took place years earlier, about a freshman at a high school who had tried out for the boy's tennis team. Standing over 6 feet tall the young boy was all arms and legs. The high school coach took a look at the boy and told him he was too tall to be a good tennis player.

"Perhaps you should try a different sport," the coach had said to the boy.

While many a boy or girl, when told that they might just not be good enough, would probably turn away and not pursue their quest, this boy continued to play tennis.

The player was reported to be Stan Smith, and he went on to become the number one tennis player in the world in the early 1970's.

* * *

To give one more example of distinguished individuals, I had a player in California who seemingly lacked any ounce of tennis athleticism. He was a Vietnamese boy named Hien Wu who had come out for my large tennis team as a freshman. Since I never cut players, Hien was the last boy on my roster, number 52 if my memory serves me. When we began working with our new players, Hien literally could not drop-hit a tennis ball. Tossing to him was like watching a movie with the sound track playing late. He would constantly swing too early or late and was lucky to hit the ball at all. While my first instinct was to cut him simply to save him the embarrassment of what others might say about him, my assistant coach talked me into maintaining our procedure of not cutting players…we kept him.

To make a long story short, Hien became the number-one ranked doubles player in the tennis-rich area of Southern California. He teamed with three different partners in three years on varsity (his sophomore year to his senior year), and went 152 – 0 in region during those three years. (Imagine if I had indeed cut him!) Hien's success can be directly attributed to his desire to become a good tennis player. He worked after every practice, begging us, and anyone else, to stay and hit balls to him.

Roger Hillie overcame his obvious physical limitations; Stan Smith didn't allow one person's opinion deter his dreams and aspirations; Hien Wu overcame questionable athleticism.Yet, *how* Roger Hillie, Stan Smith, and Hien Wu overcame what most people would label as obstacles is part of what this book is all about.

All of them acquired "Tennis Mastery" and you can too.

But first, before you can acquire any semblance of Tennis Mastery, you must have a clear understanding of its definition. Like taking a trip without a predetermined destination, your journey to reaching Tennis Mastery will be short lived without knowing where you're headed! And without knowing where you're going, determining how you will get there will be a true practice in futility and a complete waste of time!

> *Definition: Tennis Mastery is the summation of all the elements a player must acquire to compete* **successfully** *at any level, against any opponent, under all conditions, and within all circumstances.*

Notice that I have written "**successfull**y" in bold print. Notice also that the word "winning" is conspicuously missing in this definition. The reason for this omission is intentional; its absence is used to emphasize that you don't have to win to be successful. Oftentimes, people only associate being successful with winning. However, many of us who have been playing tennis a while have engaged a tough opponent, perhaps far superior than we, and yet walked away feeling like we played the best tennis of our life… even though we lost!

Success isn't always measured by trophies, medals and circled match scores on a draw sheet.

As I just mentioned, success is not always associated with winning. And, more importantly for players, winning should not be the *instrument of assessment*, especially in determining your level of Tennis Mastery. Winning is, however, a common outcome for those who have acquired Tennis Mastery. (Which is why so many people associate winning with this success!) The difference between these two mind-sets is in the objective: A player who focuses on winning will have a difficult, if not impossible, time reaching Tennis Mastery.

A player who searches, observes, studies, attempts, practices and understands Tennis Mastery will not only eventually attain higher levels of Mastery, he or she will procure more wins in the process.

A player who looks at winning as being the singular proof of success will miss out on an even greater learning tool:

LOSING.

The truth of the matter is that Tennis Mastery is only possible when a player begins to realize his mistakes.

Jim Hastings, former coach, television analyst and author, called a player who loses a match and then loses the opportunity to learn something from the loss a "Double Loser". This is an excellent description as it really does capture the sense of losing twice which these players have done in not learning from their loss. Writer Jeff Greenwald wrote this about the concept of winning and losing in an article found at www.tennisone.com:

We've all been conditioned -- by parents, by schools, surely by society -- that winning, as Vince Lombardi used to say, is everything, the only thing. It shouldn't be. When it is, I believe it's a handicap. Yes, winning is a great feeling, but there's a better feeling out there -- the feeling that you are playing the best tennis you are capable of, all the time; that you are playing full out, enjoying the drama, embracing the moment, relishing the opportunity to compete, learning something every time --- whether you are winning or losing. And a funny thing happens when you rel-

ish and enjoy and play up to your potential - - you win more. It has happened to me, exactly like that.

While Jeff's statements actually have an application in the "mental" side of tennis, his remarks clearly indicate that winning is not the ultimate goal.

Indeed, in losing, the player who is sincerely pursuing Tennis Mastery will gain from his loss. He will analyze the strengths of his opponent's game as well as the weaknesses in his own; he will look for ways to improve those weaknesses and, in the process, come one step closer to Tennis Mastery. The player focusing on winning as the ultimate goal, however, will be easily discouraged and frustrated in each defeat. This type of player will usually look for excuses and, often times erroneously, identify various circumstances that caused victory to seemingly be snatched from his grasp. (Again!) These players will undoubtedly be unable to identify the actual reason they lost. Players that often lose—or lose to players they believe they shouldn't lose to—oftentimes are overheard saying remarks such as: "If that guy wasn't such a dinker, I would have killed him," or, "I should have won. I'm a lot better player than she is. She just cheated me out of the important points."

A player who loses a match and then passes on the opportunity to learn something from the loss is called a "DOUBLE LOSER"

!

These players are in denial. It hurts to acknowledge our weaknesses and shortcomings. And yet, this failure to recognize the actual deficiency in our own game is what will prevent us from overcoming it.

Recognizing the meaning of Tennis Mastery, then creating a meaningful and logical plan to acquire it, is the first step in achieving Tennis Mastery.

Learning the true "meaning" of Tennis Mastery will, indeed, be your first step. We will talk about the elements that make up Tennis Mastery in Chapter Four.

Whether you are a beginner, a seasoned veteran of tennis, a social doubles player, or a tournament competitor, the tools that follow will help you on your quest to becoming the best!

CHAPTER 4

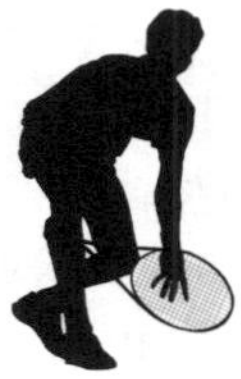

The Advanced Foundation–What makes up Tennis Mastery?

Whether you are a beginner or a seasoned veteran of competitive tennis, gaining greater Tennis Mastery at any stage of your development will allow you to pursue and successfully attain higher levels of tennis proficiency. Understanding the component parts of Tennis Mastery and how they can be practiced and perfected is the backbone of tennis success at every level. Training within the Advanced Foundation includes knowing how the component parts of Tennis Mastery are related and how they can contribute to your success on the court.

Elements of Tennis Mastery

What are all the "elements" of Tennis Mastery that I referred to earlier in Chapter Three (from its definition), that a player must acquire? You might guess them to be things like a topspin backhand, a great second serve, or a killer instinct. If these were some of the things that came to mind, you would be correct… but only partially. In reality, those are just a fraction of all the elements that make up Tennis Mastery.

Simply put, all the elements that indeed make up Tennis Mastery can be grouped within two main categories:

- *Tennis Mechanics*
- *Mental Tennis*

It has been said that tennis is over 60% a mental component. At some levels it is, perhaps, an even higher percentage. Of course, if faulty or unfamiliar strokes prevent you from being able to hit a ball over the net, tennis at that point is 100% a mechanical component! Forget knowing why hitting a crosscourt groundstroke has certain advantages over a down-the-line, or that developing techniques to block out mental distractions will help prevent choking; you're not going to win any points if you can't cause the ball to land on your opponent's side of the court! (Nor will you have much fun!)

Many books, including this one, discuss mental tennis and how it can make or break you as a competitive tennis player. However, the key word in this sentence is "Player". To be considered a "player" you must have some semblance of strokes, footwork and technique that can, at least, get you on the court with other players!

No matter at what level you are, at some point you will probably find yourself on the court playing opponents who are head and shoulders better than yourself. When this happens (and it will!), the feelings of apprehension or fear can be the same for the beginner as they are for an experienced player. However, the player who is sincere in his or her search of Tennis Mastery will come away from the match a wiser tennis player. Those who are not in search of Tennis Mastery will try to forget the loss, only to come away from the match embarrassed and humiliated. You can quickly see how, even for beginners, tennis can indeed be a mental game!

I've heard people comment on how talented professional tennis players never experience the embarrassment of a sound whipping since they are all so good. On the contrary, look at the match scores from any professional tennis tournament and you will find numerous players who lost a 6 - 0 or 6 - 1 set. Experienced and talented players will "meet their match" at some point in their career! However, the player with Tennis Mastery will learn from these past beatings and become stronger from them.

In this book you will discover the secrets to mastering both mental and mechanical tennis, and, hopefully, in the process find yourself fewer times on the losing side of one of those 6 - 0 matches! Understanding how these two integral parts of Tennis Mastery work and addressing them throughout your development will help you become not just a better tennis player, but also a tennis champion!

Let's take a closer look at these two main parts of Tennis Mastery.

Tennis Mechanics

In learning to walk each of us, as infants and toddlers, learned through trial and error how to balance and sequentially step our way into the world. (And often into walls and other precarious situations!) Now, as grownups we are accomplished walkers, barring some sort of handicap. We seldom, if ever, have to think of how to walk from point A to point B! We don't have to think which foot to start with, what part of the foot should strike the ground first, or how much we have to bend our knees before transferring the weight of our bodies onto the other leg. Imagine how inept we would be if we had to consciously think about every component of walking each and every time we decided to walk!

In reality, players who have prepared through practicing fundamentally sound strokes already know how to hit the ball – just as we already know how to walk.

This is a common problem with tennis players who have learned—but not mastered—tennis mechanics. While playing matches, they often think too much about "how" to hit the ball while trying to execute shots. In reality, players who have prepared through practicing fundamentally sound strokes already know how to hit the ball—just as we already know how to walk. And, similar to walking, all tennis players really need to do is know where they want the ball to go! (Aim!) This is perhaps an over-simplified statement. However, accomplished players seldom think excessively about how to hit the ball during match play.

We have words or phrases in tennis that we often use to describe a player who is playing great tennis. We sometimes describe them as playing "unconscious". When asked, these players often mention that, indeed, they "weren't thinking". Some players recall they were "just out there hitting the ball" or they were playing "in the zone". The fact is, when we let what we already know happen on the court, we generally play some of our best tennis! I will be discussing these concepts of playing your best tennis while in match-play competition further in Chapter 13 on Mental Tennis.

However, we must learn and master proper strokes before we can begin to let them happen "unconsciously".

We must take that proverbial first step before we walk...and before we can run.

BREAKING DOWN TENNIS MECHANICS

Obviously, strokes are the major component of tennis mechanics. However, there are actually four distinct parts to tennis mechanics—as they apply to the Advanced Foundation—which must be addressed before becoming mastered:

- *Sound tennis strokes*
- *Proper footwork*
- *Hand-eye coordination*
- *Shot-making skills and execution*

How each of these is related is important to your improvement. If you neglect any portion, your mastery of tennis mechanics (and thus, Tennis Mastery) will be inadequate. "Your training will be incomplete, young Jedi Tennis Master."

All Star Wars humor aside, understanding each part of tennis mechanics is essential.

Components of Tennis Mechanics
SOUND TENNIS STROKES

There are more books written and videos produced on hitting tennis balls than the teaching of all other areas of tennis combined! It is logical since without the ability to hit tennis balls with intention and accuracy, all the other components of Tennis Mastery will be virtually useless on the court! Simply put, tennis strokes are the heart of playing tennis.

Yet, understand that simply working on the multitude of elementary methods in getting a ball over the net will not necessarily provide you with long-term improvement.

Solid Foundation—Progressive Foundation: Advanced Foundation

Proper tennis strokes (those which will provide for continued advancement) are built from what I call a solid "Progressive Player Foundation". Because this foundation will lead players who adopt it to advanced play, I generally refer to it simply as the "Advanced Foundation". It is from this foundation that your development of spin, pace and directional control will be not only possible, but your continued improvement towards higher levels of play will be insured. In addition, this foundation will determine your ability to hit consistently as well as being able to hit a variety of specific shots successfully. A flawed foundation, one that is composed of one or more mechanical faults, can seriously hinder a player's ability to improve in these areas.

I often compare tennis to golf when I talk about building a sound foundation. Tennis and golf are both so dependent on precise and repeatable swing patterns that, often, when players try to teach themselves, they develop bad habits that are very difficult to correct and overcome. In addition, players who first develop "basic" swing patterns then fail to make the necessary changes to more advanced patterns will have a difficult time sustaining their improvement. The ability for a player to develop a correct swing pattern that can be repeated in the heat of competition is perhaps the most determining factor in that player's progress as well as confidence. If a player learns a flawed stroke pattern, or one that prevents proper evolution and advancement, then a player runs the risk of never achieving their true potential. It is no wonder that there are literally millions of very average and below average tennis players on this planet…and many of them have been playing the game for years and even decades!

As I have mentioned, a great majority of books on tennis teach a process of learning that I believe can be detrimental to all players. They tend to teach a stroke or method which they say, "is an easier way to learn to play tennis" but they go on to add, "the student will want to change to a more advanced stroke or method later," *after* they become familiar with the concept. Among the many problems this teaching philosophy presents, it does not take into account all the changes that need to take place to accommodate just one aspect of a change.

In Section 2, "The Strategies of Hitting" (Chapters 7 – 12), I will address the issue of strokes and how to produce them correctly so you won't have to make uncomfortable changes later on in your progress! In fact, when you learn strokes from this standpoint of the Advanced Foundation, the changes you might make are changes you WANT to make instead of making changes because you HAVE to! In other words, you will be in command of any changes you might want to explore within an incredibly sound foundation.

By learning proper footwork combined with the appropriate tennis stokes, the results can produce stellar strokes that will prove to be devastating weapons against your opponents

PROPER FOOTWORK

Most books, which include stroke production in their context, will also describe proper footwork. It stands to reason that if you don't get to a ball you want to hit (or if you overrun it), you probably won't be able to use that great new topspin backhand you just learned!

But footwork goes far beyond just getting to the ball. As you will learn, footwork is a vital link in the framework of hitting a ball well and effectively. You will discover how a simple step using the wrong foot at the wrong time can result in negative "cause and effect". A simple misstep can result in unfavorable strokes which, if unchecked and not corrected, can reside permanently within a player's mechanics. Likewise, by learning proper footwork combined with the appropriate tennis strokes, the results can produce stellar strokes that will prove to be devastating weapons against your opponent!

Because successful strokes are so dependent upon proper and accurate footwork, I will address all the issues of footwork and how they apply to strokes also throughout Section 2 on the Strategies of Hitting.

HAND-EYE COORDINATION

It is this topic which falls short in most books which I have researched. We all know that people possess and exhibit extreme variations in natural hand-eye coordination. Since our coordination is inherited and/or developed so early in our lives, we usually have little say over its evolution prior to picking up a racket. Nevertheless, there are ways in which you can improve your coordination as it relates to hitting tennis balls. I have developed some very simple yet productive exercises that I use with the players I teach, regardless their level. These drills help to improve everything from power to touch, from control to reaction time, as they relate to hand-eye coordination. (Most of these drills, or "tools" as I call them, will be presented in appropriate sections or chapters throughout this book.)

As with all sports that use an implement (racket, bat, stick, club or other device) to make contact with the corresponding ball, puck, shuttlecock, etc., tennis is a sport that truly requires superior hand-eye coordination. Consider, too, that unlike golf where you are hitting a stationary ball, or baseball where you are attempting to hit a ball that is thrown at least near to where you are standing, in tennis you are required to hit a ball that is intentionally hit away from you! That doesn't mean that golf or baseball or any other sport is any less demanding than tennis. The fact of the matter is that due to the demands required to play successfully, tennis players must be able to meet those demands specific to tennis with regularity and precision.

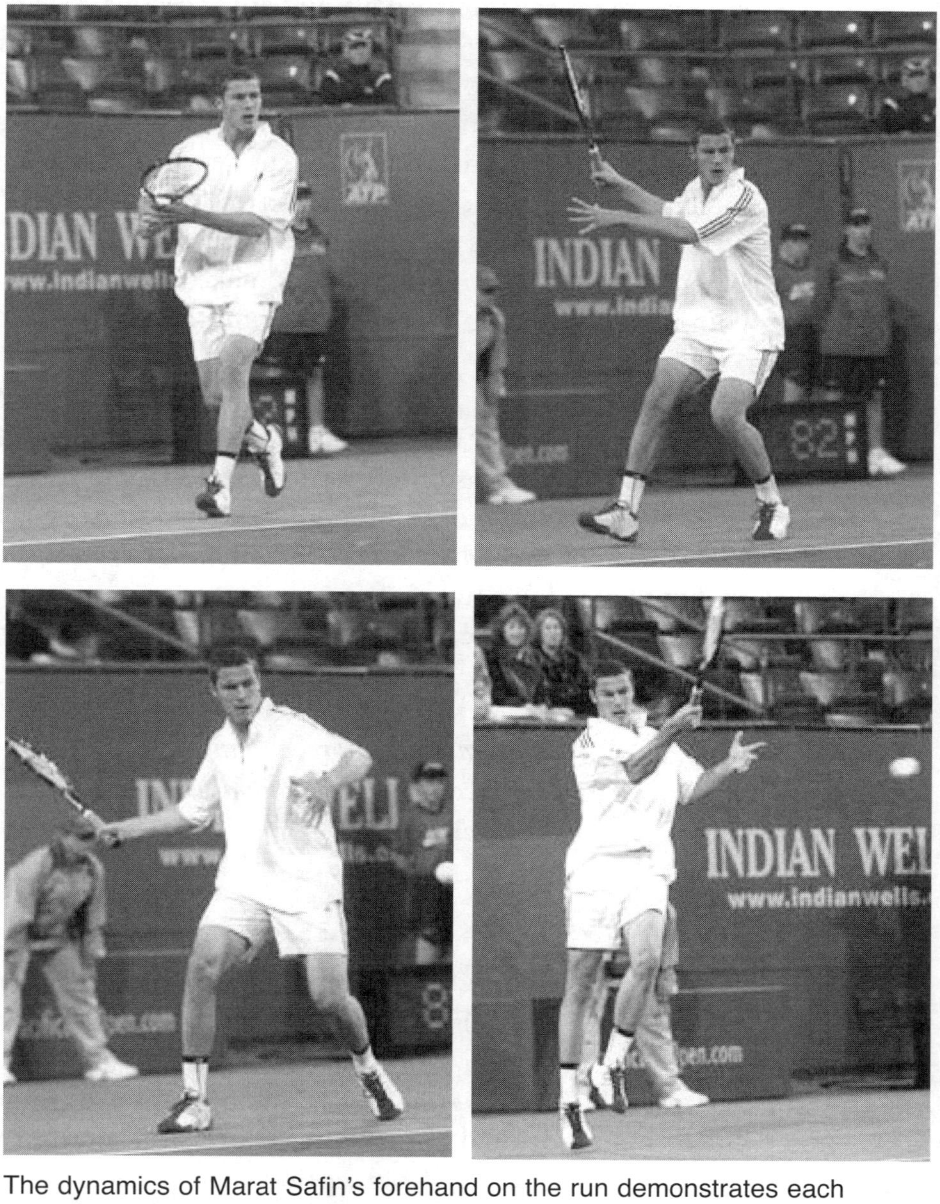

The dynamics of Marat Safin's forehand on the run demonstrates each of the first three components of "Tennis Mechanics": A) Tennis Strokes; B) Footwork; C) Hand-eye Coordination

Beginners often quit tennis after only a few attempts because many believe they are just not "cut out" to play it well because of an initial lack of "Tennis Coordination". However, I have witnessed countless players, who seemed to possess almost no natural tennis or hand-eye coordination, become extremely successful tennis players! I honestly believe, without a doubt that, any player who can hold a racket and see a moving ball can learn to play this game well.

In Chapter 6 I will discuss many of these coordination-building drills and how they can be integrated within a player's warm-up, practice, and playing session.

SHOT-MAKING SKILLS AND EXECUTION

The ability to hit the ball is one thing. Having the ability to vary, direct, and hit shots under pressure is something completely different. Many players I watch are what I call "one-dimensional". That is, they only have one style or strategy of play. Against some players, this single playing style might be fine. On the other hand, another opponent might relish this single style and proceed to dispatch the player in record time. Perhaps even more for the intermediate and advanced player, the ability to change the pace, spin, or style of play is critical in tennis today. Examples of these types of change would include: being able to play a serve-and-volley strategy in place of a baseline game; hitting slice groundstrokes instead of topspin; playing a finesse game with drop shots and angles instead of a power game that is one of depth, and other subtle and not-so-subtle changes!

Later in this book I will address these issues and how they relate both to the mechanical side of tennis as well as the mental side. Being able to hit all shots is one thing. Knowing when, where, and how to make all shots under pressure falls under the mental component of tennis as much as the mechanical.

Components of Mental Tennis

As you begin mastering the mechanical side of Tennis Mastery, the mental side of tennis will take on more and more significance. As they must know tennis mechanics, all players who seek higher levels of Tennis Mastery must know and understand the many components of Mental Tennis.

Basically there are four main parts to Mental Tennis:

1. *Mental toughness*
2. *Strategy comprehension*
3. *Recognition of personal limitations*
4. *Tennis Physics*

MENTAL TOUGHNESS

Mental toughness in tennis is, perhaps, the most difficult to comprehend and master completely. This is because it is so dependent on variables that are under control of our individual personalities—personalities that are ingrained deeply within our psyche. Those variables can include a player's natural disposition and character, his or her emotional control and expression, natural reaction to stress and adversity, as well as a player's self-perception (ego or lack thereof!). I have seen many talented individuals self-destruct (or at least, not reach their full potential) because they were unsuccessful in controlling their emotions. However, despite the fact that these variables have a foundation that is deeply entrenched in each one of us, I will teach you how to train and overcome many of the harmful mental situations that can arise. In addition, I will give you some substantial and concrete methods that will make you a more mentally tough player.

Mental Toughness can be broken down into these sub categories:

- *Playing well under pressure*
- *Playing well against weaker players as well as stronger players*
- *Avoidance of choking, tanking, and anger in the heat of competition*

The tools I teach in the following chapters will address most every aspect of Mental Toughness. It is through your off-court preparation (Chapter 5), your on-court practice routine (Chapter 6), and your match-play application of Mental Tennis (Chapter 13) that you will begin to understand and master these very essential parts! I have had countless situations, in both my personal playing and coaching careers in which the results of this preparation and application have paid off in dramatic fashion. Surviving match points and coming from behind victories (where a "momentum shift" can turn a sure loss into a sensational victory) have been common in both my playing and coaching careers! Some of my most memorable moments came while coaching, at a time when my players were on the brink of defeat. During these moments my players were able to reach down deep into the very essence of which we had practiced and prepared. Time and time again, my players turned seemingly one-sided matches into victories for themselves. These victories were where their ownership of Tennis Mastery was revealed. You, too, will experience these same thrills!

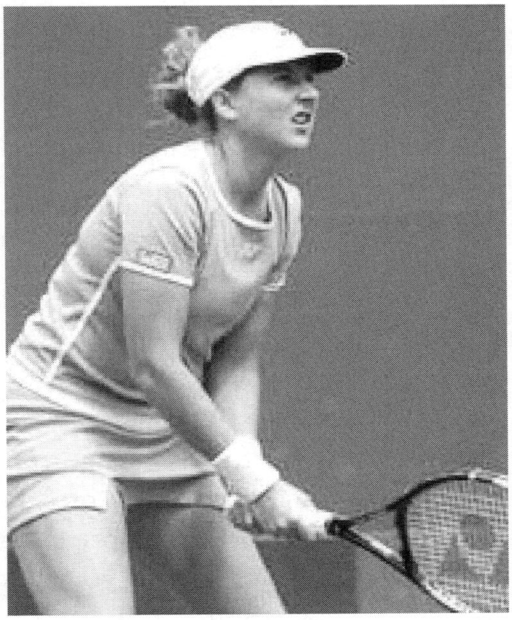
Mental Toughness: Sincere determination and a true competitive spirit

The pressures of competition bring out hidden characteristics in many of us. How we handle these pressures and their ensuing effect they have on us is what oftentimes separates the champ from the chump.

If you have any competitive spirit, each match you play will be significant. Whether it is simply for pride, or because the match has some significance, or that you simply hate losing, each tennis match should have meaning to you. How you handle the consequence of that meaning and move through the effect it will have on you will help determine whether you regularly play up to your potential.

STRATEGY COMPREHENSION

Similar to Tennis Mechanics, Mental Tennis includes the knowledge of ideal shot selections: when to use the strokes you have developed at optimal times. For example, a doubles player—after reading Chapter 8 on volleys—has learned how to hit an angle volley. This player then practices it and is now able to hit it with regularity. If that player knows how to hit the angle volley, but hits it at inopportune times (or doesn't hit it at appropriate times!) that person is lacking in strategy comprehension!

In watching tennis players compete, I quickly recognize those players who have not been taught on-court strategy. Players moving to the net or retreating at the wrong time often miss opportunities for easy shots! On the other hand, players who understand the strategies of the game can overcome some weaknesses in their game to beat those who might have better overall tennis mechanics. As you can see, strategy comprehension also includes knowledge of court position and coverage.

Like reading a classic novel, the more you learn about strategy the more interesting the game becomes. Consider how the strategy of a beginner (just get the ball over the net!) evolves into hitting angle volleys, down-the-line passing shots, topspin lobs and poaching! Tennis is a never-ending story with each chapter (match) a combination of conflict: battle between players; antagonist: your opponent(s); mystery: who will win; drama: surviving game or match point, and of course, the eventual climax and resolution. Try to enjoy each chapter of your tennis!

RECOGNITION OF PERSONAL LIMITATIONS

Perhaps second only to mental toughness, the ability to recognize personal limitations and understand them is very difficult for most people! Whether the limitations are physical or psychological, from a lack of experience, or simply from the lack of having a good backhand, recognition that we are subject to human frailties is hard for a lot of us to accept! Part of this is due to fact that this recognition is "ego-centered". After hitting a great shot many tennis players often believe that shot is now part of their permanent repertoire! However, in reality, it was more of a "lucky" shot than a "mastered" shot! Thus the player tries—and misses—the same shot over and over, not comprehending that it was indeed a lucky shot!

This concept is readily apparent with inexperienced players. Go to any group clinic where there is a mix of abilities. Often you will find the players who are the least experienced trying to hit ten times harder than the accomplished players with absolutely laughable success. Although this might be a macho thing, it still boils down to the recognition of what you can and can't do. I almost always bring this concept up at clinics as a reminder to those who are indeed trying to hit beyond their means: "Notice that the strongest player here is hitting with so much less pace than the rest of you. A strong player who is experienced KNOWS he or she doesn't have to hit strong shots to win. Be confident that you are strong enough NOT to hit hard shots!"

In Chapter 13 on Mental Tennis I will discuss the importance of playing "within oneself" and recognizing these personal limitations. This concept alone will benefit every level of player.

TENNIS PHYSICS

The natural laws of moving objects have a very important role in how and why we hit certain tennis shots. Due to the scientific approach of *Tennis Physics* (unlike mental toughness) players tend to understand the concepts and have an easier time making the connections in this area of tennis comprehension. Air pressure, velocity, and spin all cause tennis balls to behave differently while in flight. Knowing how these principles work will increase your understanding of why we hit the shots we do! Many players, especially those who have not been exposed to other sports or activities in which balls spin in flight, don't have a clue as to the effect spin has on a tennis ball. In addition, many players don't understand how the racket in their hand can make a ball spin in these different directions. These concepts are vital to your understanding and Mastery of tennis!

In Chapter 7 I will discuss the many elements of how physics plays a vital role in tennis strokes, both in stroke mechanics as well as resultant effects of those stroke mechanics. Your understanding of these principles will help you understand the purpose for many of the mechanics that are presented in this book as well as other books. At the same time, you will comprehend why certain techniques are prohibitive in terms of proper and progressive stroke development, and why you will want to avoid many of these commonly accepted, yet truly devastating pitfalls, that so many players have encountered.

Now that you have been introduced to the elements that make up Tennis Mastery, let us proceed to the methods that will allow you to experience it!

CHAPTER 5

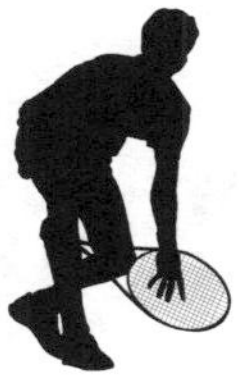

The Advanced Foundation–
Preparation "Before You Pick Up a Racket"

No matter what level of player you are or hope to become, there is some "groundwork" you should consider before you proceed to an on-court practice routine. This preliminary preparation will not only increase the productivity of your actual on-court practice sessions, it will give you an edge over players who don't prescribe to these preparatory recommendations.

Training within the Advanced Foundation includes knowing AND DOING the things that are not necessarily accomplished just on the tennis court! What separates equally matched players can often be traced to the extra things one did that the other player did not do. More than anything, the purposeful attention to these items gives a player a greater sense of accomplishment and value to both their study of the game as well as the eventual Mastery of the sport.

Proactive On-Court and Off-Court

There are two basic types of on-court players: Proactive and Reactive. The reactive player waits to see what will happen and bases his shot selection after his opponent has made his shot. This reactive player tends to stand still after hitting his shots, watching and waiting to see the result or the effectiveness. The proactive player looks for opportunities and often anticipates his opponent's shots before they are hit. For example, a proactive doubles player who sees that his partner has hit a deep return crosscourt where the opponent is moving back, will move in and begin to anticipate a weak return to the open half of the court. As a result, he will usually have an easy volley for a winner by poaching, knowing where the opponent will likely hit the ball.

The ability of being proactive while playing tennis is usually something that is developed over time and when the right types of practices are instituted. However, being proactive is not reserved strictly for on-court competition. A player can be proactive before he or she ever picks up a tennis racket!

BE A PROACTIVE OFF-COURT PLAYER!

Over the years I have given thousands of tennis players lessons. The great majority of these players are "reactive" players when it comes to learning and preparing to play tennis. Becoming a good tennis player is like becoming a good piano player. Between lessons, you should find ways to practice or the lessons themselves will produce mediocre results at best! Unlike owning a musical instrument in which daily practice is usually possible if desired, tennis players don't always have access to a tennis court or a hitting partner to accomplish this practice when it is convenient or when desired. Nevertheless, there are many ways a player can learn a great deal about tennis before and between each lesson and practice.

The proactive off-court player will look for ways to "KNOW" tennis.

When growing up I remember my father always telling me to "look for things that need to be done. Don't wait to be told to do something." This same advice is true for the tennis player. The idea of "knowing tennis" refers to understanding tennis from both a physical standpoint (for example, knowing how to utilize proper tennis mechanics) and from a cognitive one (understanding tennis rules, physical laws of spin, strategy etc.). When a player "knows tennis" on a cognitive level, especially before he or she starts to pursue the sport, the player moves through the learning process with far greater speed and over-all understanding. Thus, I recommend that all players, especially beginners, read and comprehend this portion dedicated to cognitive learning before heading out to the courts!

KNOWING TENNIS

One of the questions I ask many new players to the game is: "Have you ever seen top tennis players play tennis in person?" Amazingly, most beginners I ask this question say "no". On top of that, a large majority of junior and adult beginner players have never even watched a full set of tennis on television! Imagine if everyone who ever attempted sports such as baseball, football, or basketball, had never watched those sports played—let alone learned the rules of that sport—before attempting to play it! I remember as a kid I would try to mimic the moves I had seen by pro basketball players on my own basketball court at home. My friends and I would pretend there were five seconds left and we would shoot the winning basket. Watching the sport played by proficient players followed by a desire to play that sport allowed me to first develop those subtle images of how basketball is played. I'm sure all of us, at least those of us who have ever watched a sport on television or in-person, can relate!

The problem with tennis is that initially many kids only take tennis lessons because their parents want them to. Likewise, adults sometimes take lessons only because their friends play tennis or their spouse or "significant other" plays tennis and they don't want to be left out. Others come to realize that tennis is one of the truly competitive sports that can be played over an entire lifetime and recognize the intrinsic value of being able to do something fun for that lifetime.

Whatever reasons a player might have in order to pursue tennis, understanding the generalities of the game is vital for the player to improve. Learning tennis will be excruciatingly slow when the player has no idea what they are trying to achieve! So my first important suggestion to every player is: watch tennis!

Know what playing tennis "looks like"!

It has been proven that the vast majority of people learn best by using visual cues. For example, three groups of people who had never played basketball were used to test this theory by shooting free-throws. One group was given only auditory information; everything from proper foot position to hand position was given verbally. The second group was given the balls and told to simply find a way to shoot the ball into the basket. The third group was shown a video of top NBA players shooting free-throws with no verbalization of technique or instruction given. As you have probably surmised, the group that simply watched the pros did considerably better than the other two groups.

Imagine the frustration tennis instructors encounter when teaching people how to play tennis when those people they are instructing have never really seen tennis played well! It is a lot like trying to explain football or basketball to a person who has never heard of those sports. It is in your very best interest to watch tennis played at a high level before you begin to invest in tennis lessons!

Where to Start?

Planning to watch as much tennis as possible is a great start. The next step is going beyond watching. This means all players, from beginner to advanced, who want to excel in tennis will need to do the following:

STUDY TENNIS

During the 1999 Wimbledon fortnight it was reported that Pete Sampras did something I have been telling players to do for years. When Pete was a young player, the announcers had said he would do reports on all the top players. This research was not for school or for his tennis coach, but for himself only. He undoubtedly studied each player's game from their individual strokes to their playing strategy. From this process, as he learned more about these past champions, he learned more about becoming a champion. This might entail more work than what you might be willing to do. However, if you sincerely want to become a champion, you must do more than what other players are willing to do. Consider this as being just one more "rung on the ladder" which you can use to climb your way to the top! Perhaps this idea will be "that little something extra" which will give YOU an advantage over the others!

Here are some ways players of all levels can begin their study of tennis.

Tennis On Tape

While growing up, I can still remember the infancy of videotape! In 1973 my high school had just purchased a video camera and playback system that was absolutely huge! (And, as I remember, very expensive!) The system had to be transported on a wheeled cart, and the camera was so heavy that you had to use it on a tripod. In addition, the camera had to be attached to the recording system by a thick cable. I reminisce on this only to make this point: today, tennis players have a wonderful tool in learning that we could only dream about having when I was growing up! Players now can easily record tennis matches from television as well as videotaping themselves for stroke and strategy analysis. Utilizing this important technology will help you learn!

In this section I want to first address the idea of watching tennis on tape. Whether it is a match, an instructional video, a highlight tape, or watching yourself play, the concept of using videotapes can be applied to all levels of player and it can be a very helpful tool for tennis coaches.

Beginners:

As I mentioned earlier, I recommend that you watch as much tennis on television as possible. Record matches played when you can't watch them live and watch them when it is convenient. Become familiar with the current top players and pick a couple that play the way you would like to play. From this humble start you will have an image already implanted in your head of what playing tennis is all about...even before you step out onto the court! You will gain a greater respect for the game as well as developing a visual impression of how shots should look long before attempting to hit them yourself!

Intermediate and Advanced players:

Take the same advice I just offered to beginners. However, instead of just "looking" at recorded matches as a whole, look very carefully at the strokes and the strategies of each player. If you record a match, replay points and determine how the points were actually won. Study what shots were hit—how did they set-up the winning shot? Determine the strengths and weaknesses of each player; count the number of crosscourt shots and down-the-line shots hit, etc. If you have a slow-motion feature on your VCR, slow down each stroke while you analyze everything you can about the shot. Look at footwork (before, during and after the stroke), racket preparation and follow-through. Watch all aspects of the player's body, the non-dominant arm and hand, head position, and over-all balance the players possess through the course of each rally.

It has been often stated that when golfing great Tiger Woods was younger, he recorded previous golfing champions and studied every aspect of their play, from how they handled themselves under pressure to how they strode up to the eighteenth green with a big lead. I'm sure Woods gained a sense of what it would be like to be a champion long before he himself became one.

VIDEO TAPE YOURSELF

After watching tennis, gaining the ability to identify what "good tennis" looks like can be applied to your own game. Video taping yourself playing tennis and comparing yourself to what you have recognized as skilled performance will undoubtedly reveal characteristics in your own form and mechanics as inadequate or, at best, inefficient. Or, as has often happened with many of my beginners after establishing the makings of our advanced foundation, you might discover you are not far off at all in your pursuit of skilled stroke execution! In Section 2 on the Strategies of Hitting I will discuss further what you will want to look for in your own strokes and form. In the meantime, understanding that the video camera can become a tool in your development is critical. In fact, most of the top rated tennis camps across the country utilize videotape analysis in their teachings. They recognize the value of providing players with the ability to see themselves hitting a tennis ball. You should too.

PLAYER NOTEBOOK

This next section deals with a very important tool beneficial for every level of player: The Player Notebook. The Player Notebook is a self-motivating tool that provides an impression of "ownership" for a player in regards to his or her tennis ability. By developing a personal notebook, a player will have a "stake" in his or her improvement. The Notebook not only provides a physical record of goals and accomplishments, but the effort in sustaining it will be a source of pride and inspiration. In addition, the memories within the book will be priceless!

Although the player notebook should be very personal and individual, each player's notebook should be composed of at least five basic parts:

1. *Pictures of professional tennis players in action; Tennis Tips*
2. *Written statement of personal goals, expectations and prescriptions*
3. *Practice plan (within each set of goals)*
4. *Personal record of achievements in tennis*
5. *Daily Journal*

1. Player Pictures

Obtain tennis magazines. These can be procured by either subscribing to any one of the tennis publications that are available in bookstores and newsstands or finding a friend or neighbor who subscribes and asking them for their issues when finished. Also, most tennis clubs receive issues and usually just toss them out at the end of each month. Check with your local club's head pro and ask if you can have their past copies. After reading the magazines, cut out action shots of professionals and paste them on card-stock paper and put these pages in your notebook. It is a good idea to group the shots by category such as forehands, backhands, serves, etc. This should be an on-going project; you will continue to add more pictures as they become available to you.

What these photographs of professionals-in-action will help you do is reinforce the techniques you are attempting to master. Just as you do when watching videos, analyze what is happening in each picture. Even though professionals hit with varying idiocrasis, look for similarities between similar shots by different pros. Look at every detail such as grip, rackethead location, arm position, point of contact, etc. Pictures, as they say, are worth a thousand words! More than that, they are valuable visual references that you will be able to refer back to many times. By cutting out these pictures from the magazine, you are spending a great deal more time actually looking at the shots than if you were just looking at the magazine. This "forced" analyzing of pictures helps build a more focused mental visualization of them, also.

In addition, most tennis magazines offer "Tennis Tips". Cut these out and put them in your notebook as well. Photocopy pages from books that contain tips that you specifically find helpful and include these in this section of your notebook.

This photo and tip portion of your notebook will be very valuable to you as you continue to play. The fact that you spent time in putting these elements together in your notebook will make them more important to you than if you just read them once in a magazine.

2. Written Statement of Personal Goals

This is, perhaps, the most important part of your notebook. It is a declaration of your intentions—how good you truly want to be.

Your personal goals should be divided into two distinct sections:

a. Short term goals and prescriptions
b. Long term goals and prescriptions

Short-term goals will change as your advancements and achievements occur. These goals should include a list of accomplishments you hope to achieve within the next month to three months. For beginners, this could include things like being able to hit a slice serve or hit with topspin on forehand and backhand sides. For advanced players, the list of short term goals will be more abstract, such as winning a particular tournament or beating a particular player or playing in a higher division or age bracket.

Long-term goals should include distinct levels of play in which you wish to be within a year and within the next specific time frame. (For example, by the time you are a freshman in high school or by the time you reach college or by the time you reach your 60th birthday!) Long-term goals should be thought of as a crystal ball: How good do you see yourself at these stages? Do you see yourself as a top college player? Best in your tennis club? Perhaps best in the world? These are all worthy aspirations. Yet, as you will see in the next section, you must be willing to work as hard as it takes to make these goals a reality.

Goals must match sacrifice

Whatever goals you set for yourself, you must be willing to make the necessary sacrifices to reach them. (Or you never will!) In other words, you must set goals that match your sincere aspirations. When the desire is genuine, then the work and sacrifice will be worth it! That is, every step you take in reaching your goal will be rewarding and worth any amount of sacrifice you make along the way. Another way to look at it is this:

If you find that working hard towards your goal is boring, or that you find it difficult to set aside time to work towards your goal, then your goal is not sincere.

We can all say we want to be the best tennis player in the world, but few are willing to pay the price (in terms of sacrificing other wants or desires) to actually be the best. Those who have become the best in anything didn't get there by wasting time or avoiding the hard work that they knew it would take. Ask any champion if they didn't make serious sacrifices in their pursuit of perfection. The value of anything is usually enhanced, if not heightened significantly, by the sacrificial component taken by the person.

Your long term and short-term goals will serve as maps; they will be a constant reminder of where you want to go.

Prescriptions For Goal Attainment

Once goals have been established and players have made the commitment, a detailed prescription must be written which outlines a basic plan of attack.

Prescriptions should be written for both long-term as well as short-term goals.

However, the two prescriptions are decidedly different.

SHORT-TERM GOAL PRESCRIPTIONS

These prescriptions will change as the goals themselves are reached and reestablished. Each goal should be addressed with a particular plan describing how each goal will be reached. Here are some examples of what you might want to consider for your short-term goal prescriptions for three distinct levels of players.

For a beginner who is just starting out. **SHORT-TERM GOAL: Hit a spin serve.**

- Identify several professional players whose serves are desirable
- Take a series of lessons from a reputable pro
- Work three days serving baskets of balls for 20 minutes each session

For a senior player whose backhand is inadequate and wants to learn a two-handed backhand and be able to hit topspin. **SHORT-TERM GOAL: Rally consistently with a two-handed backhand.**

- Learn desired technique visually through video and/or pictures of players hitting the two-hander
- Take lessons followed by a videotape session to observe personal development.
- Work specific days each week on ball machine followed by live ball hitting with a pro or good hitting partner.
- Use the new backhand exclusively in match-play competition.

For a ranked junior player who wants to learn how to create an open court through greater angles on groundstrokes: **SHORT-TERM GOAL: Hit topspin angled forehand and backhand groundstrokes.**

- Identify how to hit groundstrokes with greater precision, topspin and angle
- Work specifically on ball machine or with a teaching professional on producing shots that are desirable
- Play matches in which the only groundstrokes attempted are angles to learn how the shot can be used effectively and when the shot should not be hit strategically

Short-term prescriptions should also include off-court plans:

- Join USTA
- Subscribe to a tennis magazine
- Record several tennis matches on video tape and watch
- Begin a tennis library of books
- Find a hitting partner
- Set up lessons or clinics at a club or with a pro

LONG-TERM GOALS AND PRESCRIPTIONS:

These are more general plans that should describe the player's intended level of play at specific intervals of time. These should reflect the player's combined short-term goals as a whole. Long-term goals and their prescriptions might include the following:

- Gain a 4.0 NTRP
  PRESCRIPTIONS: Play 3 days a week; attend two clinics each week or take one private lesson each week;
- Make varsity by next season
  PRESCRIPTIONS: Take lessons and clinics; set a practice schedule and stick to it for the next three months; play junior tournaments over the summer; work weaker parts of game
- Be the top player on the junior ladder at the club
  PRESCRIPTIONS: Play four days each week with at least two lessons or clinics each week; set a summer schedule of 3 hours each day of tennis and conditioning.
- Win a senior player tournament
  PRESCRIPTIONS: Work on conditioning including flexibility and speed; plan to increase practice time each week by 15 minutes; play younger players at least once a week
- Become a nationally ranked player
  PRESCRIPTIONS: Schedule the upcoming year's tournaments; plan a practice schedule that includes 3 hours of hitting five days a week; plan a workout schedule that works towards specific physical goals including strength conditioning, cardio conditioning, flexibility and agility conditioning, and mental conditioning

Actually, your long-term goals could include several prescriptions from each of these examples...and they should! Obviously, every player will benefit from greater conditioning, lessons, number of days hitting, playing tournaments, and having hitting partners! You should seriously consider which are realistic for you and your goal. If your goal is unrealistic, your prescriptions will most likely include more than you are willing to do. If this is the case, you will need to reevaluate your goals basing them on your true intentions.

3. Practice Plan:

There are many tennis books that offer basic drills and practice ideas...this one included! As a player improves, his or her practice plan will change as the need for more advanced drills, strokes and game strategies increase. Within your notebook you should have a section that you can categorize basic practice schedules. This will do two things:

a. It will help you identify those areas that you need to focus on at the present time
b. It will help you include proper drills needed to improve those areas that need work in each practice session.

Players typically go out and just hit. Even players who know they need to drill inevitably wind up driftying away from any drill pattern and end up just hitting shots or playing sets. The reasons for this are: first, they don't have a set plan to follow; second, many players are, by nature, competitive; thus, they end up playing each other in a set instead of working on weaknesses. By setting up a practice plan you will begin to look for ways to make each practice more productive.

Your practice plan will change quite a bit over time. Initially, you will be focused on the areas of basic and proper tennis mechanics that I will discuss in Section 2. Later, your practices will move to more game-situation drills, mental toughness drills, and competition. Regardless of your current level of play, this "proactive" approach, by physically writing down a practice plan and keeping it current, will add to your overall tennis growth and Mastery.

4. Personal Record of Achievements

This portion of your notebook will be the most personal. In it you should include pictures of yourself and your friends that play tennis, as well as any of the following items:

- Tournament results and draw sheets
- School match scores and team information

- Newspaper clippings of your accomplishments (If you follow the instructions within this book, you ***will*** have newspaper clippings!)
- Pictures of places you travel when playing tennis
- Ribbons or medals won playing tennis
- Anything that has a connection with tennis and you

What you will discover is that all these items you put in your notebook will build a sense of accomplishment as well as a steady source of encouragement for your future, not to mention that it will be a priceless memoir that you will value for your entire life!

One of my most prized possessions is a player's folder which my high school coach, Mason Long, put together for me. In it he included all our team match score sheets including names of players I had played and scores, tournament results, a personal letter from him to his players, pictures, and a host of other tennis memories. I would run across some of these players—those I had played against from other schools as well as players who played on the same team—and I was able to reminisce with them about playing those matches and other events associated with those years. The memories have become even more priceless as the years have passed.

5. Daily Journal

A good practice is to write down many of your thoughts following lessons, matches, tournaments, or even after watching a tennis match on television. By recording your thoughts, you put weight on each concept or thought you recall. Just the process of replaying a lesson or a match in your head while thinking of important points will add value to aspects of your play and practice. This is totally a free-form report only for you. So include anything you want and feel is important to your tennis success

The Start of Your Foundation

Creating and maintaining a notebook, watching and studying videos, reading books, watching tennis—all these things are part of what I call "Building Your Foundation." All of these elements will play a role in developing your complete understanding of the Advanced Foundation. The Advanced Foundation must be achieved not only in your strokes, but also in your on-court strategies and mental toughness. Building upon a flawed foundation in any of these areas will result in an undeveloped over-all game. In addition, a flawed foundation will make learning slow and discouraging. Spending a little time off the court will pay big dividends when it comes time to be on the court.

TENNIS LESSONS

Because tennis has so many component parts and requires many specific fundamentals to play it well, it is advisable to get some professional help before you play. Nothing is more difficult than trying to fix a self-taught player's flawed mechanics! Players who go out and try to play without at least some knowledge of basic tennis skills will usually become quite good at hitting bad shots! You basically have two choices in trying to acquire this knowledge properly: one, buy several good books and videos on tennis (one of which you have in your hands!) and teach yourself from these; or two, invest in tennis lessons from a good pro. Obviously, the ideal learning situation would include both.

As I have already stated, every player must "study tennis." That includes both the investments in good tennis books or videos, or in obtaining proper instruction. Reading about tennis will speed up your on-court learning dramatically. Nothing is more frustrating than working with a player who actually knows nothing at all about tennis and expects that a few hours on the court with a pro will satisfy this requirement! At the very least, beginning players should learn how to keep score and know basic rules of tennis. If a player really wants to learn tennis as fast as possible, the study of basic strokes and strategies prior to stepping out onto the court will be a wise decision! When a pro talks about topspin or slice, overheads or half-volleys, the student, who has a general idea of what these things are will benefit from the increased efficiency of the lesson. In fact, if you have a good understanding of your own body movements while you practice, you will have an excellent head start on becoming a great tennis player! One way to increase this self-perception is to look at yourself in the mirror while swinging a racket. So often, players on the court lose conscious control of their racket, especially on the backswing. As soon as their attention becomes focused on the ball, their racket seems to take on a mind of its own! It helps greatly if all players look at their swing in a mirror and identify key position points visually as well as kinesthetically.

Tennis lessons will, moreover, give you a greater insight to your over-all stroke production and strategy comprehension. Nothing beats having a live person hit balls to you, critique your strokes, and offer tips and feedback. In addition, and perhaps most of all, a good tennis pro will be able to give you that vote of confidence and affirmation if you are indeed hitting the ball correctly!

Understanding that lessons are a very good investment might help you make the decision to take tennis lessons. When you consider that you will most likely play tennis most of your life, the money paid towards lessons today will be insignificant compared to the countless hours you will enjoy playing better tennis! The reward of playing better tennis over those years will be immeasurable! This is especially true for children whose parents are investing in tennis lessons.

In my 30 years in tennis, I have seen what an impact tennis has on so many people.

Young or old, tennis has helped thousands of players be more productive in life, open opportunities towards successful careers, or simply provide a valuable outlet to exercise, meet other people and to compete.

Finding a Teaching Pro

If you have decided to take tennis lessons, there are many avenues to pursue. The simplest and perhaps the most affordable methods are taking lessons through your local city recreation department. However, although this is the most affordable method, it isn't always the highest quality of instruction! Often, recreation departments hire anyone that has some semblance of tennis background to teach. (To give you an idea of this, I was hired during my sophomore year of high school to teach for our city recreation department! Even though I was one of the top high school players in the city at that time, I certainly didn't possess much in the way of tennis teaching experience!)

A great source for finding quality tennis instructors is to use the Internet. The two most reliable sources are the USPTA, (The United States Professional Tennis Association, www.uspta.org), and USPTR, (United States Professional Tennis Registry, www.usptr.org). Both of these associations call for rigid testing requirements of their members (written and playing), as well as a minimum number of years teaching.

Perhaps the best place to obtain a qualified teaching professional is at a tennis club. Most tennis clubs require tennis instructors to not only be USPTA or USPTR certified, they usually only hire tennis professionals who have had a successful background playing tennis as well as a minimum number of years teaching tennis.

There are basically two criteria that all good pros possess:

a. Playing experience. (Either former or current)
b. Teaching experience. (The more years the better)

Obviously, an instructor who has competed at a high level will have a greater chance of being able to pass on information that he or she has acquired through this playing experience. This is especially true for competitive students who are looking to be exposed to these experiences.

Teaching experience is, in my opinion, one of the most important criteria for a qualified instructor. Through teaching many players, instructors gain understanding on how students learn differently. They also discover how certain phrases, analogies, and visual cues can be helpful for their students.

Tennis instructors who are certified are more likely to have read, studied, and communicated tennis (with other teaching pros) than those who are not certified. Many certified pros attend yearly conventions and clinics which help them learn the latest ideas in tennis instruction as well as discover new teaching methods, drills, motivational techniques, etc. These tennis pros certainly have the potential to provide you with the best possible instruction that reflects the current thinking and philosophies accepted within the profession. It is wise to ask your potential tennis professional what background they possess in both areas of teaching and playing. (It is also advisable to ask for proof of these qualifications. I will discuss this a bit later.) Understand, too, that many of these certified pros only become certified to say they are certified! In other words, many of these instructors have never attended conventions or seminars to broaden their field of expertise. This is unfortunate as it lowers the respect and reputation of those of us who are true professionals within our field. I highly recommend that you inquire the extent of a prospective pro's involvement in professional development. Most active pros that partake in such personal development will have a file of certifications showing attendance and completion of such instructional course work.

In addition to these two basic criteria, (playing and teaching experience), tennis instructors should be personable and approachable. It is advisable that you ask to watch a potential pro teach a lesson before you spend your money. Look to see if the instructor has the personality that you expect in someone teaching you. There are many pros that know their stuff but have the personality of a brick. For some students this is just fine. Other players might want to have a pro that will push them by both words and actions.

Also, look for an articulate professional. This might not seem important at first, but I have found that professionals who possess a greater education and/or vocabulary maintain a greater arsenal of phrases, key words, visual cues, and terminology to help get their point across! In addition, I have found that tennis instructors who possess a working foundation of basic human anatomy, physiology, physics and biomechanics are better suited to relate tennis processes to students in ways that the student will comprehend.

I have seen a few good tennis pros that didn't necessarily meet the criteria I listed above. However, you will be much more assured of receiving sound tennis advice if the pro from which you are taking lessons meets one or more of these standards. Be especially wary of "pros" that put up fliers around tennis courts or hand out their business cards to attract potential students. Check to see if these pros meet any of the criteria I listed before paying for lessons. These "renegade" instructors seldom have met the qualifications I have listed and, as a result, have been unable to get a job teaching tennis at any reputable tennis facilities due to their lack of credentials. Often, these pseudo pros talk a big game and may claim to have many tennis accomplishments. If you encounter an instructor like this, ask them for some documentation such as newspaper clippings or letters of reference. Every player who has had success either teaching or playing should have something that can verify these claims.

"Rules of Taking Lessons"

Students who take tennis lessons often feel that the instructor is the one responsible for their learning. This is half correct. The student has, perhaps, an even greater responsibility, both during and after a tennis lesson. There are some "rules" which the student must understand and adhere to in order for any tennis lesson to be effective.

First, players must be ready for change. Obviously, if a player is taking lessons, they must know that they need to change elements of their game. It amazes me to this day that people will dish out forty or fifty bucks and basically say, "don't change my game!"

Second, the student must be willing to attempt the strokes or tip prescribed, over and over. Typically, a player will try a new stroke once or twice and believe they should be cured of all their tennis woes. After a couple of tries, they tend to remark, "hey, this stroke doesn't work." I always remind the player that they have been hitting their flawed stroke pattern/grip/stance, etc., for X-number of years. Then I remind them that they have only been working on the correct stroke pattern, grip/stance, etc., for only three minutes! Players tend to expect quantitative results from a definite qualitative human body!

The success of every tennis shot depends on how well the body can emulate the necessary tennis stroke combined with the proper timing and hand-eye coordination. Because of this any student who has a flawed stroke pattern must change the way his or her brain sends signals to the muscles. This change in the sequence of signals and the physical adjustment needed to make the change is almost always uncomfortable. As I have mentioned many times, it is this discomfort that prevents so many from attaining the desired improvement they seek in tennis!

Usually, for those players who have faulty strokes, the reality lies in the sincere desire to work through the discomforting feeling of being worse before becoming better!

Here is something else to consider. Oftentimes players who are attempting to use the correct form actually hit better shots, more consistent shots, and more effective shots… yet, they feel like they are playing much worse than when they played using their old, ineffective form! That is how powerful the discomfort of change can be! Players often focus on the one shot they missed and quickly reason, "the new way just isn't working." These players have a hard time acknowledging (to themselves or to their pro) that the new method did indeed, meet with success. Even a well-hit, proper stroke can feel improper to a student making a change. Thus, as is so often the case, these players inevitably go back to their old, comfortable, and basically ineffective strokes and wonder why "that darn pro didn't teach me anything!"

TENNIS TEACHING IGNORANCE AND EXPERIENCE

Today's tennis has seen an amazing transformation over the past thirty-plus years. Some might argue it has been an ongoing transformation since the beginning of the modern game. Whatever the case, tennis today is far different than it was forty years ago. Just twenty years ago, most knowledgeable tennis enthusiasts would surely have looked at someone hitting a two-handed forehand as a beginner who hadn't been taught correctly. Today, we are seeing more and more prolific players hitting a two-fisted forehand. Monica Seles certainly has made the shot a recognizable weapon over the past twelve years and more recently American Jan Michael Gambill has shown a two-handed forehand can be hit successfully on the men's side of tennis. In fact, there are many others on the men's and women's tour that posses a two-handed forehand; Fabrice Santoro and Marion Bartoli both from France, and Raemon Sluiter of the Netherlands all have versions of the two-handed forehand and all are now among the world's top fifty. Several of the top ranked boys and girls in the U.S. also are demonstrating the effectiveness of this relatively new shot. However, ask 95 percent of those currently in the tennis teaching profession if learning to hit the two-handed forehand should be explored, and you will get a resounding NO.

Why?

Before I provide insight to this question, consider these interesting historical facts about a stroke that was considered an anomaly only three decades ago: The two-handed backhand was almost a non-existent stroke on either the men's or women's tour. We can even see how top players of a generation or two ago could not have guessed how the game would evolve. Legendary player Jack Kramer had this to say about the two-handed backhand in 1949:

"The use of two hands not only weakens your strokes but robs you of confidence and gives your opponent a psychological advantage."
Jack Kramer, 1949

With over 90 percent of the top women players using the two-handed backhand and nearly 70 percent of the top men using the shot, it would appear that even Jack Kramer was completely ignorant of the potential of what players could do with a two-handed backhand!

It is this kind of ignorance that provides us with the answer to the question of why so many pros today will not teach the two-handed forehand. Clearly, ignorance would prevent any pro from teaching something they know so little about. However, many pros overstep their ignorant ways and proceed to denounce such a method of hitting the forehand as "stupid" or "ludicrous!" Yet, amazingly enough, every single pro that has stated such distaste for the concept of hitting forehands with two hands has never ever attempted to teach the shot! (If they first studied what methods are best suited for the shot and then proceeded to try teaching it to any number of players, I guarantee every pro would quickly recognize the value of this shot!) While the shot may not be appropriate for every single person, the two-handed forehand has great value for a large percentage of students, especially for those who might have trouble hitting a conventional forehand. I have seen pros teach the forehand to individuals and make absolutely no headway in helping the individuals improve their forehands because they knew no other methods to prescribe. This is where both ignorance and a lack of experience can cost students time and money in their quest for tennis success.

Such ignorance is still being demonstrated day after day in today's tennis teaching forum. The root of today's ignorance can be found in the deeply troublesome aspect of some ineffectual tennis-teaching professionals. While the number of pros who are ineffective is low, those few that are ineffective can influence many unwitting students. This ineffectiveness, (or we could simply say ignorance), stems from several key inadequacies. These would include:

- Uneducated
- Inexperienced
- Untrained
- Lack of competitive experience

Such inadequacy ends up producing only subjective teaching methods based usually on individual perception of what worked for them as a tennis player (if they were really ever "players" in the first place!) instead of what will help most players to develop skilled tennis strokes.

The result of this process has created tremendous conflict even among the "respected" teaching establishment. The problem is not that all teaching "styles" are bad. In fact, many pros attend conventions and workshops each year to hone their teaching skills and improve their effectiveness. However, even in these environments you would be surprised to know the amount of disagreement that exists among even the most respected teaching professionals. Unfortunately, many of the most well known pros have seldom, if ever, taught large groups of players or taught players for any significant duration of time. But because they were funny, or they touted impressive sounding research, or they were just in the right place at the right time, many recognizable names in the industry were successful not because of producing results, but because of other extrinsic instances.

The importance of teaching large groups is that pros can learn what effect certain teaching philosophies will have on players as a whole, such as recognition of what players will respond to and if the applied methods are producing recognized progression within all players' ability and desire.

The importance of teaching individuals for a significant period of time provides the pro with a true picture of player progression over time.

There are some pros that only teach players for 3 days and never see them again! How can such pros know for sure that the methods presented in those three days are beneficial in the long run for any of their players? They can't! (Unless they have seen such methods presented to others who have indeed accomplished skilled play through over time.)

It is very important to understand that these limitations exist within the tennis teaching profession. If a student is educated in these areas, they will be able to ask more educated questions of their teachers and be able to better evaluate the potential of all teachers in helping them.

Student Responsibilities

In order for lessons to have an impact, the student must meet the following criteria:

1. THE PLAYER MUST RECOGNIZE HE OR SHE HAS A NEED FOR HELP

There are players who actually take lessons only to tell the pro that they already know how to hit! These players proceed to ignore any advice and hit the way they want to hit. I've had students who insist they are hitting a topspin forehand when they are actually hitting a slice! The student must forgo the ego during any lesson and realize that they might not be hitting the ball as well as they could!

2. THE PLAYER MUST RECOGNIZE AND UNDERSTAND HOW THE LESSON (OR NEW STROKE) CAN HELP THEM.

Understanding how certain shots are more desirable and offer a greater chance of success is very important for improvement. Oftentimes, players who use form that is hindering their improvement fail to realize how making certain changes will allow them to not only improve immediately, but how such changes will help them continue to improve over time. Players must listen carefully and understand not only ***what*** the pro is suggesting, but also ***why*** the pro is suggesting it.

3. THE PLAYER MUST WANT TO MAKE NECESSARY CHANGES.

Players often know they have a weakness but aren't always willing to make the necessary changes to improve it. As I have mentioned, this is because making changes are, most of the time, uncomfortable. Examples of this can include changing from a one-handed backhand to a two-handed backhand, or a player trying to make the change from serving with an eastern forehand grip to serving with a continental grip. Any of these changes will require time and commitment on the student's part to make them permanent. For the student to be patient and committed enough to make the change, the student must really want to make the change! In addition, any player making necessary changes in their game usually will need to do "extra" things to complete the change. These extra things might be anything from doing bouncing drills several times a day between lessons to gain comfort in a new grip or shadow swinging hundreds of times in front of a mirror to develop a new swing pattern. Discipline is the key in making any change in a player's game.

4. The player must be willing to employ the new form in competition.

This is the hardest part for the student to comply with. Because new strokes and mechanics are uncomfortable, wanting to employ them in match-play competition might feel a little like contemplating suicide! Players know they are not going to feel comfortable, so they feel they won't be successful. Yet, if a player continues to fall back on old habits in competition, then they will never be able to master the new stroke at all. A classic example of this is a player developing a spin serve instead of a dink serve. If the player always goes back to the dink serve in competition, they will never be able to develop an effective and consistent spin serve under the pressure of competition. Sadly, I see players revert back to these old ineffectual serves after a single double fault attempting the more advanced serve. Ironically, these same players hardly blink an eye when they double fault using their old dink serve! If you are going to double fault, gain something from it!

When a player incorporates new methods in competition, the body, mind, and muscles learn faster due to the added importance competition puts on the shot each time it is attempted. During a lesson or in practice, shots don't have the same emphasis as they do when they are attempted in competition. This is why students who make a conscious effort to employ new techniques in competition will be quicker at mastering the needed change, and will reap the benefits!

Personal Limitations

Every player will have certain limitations that can slow down the learning processes. Older players who are just starting out need to understand that although tennis can be played at a leisurely level, it still requires elements of endurance, strength, quickness, and agility. The better the physical condition of a prospective tennis player, the better suited the player will be for these demands. Doing some preliminary work prior to stepping onto the court can be very beneficial to all beginners.

Older players can prepare by doing some cardiovascular training such as brisk walking or cycling. Find comfortable tennis shoes and break them in during this training. (Nothing is more frustrating than the player who gets blisters on their feet the first time on the court!) Strengthen your hand and forearm muscles by doing squeezing exercises. Use an old tennis ball or one of those grip-strengthening tools to work your hands. (Both hands!) Work up to doing several sets of these exercises each day for at least a week before heading to the courts. (This will also condition the hands to help prevent blisters.) Pushups, sit-ups, and any large muscle group exercises will also be a big help. Pushups are excellent for preventing tennis elbow.

Young children are also susceptible to the same conditions an older person might encounter. Because kids are so much more resilient and have an abundance of energy than older people, it is sometimes harder to get kids to recognize this need. Yet, they, too, will benefit by taking the time to be prepared to play.

ARE YOU DOING EVERYTHING YOU CAN?

This entire chapter deals with concepts that are designed to help players become better players before they step onto the court. However, any player who hopes to excel at tennis must look beyond the concepts I have just stated.

I have coached junior players who claim they want to be the best in the world. When I ask these kids if they have done everything they can to reach this lofty goal, they shrug and reply, "I think so." Then I run the following list by them and ask them to answer each question. I will run it by you, too. Get a pencil and fill in the blanks and let's see how dedicated you really are!

1. Have you purchased an USTA card? _____
2. Do you have a subscription to a tennis publication? _____
3. How many tennis books do you own? _____
4. Do you have a basket of tennis balls? _____
5. How many tennis videos do you own? _____
6. How many tennis tournaments have you entered? _____
7. Do you have a tennis notebook? _____
8. Do you have a hitting partner? _____
9. Do you take your tennis racket with you on trips? _____
10. Do you know how many inches a tennis net is at the center? _____

<u>These ten questions are extremely important to any player who sincerely wants to become a great player. Here is why.</u>

1. Owning a USTA card insures that you will receive tournament information in the area in which you live in. It provides you with several additional tennis paraphernalia including a tennis magazine subscription and a rules book, (something every tennis player should carry with them whenever they play!).

2 Subscriptions will guarantee that you will get a steady supply of tennis literature sent to your home. If you follow my advice regarding a Tennis Notebook, having a monthly tennis magazine sent to you will help you build your notebook. Most tennis magazine subscriptions run less than $20 per year. This is a tiny investment in your tennis future!

3. Tennis books are like tennis teaching professionals—there are a lot of them out there and you never know which one will offer the advice that clicks for you! I try to encourage all my students to take lessons, or camps, or clinics from other pros in addition to myself. No matter how good a pro is, there might be a word or phrase that another pro or player might mention that makes all the sense in the world to you. Tennis books offer this same approach. All of them offer tips and strategies that obviously have worked for someone! So read up and learn all you can from the printed word.

4 A basket of tennis balls is critical. If you can't hit a ton of balls in succession, developing "grooved" strokes will be slow and nearly impossible. Most all tennis clubs and sporting goods stores can order a good ball basket. Make sure to get one that can stand up and fold down for storage. And get one that holds at least 75 tennis balls. As for filling up a basket with tennis balls, there are several ways to do so. You can purchase a case of balls, (24 three-ball cans come in one case), and fill it up with new balls, or you can find used

balls. Most tennis clubs collect used balls from club use, tournaments, or from lessons and donate them to members, schools or individuals who request them. Call up your local club and let them know you would like their used balls which they are no longer using.

5.Like books, tennis videos can offer many tips and technique strategies that might be more meaningful to you. The visual component of videos alone makes them a valuable resource to almost every type of player. Don't forget to record tennis matches on video. You never know when a match will be a classic!

6.Tournament participation is an absolute must for every player who wants to be the best. No amount of practice can simulate the pressures and emotions a tournament presents. By competing against a variety of unknown players, you begin to develop your true playing style and char-acteristics. It is also here, in tournaments, that you will discover your playing weaknesses and strengths. Without playing in tournaments you will not learn what you really need to practice.

7. I have already described the value of a personal tennis notebook. By subscribing to the importance of building a player notebook, you will have a far more valuable resource that will have personal meaning to you.

8. Finding a hitting partner that is right for you is like finding a spouse! Finding a hitting partner who is near the same level as you, has the same dedication and, perhaps, aspirations, and someone who is willing to work hard with you is perhaps the hardest thing to do from this list! Yet, finding a player with which to work is worth the time and energy! Many players who do find such a partner go on to become world-class doubles teams.

9. Taking your rackets everywhere you go (when possible) is a wonderful way to not only improve your game if the opportunity arises, but it is a great way to meet new people! I remember my father and I taking our rackets on a cruise when I was in high school. We would find some public courts or simply a parking lot or grass area and hit volleys to each other. While in Puerto Rico I ran into the top junior player on the island. I was invited to play at his home which happened to be the home of the president of Puerto Rico! Talk about a great opportunity! You never know who you might meet or where you will get a chance to play!

10. It is actually irrelevant knowing how many inches a tennis net is! However, any player who has studied the game of tennis knows that the center of a tennis net is 36 inches! So, if you didn't know the answer to that question, you certainly haven't studied the game of tennis to any degree! Learning the rules of tennis is something you don't have to pay a pro to teach you. There are countless books on the sport and the rules. It also pays to know the rules when it comes to competing!

What's Next?

If you have read this chapter carefully, you realize there are responsibilities on your part which will help insure your reaching tennis mastery! The next chapter is designed to teach you HOW TO PRACTICE. Whether you are working with a teaching pro, or heading out with a hitting buddy, or going to hit against the wall at the local high school, the methods and philosophies in Chapter 6 will guide you to the most effective practices you can achieve.

Above all, remember that tennis is hard; if it were easy everyone would be a pro! To play tennis well does require time, patience, effort, and sacrifice. Yet, I promise you, the reward of such commitment is actually life changing! Personal enjoyment and satisfaction are just two of the innumerable rewards you will experience.

CHAPTER 6

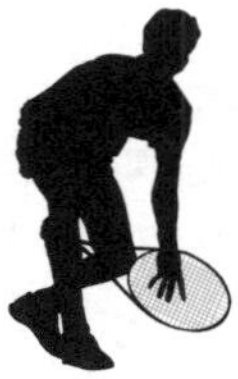

The Advanced Foundation– Making Practice Count

Practice Philosophies

Whether you are a beginner or a tournament competitor, your on-court success and over-all Tennis Mastery will come primarily from the way you practice. Obviously, if you practice poor form and improper technique, your game will be composed of faulty and unreliable strokes. Therefore, it is paramount that your practice routine be centered on proper form and systematic procedures. This will allow you to achieve not only on-court success, but to accomplish this success in a timely manner. Obviously, nothing can replace experience...and gaining experience will take time. This time of gaining experience includes practice experience, competitive experience, and one other form of experience: "thinking experience"! In Chapter 5 I discussed ways in which you can prepare even before you set foot on a tennis court. If you want to speed up the experience-gaining time frame, you must interject tennis into your thoughts often every day.

In the context of this book you will gain precious time in learning the right methods at the very beginning. (As we have discussed, there are ways to successfully execute tennis strokes as well as many methods that thwart progressive learning!) You will also learn tips, cues, strategies, and practice principles that will help you play tennis effectively as quickly as possible. It will serve you well to identify these concepts often during your waking hours. (It probably won't hurt to "dream" about these concepts in your sleep, either!)

In this chapter I offer my proven practice principles that will ensure tennis improvement and over-all growth towards Tennis Mastery when practiced with the proper stroke mechanics. (I will discuss these mechanics later in Section 2.)

PRACTICE PRINCIPLES

Every level of player must recognize that each practice must encompass many diverse procedures, each specifically designed to meet very distinct tennis goals and particular tennis abilities. Obviously, practice programs will be different for each player based on current ability, current strengths and weaknesses, and specific shots as needed.

Within the processes of developing proper tennis strokes, there are three basic practice principles that should be included in each practice session. They are (a) targeting; (b) counting; (c) working weakest shots first.

1. Targeting

When drilling with a coach, pro, or fellow practice partner, or even by yourself, the use of targets gives each shot value. By value, I mean importance as well as instant feedback. While practicing hitting shots at targets should you miss, you naturally will make adjustments to come closer on the very next shot. This "fine tuning" makes the mind/muscle collaboration learn necessary timing and correct motor mechanics faster than just aiming for a broad part of the court.

Considering that the game of tennis can often be truly a game of inches, you must make your practice as precise as you expect your game to be. (Check out how many times in a professional match the ball lands on or very near the lines!) Obviously, if you are a beginner, aiming for the lines would be sheer suicide in terms of winning and losing! Aiming for the lines doesn't offer much leeway especially if control is minimal. Yet, using specific targets in practice does offer increased value to each shot, whereby aiming for general areas of the court does not.

I've heard players comment, "I use the corner of the court as my target. I don't need a cone." Consider this: a target is very precise; either you hit it or you don't. The corner of the court is somewhat nebulous. You could hit a ball within 4 or 5 feet of the corner of the court and feel like you hit your target. Thus, your desire to improve this 4 or 5-foot difference in location might not be critical or immediate. The fine-tuning corrections that you would normally make if aiming for a cone would not be utilized to the same degree if only aiming for a particular portion of the court.

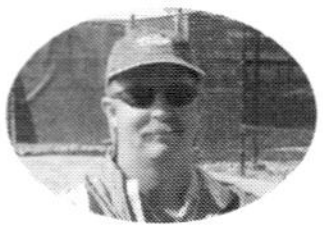

Author's Note

We know that "muscles" actually can't "learn" anything! The motor-learning components required for muscular replication and over-all accuracy include specifically the brain and its ability to command desired muscular movements. Thus, training increases the precision in which the brain "communicates" these commands. A well-trained athlete "allows" the brain to make the muscles repeat or execute a desired movement on cue without thought, (or at least without letting the mind get too much in the way!) Hence, the phrase "muscle-memory" has been used for years to describe a player's ability to repeat desired movements. When the phrase "muscle-memory" is used in this book, it refers to the overall understanding of this concept.

Targets can be anything from cones, towels, racket covers, a wad of paper, or even another tennis ball. As long as the target can be clearly seen by the student, it will serve this valuable purpose!

Beginners often feel they are not good enough to use targets. This is far from the truth! The fact is, when you are attempting to hit a target using new form which you are trying to master, your muscles make a more "conscious" effort during the course of the stroke. There are times a pro will have a player literally aim for nothing so the student can focus only on trying to accomplish a particular stroke. But once the stroke becomes repeatable, utilizing targets will increase the learning process.

Obviously, advanced players benefit even more when targets are used. In match play, advanced players must pinpoint very specific areas on the court to pass opponents, to hit service winners or aces, to open the court up, etc. Advanced players can almost envision imaginary targets during the course of their swing when trying for such precise shots. This imagery is enhanced by the use of targets in practice.

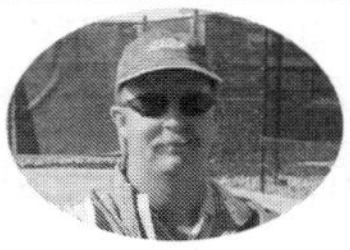

Author's Note —Targeting versus Stroke Development

Both players and instructors must be consciously aware that hitting the cone/target is NOT the ultimate goal of a player trying to develop proper and effective strokes. ATTEMPTING to hit the target while using proper form is paramount in terms of player development. Oftentimes, a player will change their form to something more familiar or comfortable in attempting to hit the cone. This type of practice happens a lot in group clinics where the target is sought by each player in an ego-gratifying reward if hit. Players must be reminded of the goal of BECOMING A BETTER PLAYER: if dinking the ball or using questionable form allows a player to hit the cone in an exercise, the player is not progressing within the bounds of true player development. However, when a target is used in a conscientious effort to hit with proper form, the player is provided immediate feedback as to the directional control provided by the shot. If a player adjusts the aim/spin/timing while maintaining proper form, then the player is truly developing into a more skilled player.

2. COUNTING

This is the actual vocalization of counting consecutive shots players hit when working on a particular shot. For example, when two players working on backhand-to-backhand volleys crosscourt; they count how many in a row they can make without the ball bouncing, being hit in the net, or hit out of the reach of the other player.

By counting, players will reach a particular number of consecutive shots. This number becomes the "target number". By establishing a target number each subsequent attempt to surpass it establishes a higher level of importance and game-like intensity on each shot as well as on each player. By counting out loud, both practice partners know exactly how far they are from the target number. In addition, the "word association" that develops (by counting out loud) with higher numbers of shots made without missing, increases the mind's ability to stay focused. Such counting increases each player's "mental toughness," or the ability to stay focused longer.

When we talk about mental toughness in Chapter 13, we will talk again about the importance of this drill. No other practice method or strategy can effectively emulate this type of mental practice.

Counting increases the effectiveness of many facets of your practice:

a. It makes both players focus more acutely on hitting the ball cleanly.
b. Aiming is increased as both players work in cooperation to control each shot in keeping the rally going.
c. When a rally approaches the target number, concentration automatically increases as both players work to surpass their previous best.
d. Once the target number is reached, both players now work even harder to see how high they can get their new target number.
e. Muscle strength, conditioning and endurance are increased, especially for advanced players who can get rallies to last from 50 to 150 consecutive hits. The players are "willed" to continue rallies even when they feel muscle fatigue on longer rallies.
f. Mental toughness is dramatically increased as you increase the target number in later rallies.

The results of using counting to increase this aspect of mental toughness can definitely be seen in match play. Players who use this practice tool begin to expect longer rallies and are mentally prepared to hit many more shots. I've had students who have used counting in practice tell me after matches that they were actually disappointed that their opponent couldn't hit more balls in play!

Counting is an excellent practice technique for literally every level of player. Beginners will find it fun and personally rewarding when they can beat their previous best target number. Advanced players will find it quite the test to reach a "projected" target number as their goal. In college my doubles partner and I had to reach 250 consecutive shots on both forehand and backhand volleys before we could move on to the next part of our practice routine. Talk about building up those forearms!

3. Working weakest shots first.

This is a discipline that players must force themselves to perform. Warm up by hitting your weakest shots first, then continue this theme when it comes time for drills. If your backhand is your weakest shot, start with the backhand before moving on to your forehand. We tend to spend more time on initial drill sequences and shorten the time we spend on the concluding drills (especially if our last drills are working our weakest shots!). By starting on your weakest shots first, you will get the much-needed time required to make those shots better. For those of you who "run around" your backhand, this practice technique might make that backhand a weapon instead of a handicap!

Practice Schemes

There are five areas that you must include within your practice routine. They don't have to be practiced every day and they don't have to be given equal time. You (or your coach or pro) will have to identify which of these areas need the most work and adjust your practice time to accommodate them. The duration and regularity of each will also be dependent on your level of play.

FIVE AREAS OF PRACTICE:

a. Stroke Grooving Drills

These are drills designed to allow the player to work a very specific stroke repeatedly. Once players learn the correct stroke mechanic and can emulate it without breakdown, then these grooving drills can be instituted. These drills include hitting the same shot with the same footwork and speed over and over until the stroke becomes permanently ingrained and can be repeated successfully. Every possible shot should be practiced this way—from simple forehands and backhands to angle volleys, overheads, drop shots and passing shots.

The idea of stroke grooving is to teach the body (and the mind) how to reproduce the shot without thinking—much like being able to do what we call "everyday tasks". Imagine if we still had to think about how to walk, or to open a door! Yet, many tennis players, even after years of playing and practicing tennis, still attempt to "think" their way through each shot!

There is a time and place to think about each shot. It is during this practice of grooving our shots that identification and isolation of certain moves or mechanics occur upon which we should think and concentrate. This is the "fine-tuning" of our strokes. As we get better, these subtle adjustments are necessary to facilitate the continued improvement of our mechanical foundation. Modifications to our strokes can include things like adding that extra top spin for a dipping passing shot, or hitting inside-out ground strokes for more angle to open up the court. Or, modifications can simply include working to hit deeper approach shots or volleys.

b. Game-situation Drills

These drills include the sequencing of shots which players will want to successfully hit in match-play competition. Serve-approach-volley, baseline to baseline ground strokes, closing-in volleys followed by an overhead, blood-and-guts movements, and poaching are but a few of these drills. Unlike grooving drills, game-situation drills focus on several different shots that are sequenced based on sound singles or doubles strategy. Like grooving drills, game-situation drills "program" a player to hit the right sequence of shots when needed. Also like grooving drills, the repetitive nature of hitting a series of desired shots would increase the likelihood of being able to repeat them under pressure of competition.

c. Rounding-out Drills

These are unique drills that do not necessarily feature shots hit regularly in competition. They are, however, drills which can increase a players hand-eye coordination, agility, anticipation, and the ability to react to and hit shots from unlikely positions on the court.

For example, without developing hand-eye coordination, having the greatest strokes in the world will be useless to you. Your lack of timing and spatial relationships will result in errant shots despite having perfect form.

A player who has truly mastered the game of tennis can react to situations that don't necessarily fall within the norm. Tennis players have all been faced with that freaky frame shot by their opponents that defies the laws of normal shots. Players often react to these anomalies in what seems to them as slow motion! Sometimes we panic while at the net and our opponent's shot clips the net tape, the ball jumping up and over our racket. Great players seem to be able to relax under these and other uncommon conditions by not only getting their racket on the ball, but also in their ability to turn these potential disasters into winners!

By incorporating as many "rounding-out" drills in your practice, you will learn to be calm and have the presence of mind enough to hit the right shot when these occasions do arise.

Examples of rounding-out drills that I often use in my teachings include: fast-hands drills, overhead reaction drills, sharp angle volley drills, the "oh-so-close-to-the-net" drills, "volleyball" tennis games, and even trick-shots such as behind-the-back shots and between the legs shots! (Yes, there is some value to those shots as well!)

One of my favorite rounding out drills is learning to catch the moving ball on the racket strings. You probably have seen pros do this, and thought, "How do they do that?" It isn't as hard as it looks! Not only is it fun to do, but by learning the technique, hand-eye coordination, and timing needed to accomplish it will help your tennis!

Ply metrics is another method of training. This is a training technique that does not change your mechanics, but changes the essence of power, speed, rhythm, and timing of your strokes through distinct practice routines. These, too, don't necessarily follow stroke patterns or strategies of match-play or competition. They do, however increase the players "holistic" being. That is, they exercise specific stroke segments through repetitive and magnified drills creating a more complete stroke pattern.

Ply metric drills include jumping drills onto and off of steps, lateral shuffles and grapevine footwork patterns, and many other footwork and quickness related drills. There are many ply metric information sites on the Internet that can provide better you with more in-depth understanding of this training benefit.

d. Endurance and Conditioning Drills.

When players develop a good foundation of tennis strokes, it is important to begin pushing the body in drills while maintaining solid mechanics. Player's strokes tend to break down when fatigue sets in. Like any other sport, as a tennis player gets better the demands on their body are increased. Beginners first learn to simply get the ball over the net and in the court. Consequently, the majority of their shots land near the middle of the court. Not too difficult for the beginner on the other side of the net! As a player improves directional control, balls now are hit further away from the opponent and thus, more movement takes place.

Advanced players must increase this area of practice. At high levels of competition with all things being equal, the player in better shape usually wins. Thus, advanced players will want to balance their practice with drills that also include extra movement. Look what conditioning did for Andre Agassi in 1999! And in 2001, Jennifer Capriati took the first two major championships of 2001, the Australian Open followed by the French Open, acknowledging that her aggressive conditioning and training regiment had a huge impact on her comeback.

Composure

In addition to the endurance and conditioning qualities, these types of drills teach players how to reach difficult shots and still have the composure to do something productive with them.

Generally, when beginners attempt to hit shots for which they have to move, any semblance of the strokes they may have learned goes out the door; arms go flying, footwork is entirely out of sync, and balance is completely lost!

The hardest part for beginners when having to rush to get to a ball is controlling swing speed. Most beginners get to the ball only to swing so hard that even if they make clean contact, the ball is hit a mile out! There is a golfer's phrase I've heard which I ascribe to these players who swing too hard: "It's a hard shot; hit it hard." Of course, this is the worst thing any player can do! By swinging hard on a difficult shot, you multiply the chances of error almost exponentially! Watch as good players rush to a ball only to swing with a simple motion. They make it look easy.

In reality, it is!

Top players get to these tough shots and literally make it as simple for themselves as possible. They take a shorter back swing, they use their body's momentum for power, and usually take pace off the ball by the addition of extra slice or topspin. The follow-through is shortened and, consequently, by using all these means they cut down the likelihood of missing the shot.

Most players improve in gradual increments usually learning first not to overrun shots. Once this is accomplished, a player learns how to slow their body down just prior to contact to maintain balance and control. Finally, accomplished players begin turning these difficult shots into offensive shots (for example: hitting winners on the run or controlling a tough shot for a good defensive or offensive lob).

To improve controlling swing speed, your practice should include drills where the player must move to the ball. A "single shot" drill is where players move from one spot and attempt to get to a ball hit to another spot. An example of this is where players stand against the back fence and must hustle to reach a ball hit near the net. Players work on not only getting to the ball, but also maintaining enough control to hit the ball back to a specific target.

"Multiple shots" drills include a series of movements that are more game-situation in design. "Blood and Guts" is one of my favorites where the pro or coach feeds random forehands and backhands to an individual. Usually 10 to 20 shots are used depending on the severity or difficulty of the series of shots. Players try to hit each shot to a target under control (usually all down-the-line or cross-court). This drill can be used at the net as well. Players are fed shots at the net and are directed to hit the volleys down-the-line, crosscourt, or to hit drop shots or angle volleys off difficult shots or reaction shots hit by the pro or partner.

e. Match-Play Competition

All players MUST learn to play under pressure. Basic drills can't simulate all the real pressures of competition, mainly because drills don't offer the same intrinsic reward (or penalties!) that tournaments or other forms of competition do. However, different types of competition "scenarios" can be instituted in practice to help players learn to handle tournament competition. Coaches can utilize these "mini competitions" in the form of ladder challenges to further impress their significance.

An example of this can include playing a "deep court set." This is a situation in which players must hit all shots following the serve in the back half of the court. Other examples include a "single serve" set, (to work on second serves); volley-only set, (where both players must come to the net after the serve and the return); short-court set, (players play only in the service boxes and can only hit under the ball with no topspin.)

Although I don't encourage betting, some kind of reward between players who challenge one another is another way to increase the pressure of practice sets. It can be as simple as the loser buying a coke for the winner or the loser having to do something for the winner such as washing their car or mowing their lawn.

PRACTICE TOOLS

While there are hundreds of books that offer hundreds of practice drills, few offer what I call "Practice Tools." Practice tools are specific swing and training tools to help players develop an affinity for components of the Advanced Foundation. These components can include grips, swing patterns, racket head control, balance, footwork patterns, racket head speed, and touch. While I will be mentioning many of these tools throughout the next section (The Strategies of Hitting) as they apply to specific shots, there are some general tools that I will include here in this chapter. It should be kept in mind that these Practice Tools are designed for both players learning the Advanced Foundation as well as advanced players searching to improve certain areas of their game.

Segmented Swing Tool (For Ground Strokes)

This tool helps players in many of the components I just mentioned. Player development has a lot to do with player perception as it deals with the racket and the ball in relation to the player's body. Many players, even advanced players, get into a "swing rut" where they can't seem to generate power, have control problems, or have trouble with specific shots such as the serve return or passing shots.

The Segmented Swing Tool is an excellent means for beginners to gain perception of the proper swing pattern, and in limiting their swing if they, indeed, swing too big. Here is how it works:

From the contact point on a forehand or backhand groundstroke, divide the backswing and the follow-through into 5 equal segments with a "5" being a full backswing or a full wrap follow-through. Practice swinging within specific backswing and follow-through patterns. For example, practice a "2 – 4" pattern for service returns. The first number, the 2, is a very short back swing, two of the five segments that would make a full back-swing. The last number, the 4, represents nearly a full follow-through just short of a full wrap follow through.

For beginners, practice a "1 – 3" swing pattern where they barely take the racket back and swing about half of their full follow-through.

Players have much greater comprehension when they associate these numbers with their swing. Teachers can call out specific swing numbers and have players hit balls in virtually any hitting drill and develop greater racket control and swing mechanics due to the intentional swing path each player attempts. Ironically, players discover that they often gain greater power and much greater control through shorter back swings. Such practice increases power through the confidence of greater control.

Exaggerated Angle Drills

Too often players develop a one-dimensional game. That is, they tend to hit balls relatively straight ahead, varying perhaps the depth only on ground strokes or volleys. Higher levels of tennis include learning to hit shots that create greater angles that open up your opponent's court. Typically, the beginner methods of volleys, serves and groundstrokes promote the inability to create greater angles. Eastern forehand and backhand grips on the volley and the Eastern forehand grip on the serve usually prohibit players from hitting angle volleys or creating the spin and racket head angle necessary to place serves out wide in either service box.

The "Exaggerated Angle Drill" provides a practice drill that encourages the use of proper grips and helps players learn what is possible in the way of angles. Here are some examples of the Exaggerated Angle drill:

1. *Angle Volleys: Players stand near their alley and aim not for the court itself, but for the opposite net post. Working on inside or outside volleys crosscourt, this drill teaches the player to "Set the Racket" to the angle necessary to hit the sharp angle volley. Too often, players "swing to the angle." That is, they have a relatively large backswing and attempt to swing the racket to gain the necessary angle. This makes the sharp angle almost impossible due to the fact that the player can't decelerate their racket enough prior to contact. Such a volley will almost always be hit too hard. In addition, the racket seldom gets to the proper angle necessary for the sharp crosscourt angle volley. This drill promotes the concepts of both the continental grip and the player keeping the racket head up during the volley. I will address this topic of angled volleys in greater detail in Chapter 8 on the volley.*
2. *Angle Groundstrokes: Using the same concept as the above Angle Volley drill, players aim for severe angles in hitting crosscourt shots. By aiming at severe angles players learn not to open up their body too soon. This practice allows the player to feel the racket head hitting the ball out in front of their wrist to generate greater topspin as well as learning how to hit up the outside of the ball. (This will allow a player to learn how to hit better crosscourt passing shots and to open up the court with severe crosscourt angles on groundstrokes.)*

3. *Angle Serves: Learning to create greater spin and angle on the serve is important to the development of a high-level serve (especially a good second serve!). Players should try to remain facing the opposite fence while serving to the diagonal net post, or put cones up very close to the net on the opposite side of the net near the alley. Players who work to hit such an angle learn to gener-*

ate greater spin and racket head speed by learning to get the racket head out in front of the hitting hand at contact. Many beginners to intermediate players hit the serve using the arm as the majority of the swing speed. While the arm contributes to the overall service swing, if a player swings too much with the arm, the racket head must slow down to hit the ball towards the target. This drill used for serves will have a terrific effect on learning how to serve the ball well.

There will be many more practice tools offered throughout this book. You will also want to refer back to these particular practice tools when you begin working towards the Advanced Foundation.

Practice to your level of play

Understand that each level of player will require different levels of practice. Advanced players who have good stroke mechanics should focus on game-situation drills, conditioning drills, and Mental Toughness drills. Beginners should be working more specifically on stroke grooving drills; drills that develop correct mechanics and form.

Above all, push yourself. If you want to be the best tennis player, you have to do more than "the other guy"! Certainly, some players are more naturally "gifted" and pick up concepts faster than others. However, in my experience, every single player who has made the leap from average to superior in terms of tennis performance, has had to apply themselves, regardless of any natural abilities they may or may not possess! This should be an incentive to every player who might have thought they weren't good enough…the great players all started with nothing and had to sacrifice, struggle, and simply work harder than everyone else!

Go beyond each previous set of practices in a coordinated and planned effort. Design your workouts to incorporate more intensity while allowing for proper rest, revitalization, and rebuilding.

Remember what I wrote at the beginning of this chapter: Your on-court success begins with the way you practice.

Make every minute count.

Section Two

The Strategies of Hitting

Beginning with this chapter, we will examine the actual methodology and technical aspects to playing tennis within the Advanced Foundation. Section 2: The Strategies of Hitting are exactly that…how best to learn, improve and eventually excel at the actual art of hitting a tennis ball.

Like many parts of this book, you will want to review, reexamine, and reevaluate your progress and compare it to the concepts presented. Because we are all human, our abilities to emulate stroke patterns will vary. (Which is one of the reasons why there is so much diversity even among those considered skilled players!) Our ability to combine the desired mechanical movements of our body with the coordinated hand-eye requirements necessary to find and hit a moving tennis ball will be tested time and time again. However, through educated practice and a dedication to the task at hand, each individual, regardless of their athleticism (or any perceived lack thereof!), will find excitement and success through continued progress and individual improvement.

CHAPTER 7

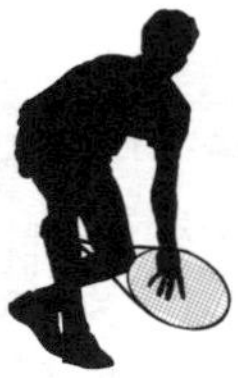

Technique and Form within the Advanced Foundation– The Mechanical Side of Tennis

Introduction of Mechanics

More books are written on the form and mechanical side of tennis than of any other aspect of playing the game. Perhaps more than any sport, more energy has been consumed by individuals in the pursuit of tennis techniques and form through videos, workshops, camps, and professional instruction. No other sport, with the possible exception of golf, offers the kinds of opportunity for players (and instructors!) to learn (or teach) the game of tennis.

This book is a culmination of many instructional texts, including tennis research and basic biomechanical education that I have studied for over 30 years. From three decades of playing, teaching, and coaching tennis, I have found quintessential techniques for every player who wants to learn this game. For those of you who are in pursuit of that edge, that elusive shot, or a way to develop an all-around game, these next few chapters will help propel you to a higher level of tennis mechanics, and, thus, one step closer to that pinnacle called Tennis Mastery.

Many fallacies and myths have permeated the learning and teaching aspects of tennis. Some of these inaccurate techniques have evolved through tennis pros that are trying to teach a player to break a serious detrimental habit. Obviously, not all techniques heard on the teaching court are designed for all players! Another reason for these myths is that some players, even good ones, think they do one thing when in reality they are doing something quite different. Another instance of mistaken methodology is when teaching pros base their teachings on one specific technique by one particular player who might be good at what he or she does. For example, one noted tennis researcher bases his volley technique and teaching on Ken Rosewall. As good as Ken Rosewall was in his day, his volley technique is generally not what top players follow today, nor what I believe should be taught to any player trying to learn or improve his or her volley. The reason for this opinion is simple: Rosewall used a "rolling racket" from almost completely horizontal on the backswing to a nearly perfectly flat, vertical racket face at contact. This move requires perfect timing and superb hand-eye coordination. Even today's top pros don't adopt such a unique stroke! Such a technique invites undesirable wrist movements and, typically, players tend to roll the racket over the ball at contact and end up hitting a great number of balls into the net! (These comparisons will be discussed later in Chapter 8 on the Volley).

One additional source of these tennis fallacies comes from watching pros playing tennis. Often a pro will hit a shot using a unique swing pattern or technique. Observers might equate this method to proper form. What many average players fail to recognize is the fact that not only are the players on the professional tour quite good athletes, they put in a tremendous amount of time on the court in the form of practice and competition. Tennis is these players' lives. These two facts in themselves can explain why a professional can, and often does, get away with hitting a shot that is not necessarily recommended by instructors to their students. Just because Venus Williams comes to the net and hits a swinging topspin volley doesn't mean that you, a student of the game, can come up with the same shot when you play! Likewise, if by chance you did attempt a low percentage shot such as a swinging topspin volley (low percentage for the vast majority of recreational players) and actually accomplished the feat, you certainly better not believe you can do it regularly! (For most players, we call it a "lucky shot"!) For many of my ranked players, YES, we do work on that very shot! However, beginner and intermediate players would have a most difficult time evolving their net game if this shot was both taught and practiced BEFORE the more fundamentally sound Advanced Foundation volley pattern was mastered.

A CHANGING GAME

If you have watched professional tennis on television, you have probably thought one of two things: "Wow, every pro hits seemingly the same." Or, "Wow, every pro has uniquely different form."

Both of these statements are accurate… depending on what you are looking for when watching the various tennis pros play the game. If you are looking at the "big picture,"—over-all stroke patterns, placement, and actuation of spin each player places on the ball—then, all in all, most pros indeed look very similar. They all hit powerful topspin forehands and backhands, the majority hit warp-speed serves, and they all move with the smoothness of a well-bred thoroughbred.

However, among all the top players there are variations in how they achieve that spin, that power, and that movement! From basic swing patterns, to grips, to footwork, players have unique form that suits them best. Do some pros do it "right" and others do it "wrong"? No.

It would appear on the surface that there are many ways to hit a ball correctly.

> *I must clarify this statement. There is more than one way to produce proper shots with a variety of grips, stroke sequences and footwork. It should be very clearly understood that, depending on the shot, stroke or footwork used, the racket will always need to hit the ball within the bounds of basic laws of physics, no matter what grip. Thus, a specific topspin forehand*

hit at waist level and hit to a specific height will have to have the racket strings moving up the back of the ball with the racket plane or face at a specific angle, no matter what grip, stroke pattern, or footwork is used!

> The myths, inaccuracies, and fallacies that have been perpetuated through inexperienced teaching pros, misinformed coaches, ego-centered "gurus" and players themselves, are many of the reasons why inadequate tennis continues to be played by so many adequate players
>
> !

This diversity and recognition of how the game has changed in some ways (and how some aspects of the game have not changed!) over the years is one of the motivating reasons I wrote this book. The myths, inaccuracies, and fallacies that have been perpetuated through inexperienced teaching pros, misinformed coaches, ego-centered "gurus" and players themselves (many who unsuccessfully tried to teach themselves without the help of accurate information!) are many of the reasons inadequate tennis continues to be played by so many adequate players! Go to any public tennis facility and witness the vast number of players who have not had the proper instruction (or have had questionable instruction), and see for yourself the differences. In my opinion, the chasm seen between those players who have some semblance of the Advanced Foundation and those who try to learn without the benefit of proper tennis tutoring is very wide.

Hitting a tennis ball basically refers to the action of the strings making contact with the ball. Hitting a ball correctly means that for any specific shot (i.e. volley, topspin forehand, slice backhand, overhead, etc.), the strings must make very specific contact and move in a very precise direction just prior to—and during—contact with the ball. Obviously, if we are going to be able to hit a tennis ball correctly many times in succession (as in a rally), we will have to have the strings make contact in the same manner each time we hit the same shot. Indeed, it is this ability that separates the "hacker" from the skilled, the "Mr. Choke" from the "Mr. Clutch".

A few months ago one of my students, when asked how he played in a previous match, responded, "Coach, I choked on the last point." He went on to describe the scenario: in a short match format he was playing a 9-point tiebreaker (instead of the regular 12-point tiebreaker). At 4 all in the tiebreaker (where the next point wins the set) my student said he went for a backhand passing shot down the line. I asked him if he tried to push the ball due to the pressure of the point or if he tried to hit the good topspin as we had worked on in practice. He said he hit the ball really well with topspin but that he hit it about a foot long. I told him, "you didn't choke, you hit the right shot. Next time, you will make it." This was an eye-opener for him as he associated choking with missing. What he did do, by attempting to hit the shot correctly in that match, was increase the likelihood of making that same shot under pressure the next time that occurs. Players who change their stroke due to pressure of match-play competition are the ones who indeed choke. Players who keep working to hit the shots in competition that they have practiced will learn and develop their strokes quicker than those who continuously change their strokes under pressure.

FOUNDATION

Building upon an Advanced Foundation is easier than adjusting, correcting, reevaluating and changing inadequate swing patterns.

The ability to hit the ball successively with repeatable, reliable and effective strokes is dependent on what I call FOUNDATION. The "Advanced Foundation," to which I have alluded to several times throughout this book, teaches the player to develop strokes that are not only repeatable and reliable, but also effective within the essence of advanced progression. Players who practice inferior stroke patterns tend to develop the repeatable and reliable qualities, but can't produce continuously improving "effective" strokes as the player develops. In other words, as the player begins to play opponents of increasing abilities, those players who develop inferior strokes will seldom, if ever, be able to compete against such players.

Players who develop repeatable swing patterns within the Advanced Foundation are able to progress rapidly in building upon their foundation as well as in the ability to improve direction—or aiming—much faster.

Building upon an Advanced Foundation is easier than adjusting, correcting, reevaluating and changing inadequate swing patterns. I have found that those players who start with grip, footwork, and stroke mechanics associated with the Advanced Foundation are not only faster learners of higher level stroke mechanics, they are also much faster at being able to actually begin playing the game, both recreationally as well as competitively. Juniors and adults alike have shown great strides when first taught stroke mechanics based on advanced principles. Extra spin, speed, and variety are then taught once the foundation of these stroke mechanics is achieved.

There are exceptions to this. Some players develop the Advanced Foundation of swing patterns very quickly and, thus, can begin to augment these patterns with individual style earlier. For example, often a player comes along with terrific athleticism. Generally, these players have previously played other sports such as baseball, softball, football, etc. Due to the natural carryover that many of these sports lend to each other, a gifted athlete can often incorporate higher advanced swing patterns from the start. Large loop groundstrokes, open-stance footwork, and extreme grips are but a few of the idiosyncratic building blocks that these advanced athletes might incorporate early on in building their foundation. However, I might add that gifted athletes tend to improve even faster when building upon a solid Advanced Foundation as opposed to trying to adopt, too soon, the very intricate advanced patterns they may have seen some pro execute. They are not only able to master the fundamentals quickly (allowing fast entry into competitive tennis), but they can soon add even higher-level stroke patterns to these essentials without frustration or confusion.

The Advanced Foundation deals with many aspects of playing. These aspects include footwork, touch, speed, rhythm, and strokes. The last aspect, strokes, is usually the first area players attempt to develop. Since the game of tennis revolves around hitting a tennis ball, players rightfully should develop their ability to correctly create those repeatable strokes I mentioned earlier. Building a solid Stroke Foundation begins with some basic understandings about spin and body mechanics. Before we begin our discussion on how to hit the ball correctly, understanding why particular strokes are beneficial, as well as important, will help us develop those correct swing patterns we desire.

Physics of Spin

Virtually every time you hit a shot in tennis, the ball will have some amount of spin. This is because of three things:

1. It is almost impossible in the course of a swing to have the strings hit the ball perfectly flat.
2. It is almost impossible to create a swing pattern that is perfectly flat.
3. If a ball hit from your opponent has spin, it is almost impossible to hit a shot that completely negates the spin of the oncoming ball after it hits your strings. A ball that bounces towards you off the court surface will always have forward spin in the direction it is traveling after the bounce. (With the possible exception of a perfect drop shot that has a great deal of backspin. Try it. See if you can hit a ball over the net with enough backspin that the ball won't have some forward topspin after it bounces!)

With the exception of some overheads, it should not be your intention to hit any shot perfectly flat. (Even a "flat" serve should have a great amount of spin. I will discuss this concept later in Chapter 11 on serving.) Shots that possess spin offer many advantages when used correctly.

SPIN: TOPSPIN, SIDESPIN AND UNDERSPIN

In every beginner lesson I teach, I first ask the student if they know what spin does to a ball in flight. A vast majority of beginning tennis players—young and old alike—doesn't fully understand what effect spin has on a tennis ball! In addition, many players don't know what effect hitting with spin has on a stroke. Without this understanding, a player will move through the motions of hitting strokes prescribed by an instructor without making the connection (both intellectually as well as visually and kinesthetically) as to why the shot should be hit in such a fashion. One of the most important ingredients in player development is their ability to connect the "why" to the "how" of any athletic movement. A player who has been taught how to hit a topspin forehand without the understanding of what effects that spin can have is missing a prime ingredient in their development. Without knowing what effect the spin will have on the ball's flight or how the spin will effect an opponent's shot, a player will give little or no value to the connection of what his or her strings are doing to the ball during the stroke! By understanding the connection of spin to your tennis strokes, you will have a much better perception of not only how the stroke should be accomplished, but also why the stroke is being accomplished in that particular manner!

Topspin

Topspin is when the ball is rotating forward in the direction it is traveling. That is, the top part of the ball is "rolling" forward in relation to the direction it has been hit. If this is confusing, simply roll a ball on the ground away from you. The ball is rolling with "topspin" in the direction it is traveling. This might be a very simple concept for some players. However, in my experience, a vast number of players, both adults and kids, don't know or understand what topspin is or how it affects the flight of the ball.

The "physics of topspin" is true for every sport that uses a ball. For many, the most recognizable spin associated with a sport is the "curve ball" in baseball. The pitcher throws the baseball with spin so the ball curves out of the "line of trajectory". If a pitcher always threw the ball straight, it wouldn't take long for a batter to start recognizing where the ball would be when it reached him. In other sports, volleyball, for example, skilled players will hit a ball with spin to control its direction or to have the ball "dip" down after it passes the net. Being able to hit a serve with this kind of spin is an obvious advantage: It allows a player to actually aim higher or hit the serve harder (or both!), and still get the serve in. Since so many people now play golf, another analogy to this idea of spin is the "hook" or the "slice" in golf.

In terms of scientific explanation, the spinning action of a tennis ball causes a change in air pressure on two sides of the ball. A ball with topspin will have slightly lower air pressure below the ball and higher air pressure above the ball. This differential in air pressure causes the ball to dip or drop. In addition to this pressure change, air-friction also plays a part in the movement of a spinning ball. As a topspin shot moves through the air, the forward spinning action causes air to "bunch up" above the ball. Conversely, the bottom of the ball is having the air below it literally spun out of the way. Likewise, if a ball is spinning sideways with the rotation of the ball to the left or right of the ball's direction of travel, the ball will curve left or right accordingly. The more spin applied to a ball, the greater the effect that these factors will have on a moving ball. Generally speaking the more the spin, the more a ball will curve out of its line of trajectory. (Velocity and gravity both will have an effect as well.)

Sidespin

A visual analogy to the sideways curving action is to watch a professional bowler throw a "hook". The ball, because of the spin created by the bowler and its friction with the lane, will curve dramatically as it approaches the pins. The ball curves from one side to the other because the spin placed on the ball is sidespin. However, unlike bowling, (where the curving movement is caused mainly by friction between the spinning ball and the surface of the bowling lane), in tennis the ball curves mainly due to air friction and air pressure. Also notice that as the bowling ball slows its forward velocity, the action of spin on the ball becomes more dramatic, causing the ball to curve more at the end of the lane near the pins rather than near the bowler who threw it. This principle is the same for tennis shots with spin. A hard hit ball with topspin will tend to stay in a straight line until it slows enough for air friction and air pressure (and gravity) to exert their effect on the ball and cause it to curve downward. This principle alone can explain why a player who tries to hit the ball too hard will inevitably make the ball go out, even with topspin.

A simple analogy in describing sidespin is the spinning nature of the earth on its axis. If, for example, on the serve, we picture the ball as the earth and we hit it along its equator, we will spin the ball with sidespin, or what is called slice as it applies to the serve. (Slice in groundstrokes or a volley usually represents underspin which I will discuss in just a moment.)

Sidespin in tennis will cause a tennis ball to move left or right, depending on the spin direction. For right-handers, a slice serve (brushing the strings across the right side of the ball) will cause the ball to curve to the left. This, obviously, can be a big advantage in moving your opponent off the court with your serve!

Underspin (or slice as it applies to volleys and groundstrokes)

For an under-spin shot, these same principles cause the ball to do the opposite: rise. You have probably heard the baseball term "raise pitch". This is a baseball that is thrown with a great deal of under-spin causing the ball to "move up" or rise on the batter. This rising action will continue until the forward velocity of the ball slows enough for gravity to negate the rising action of the ball produced by the spin and its forward velocity. This idea of higher and lower air pressure causing an object to rise or dip is the same principle that describes the lift needed for airplanes to fly. As air travels faster over the top part of the wing (due to the shape of the wing), there is less air pressure above the wing than below. Thus, the wing rises. The faster the airplane's velocity, the lower the air pressure above the wing…and the more lift potential. You can see how these principles are related.

In tennis, topspin shots are oftentimes favorable for groundstrokes. This is because a topspin shot can be hit harder and higher over the net than flat or slice shots of the same velocity. A topspin shot will tend to drop quickly allowing for a higher margin of error over the net. If you have ever seen a professional tennis match, you undoubtedly marveled at the power that these players possessed. In order to keep this kind of power in the court, a great amount of topspin is required!

In addition to the dropping action topspin produces on a tennis ball, keep in mind that topspin tends to make the ball bounce higher when it hits the ground. It will also make the ball "hop" forward. This can be a useful tool as well in terms of keeping your opponent deep on his side of the court.

However, topspin certainly should not be your only weapon! I have seen junior players who can hit topspin groundstrokes like the pros, yet who haven't spent one minute learning and mastering the slice. Underspin or "slice" shots have a purpose and, in some cases, are better suited for particular situations.

Here are some advantages that a slice shot can have over topspin:

1. Slice shots stay lower after the bounce. This feature makes the slice a good approach shot as well as a good drop shot. By keeping the ball low, your opponent will have to hit further up on the ball to get it over the net.
2. As a general rule, slice shots are easier to hit especially when a ball is hit hard to us. There is not as much emphasis on back swing on the slice allowing us to handle a hard hit ball with more control. Likewise, a ball hit to us with little pace tends to be easier to con trol with a slice shot.
3. In general slice shots tend to be easier to control especially when attempting to hit low balls that have not bounced very high. A low ball is very difficult to hit with topspin due to the fact that

a player can't get the racket down low enough to still hit up the back of the ball. Physiologically, it is easier to time and stroke a slice than topspin for many players.

Spin Advantage

There is one additional aspect of slice that helps explain why it is often easier to hit for most players. When a ball is hit to your side of the court and bounces, the spin the ball will always have is topspin after the bounce. When you slice a ball coming to you after a bounce, you are applying the same spin to the ball as the ball already possesses. Thus, the ball comes off your racket with less friction upon the strings! In other words, your racket does not reverse the spin of the ball, only the direction of the ball in flight. There has not been any study that measures the actual effect this has in comparison to the action of a topspin (in which the ball spin is reversed as well as the direction). However, it is very apparent that when a ball is hit with slice, the feeling of the shot, as well as the control of the shot, are better for most players.

A slice can also be used to keep a low ball in play without resorting to "dinking". (Please refer back to chapter 2 for detail on "Dinking".) An example of this can be seen in hitting low volleys. If we apply backspin (or slice) to the ball, the velocity of the ball being hit up (in order for it to clear the net) will be diminished. Because some of the ball's velocity is changed to underspin, gravity will be able to have a greater effect on the ball's flight, more than if the ball was hit flat with the same force flat. A flat ball hit at an upward angle, high enough to clear the net will need to be hit softer than if the same ball was hit with slice. (More will be discussed on the effect of slice on volleys in Chapter 8.)

Now that you understand what spin can do for your shots, as well as the advantages of both the topspin and the slice, let's look at the fundamentals of building your Advanced Foundation in producing tennis strokes.

KEEP THE PLANE THE SAME

As far as I know, this statement is my personal invention. (I know of no other book, instructor or video using this phrase. I apologize to anyone who may have coined the phrase before me!) I have used it for over 15 years in every lesson, camp, clinic, workshop, lecture and conference I have conducted. The reason I use it so much is that it literally describes the correct racket-head motion for virtually every shot in tennis.

For sake of definition, the "plane" of the racket is the hitting surface of the strings. Whether you are hitting topspin or slice, volleys or groundstrokes (and spin serves to a certain degree!), if you can produce strokes (from back swing to follow-through) that mimic the phrase, "keep the plane the same," you will be well on your way to making quantum leaps in improvement! It is that important!

Many players feel that in order to produce topspin, the racket needs to "roll" over the ball at contact. This changing of the racket face at contact will disrupt the player's ability to hit with consistency and accuracy. A player's ability to aim greatly depends on their ability to maintain the racket in a fixed plane through the contact zone. Even among the best players in the world, close scrutiny of high-speed videotape shows that these players keep the plane of the racket the same for the majority of the stroke.

As we discuss each stroke in the ensuing sections, I will often refer to this statement.

I bring it up here as an introduction to this important component of each stroke. The more you can institute this concept in your practice, the faster you will master each stroke.

Starting the Foundation Right: Ready Position

In order to have a good foundation players must have a good starting point. Because it is difficult, if not impossible, to predict exactly where our opponent will hit his or her next shot, it is important to get to a ready position as quickly as possible after you have completed your last shot. (Or, when your opponent is serving, be in this ready position prior to the serve.) Being in a ready position will give you the balance needed to react and move to the next shot. If you are favoring one side (such as having your racket back in anticipation of a particular shot), you will have a very difficult time making the correction if the ball is hit to the opposite side. (Especially if the ball is hit hard and you have even less time to react!)

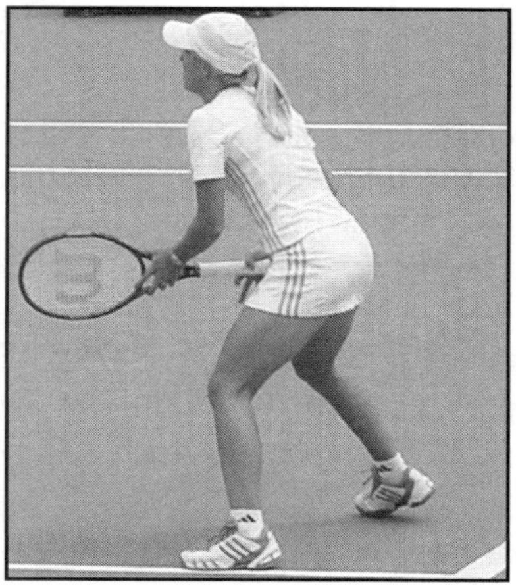

Figure 1
A neutral ready position provides for equidistance between both the forehand and backhand sides.
Photo by David Smith

The ready position consists of the following: (Figures 1-3)

A. Feet spread comfortably, about shoulder-width apart
B. Racket held in both hands, the non-dominant hand resting above the dominant hand on the grip. (There are some minor exceptions to this, which I will discuss later on.) I recommend the "two-handed" backhand grip as a ready position when rallying groundstrokes.
C. Racket head: I generally recommend holding the racket head up, especially when at the net. When at the base line, current theories include holding the racket head up, out or even pointed down.(Figures 1 & 2) The idea behind pointing the racket head down in the ready position when at the baseline is that when hitting topspin, the racket must move down below the ball prior to contact, thus saving time by having the racket down to begin with. However, there are many instructors who teach keeping the head up, especially when the "Loop Backswing" is incorporated. I will discuss this in depth when groundstrokes are discussed. What is important at this point is that the player keeps the racket centered at the mid-plane of the body that it can be swung equally in either direction as needed.
D. Stay on the balls of your feet.

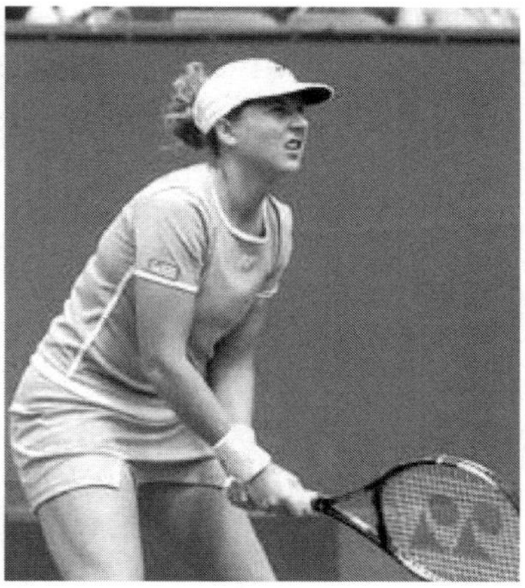

Figure 2
Monica Seles holds her racket pointed slightly down in anticipation of a serve

As you can see, from this position you can move or swing the racket to the left or right at an equal distance. Also, if you have a two handed backhand, you are already holding the racket with this in mind. One thing I have seen a few beginners do is to hold the racket only in the dominant hand and attempt to take the racket back for a backhand with one hand. At some point in this motion, they try to grasp the second hand at the right place on the grip before they start their forward swing at the ball (when attempting a two-handed back-

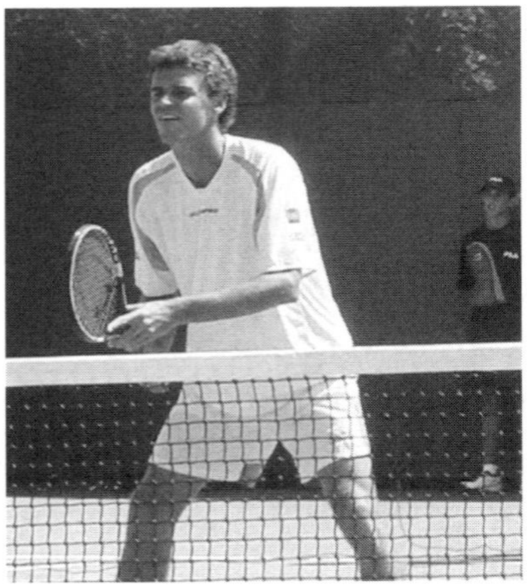

Figure 3
Ready position at the net by Gustavo Kuerten is similar to a backcourt ready position with the racket head held a bit higher.
Photo by David Smith

hand). This will produce very inconsistent swing patterns. Keep both hands on the racket in your ready position and you are all set to take the racket back for the backhand with two hands if that shot is needed. Most players who use a one-handed backhand still take their racket back with two hands usually moving their non-dominant hand up to the throat of the racket during the backswing. For the forehand, most players take the racket back with the dominant hand, letting go of the other hand at some point during the process. (The exception to this would be using a two-handed forehand where the player would take the racket back with both hands, in which case the two-handed ready position is again ideal.)

The Ready Position when playing the net is the same with emphasis on keeping the racket head up. One of the biggest errors a player makes when at the net is letting the racket head droop down. When a ball is hit to them, not only do they have to turn to hit the volley, they first have to raise the racket head up from this lower position. Because we have so little time to volley, this extra move notoriously makes player hit the ball late. In addition, a low racket head ready-position tends to make a player hit topspin volleys. This is because the racket is late on getting behind the ball and is still on the way up at the point of contact.

Footwork: The Key to Balance

Footwork is important on several levels in tennis. The most obvious of footwork patterns is simply propelling oneself to the ball. Even in this simple context, there are many intricate concepts that can increase a player's ability to get to the ball and maintain balance when arriving at the ball. In addition, proper footwork can aid in the development of proper strokes. Likewise, students who use improper footwork can hinder their acquisition of solid stroke mechanics and delay or prohibit development.

Proper tennis footwork involves a series of coordinated movements that must be mastered just like any other proper movement that are required of skilled tennis strokes. Advanced players almost flow within these movements, creating nearly the same seamless precision one might associate with dance or martial arts. In fact, it is this seemingly fluid movement that makes the uneducated assume that there are no distinct movements or transitions between movements in skilled or professional play. This assumption is furthest from the truth. After your study of this section on footwork, you will know what to look for when watching the pros as well as knowing what you, yourself, will need to work on.

With few exceptions, all the footwork patterns discussed in this section can and should be applied to all groundstrokes. Footwork for volleys, serves, and specialty situations will be discussed in the appropriate chapters.

SEQUENTIAL MOVEMENTS

During any rally there will be preparatory movements, movements to the ball, transitory movements while hitting the ball, recovery movements following a shot, and recovery movements in regards to court position. Each of these movements has a specific role and implementation format. Subtle key position points are involved with each, and they must be done in harmony and in balance.

First Move

Other than the server just prior to serving, all players will have a period of not knowing where the ball is going to be hit. While experience provides players with a sense of anticipation and awareness, nevertheless, before the opponent has hit a shot we don't know for sure where the ball is going. This unknown demands a moment of balance from which we are able to respond correctly and efficiently, in any necessary direction, when it is recognized where the shot is going. This balance point is achieved by what is called a "Split-Step."

Importance of a Split-Step

A proper and effective ready position is determined by one most important concept: balance. Because tennis is played with constant movements once the ball is in play, each player must be able to both respond to opponent's shots and be in control of their body when they do. This requirement is accomplished within a series of movements and balance checks called "Split-steps". A split-step is a momentary pause in our movements just as our opponent begins to hit a shot to us. Failure to incorporate a split-step during a point will usually result in a player's inability to respond correctly to even ordinary shots hit by an opponent. The reason for this is simple. We seldom know exactly where an opponent will hit a shot. Thus, if we are moving—or even leaning—in the wrong direction of an incoming shot by our opponent, we will not be in the best position to make a competent response. Players who fail to perform proper split-steps are often caught "wrong footed" or "leaning the wrong way." While it is impossible to retrieve some very offensive shots by our opponents, a proper split-step will insure the best possible balance and position for those shots that are within our reach.

The split-step should occur literally every time our opponent makes contact with the ball. (Actually, the point at which the split-step occurs will be very dependent on our current ability. Beginners should split-step early, usually when their opponent is starting their backswing. Advanced players will split-step later, usually when their opponent starts to make contact with their shot.) Whether we are returning serve, playing the net, or returning groundstrokes, a split-step must be executed by those players who hope to advance to high level tennis. (At beginning levels of play we tend to see less of an impact of the use of a split-step because beginning opponents don't necessarily hit the ball very hard. However, just as in developing good strokes, the beginner must incorporate proper footwork as it relates to movement, not just as it relates to accomplishing a shot.)

SPLIT-STEP MOVEMENTS

Regardless of circumstance, the split-step is utilized virtually the same for all shots and from all positions on the court. Anytime our opponent is about to hit a shot, our movements must pause and allow our body to become balanced. Since we are usually moving from a previous shot to a recovery position, we will have some movement of our entire body during most rallies that must be addressed. This pause is accomplished when we stop moving in any previous direction and "split" our feet apart. This split-step resem-

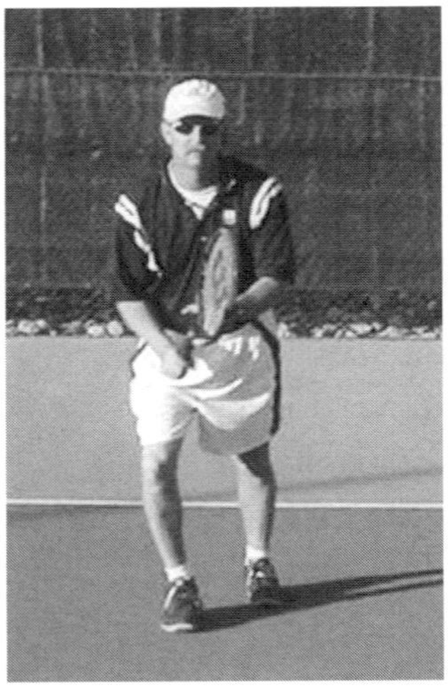

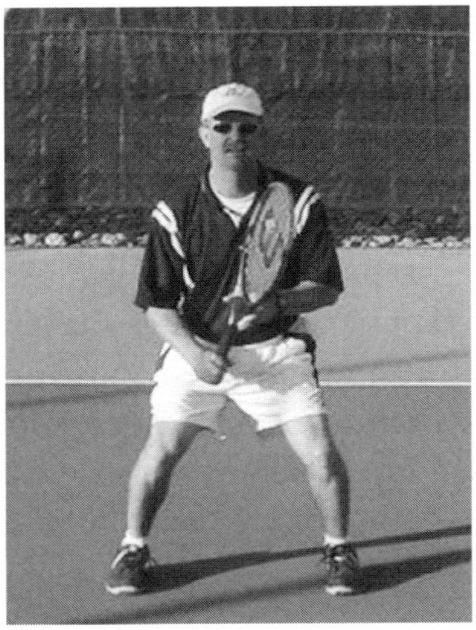

Figure 4 Figure 5

The Split Step is a momentary pause of the player's center of gravity when a player is in motion. When an opponent begins to strike the ball, any movement by a player must be under control in order to react and initiate movement in the direction of the opponent's shot.

bles the ready position I described in the previous section of this chapter. The split-step allows our body to become balanced, ready to respond to the unknown shot forthcoming by our opponent.

The execution of the split-step is simply bringing your body to a momentary balance point in relation to any previous movements. It can be analogized to a miniature hop or jump with both feet landing lightly but evenly about shoulder width or more apart. The legs will give with this landing, bringing the center of gravity to a more stable or controlling position. (See Figures 4 & 5) Obviously, if one stops suddenly, it will be difficult to maintain balance in any movement if the center of gravity is not stable. Generally, the racket should be held in a neutral position, similar to a ready position. When players are moving towards the net, it is imperative for the racket to be held with the head up. Players who notoriously drop the racket head will invariably swing up to hit the volley producing topspin volleys. (More on racket position for volleys in Chapter 8 on Volleys.)

With the exceptions I mentioned for beginners, a player should always execute a split-step just prior to any contact of the ball by the opponent. Even running from one side of the court trying to get back to the middle, a player should split-step just before their opponent makes contact. Even as this split-step will perhaps hinder your ability to return to the very middle of the backcourt, you will be in far better balance in case your opponent hits the ball behind you. Also, in running towards the open court, you will decrease the probability of overrunning your opponent's shot by making a split-step. Certainly, you might give up a small portion of open court by making the split-step at a point away from the dead center of the court. However, this consideration is far less pertinent than those shots you would probably miss from being off balanced because you didn't complete a proper split-step.

Many beginners watch a pro match and remark that the pros don't appear to be executing split-steps. This is because the pros incorporate much more subtle split-steps with well-developed anticipation skills. Even as the pros have much greater ability to anticipate shots, they still must (and do!) integrate proper split-steps prior to almost every shot. Although their anticipation skills are better than that of beginner players because their opponent's weaponry is significant, all pros must employ split-steps to counter such offensive shot-making skills. Watch closely and you will indeed see the split-steps by the pros.

MOVEMENT AFTER THE SPLIT-STEP

Following a split-step, when the player recognizes the direction of travel needed to intercept the next shot, the next issue is executing the quickest way to get from the split-step position to where the ball is—or will be—on the court. For most players this concept may seem simple enough. However, at higher levels of skilled play when reaction time is diminished by the speed or quality of the shots themselves, players must try to gain every fraction of time they can. There are three ways in which a player can initiate their movement to their right or left.

Crossover Step:

This movement involves the player stepping across their body with either their right or left foot, depending on direction. To move to a player's right, first the player will rotate the hips to the right. This is followed by the right foot crossing over and in front of the left foot. (Fig. 7)

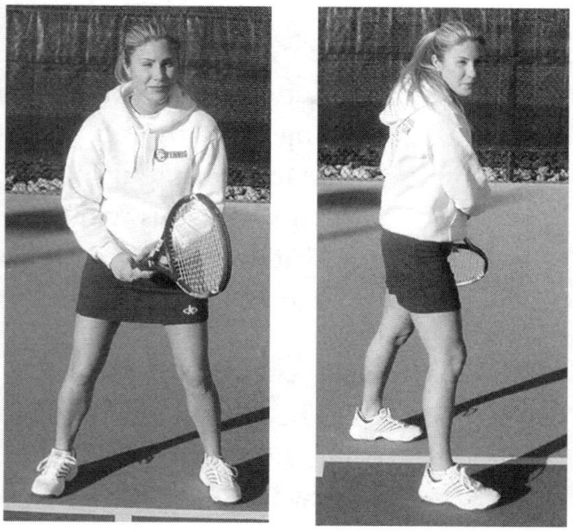

Figures 6 & 7 "Crossover Step" in these two pictures, the player moves to her left by stepping across her body with her right foot.

Jab Step:

In moving right or left, the player will simply lead with that foot. In other words, to move right the player lifts and steps with the right foot towards the player's right. (Figures 8 & 9)

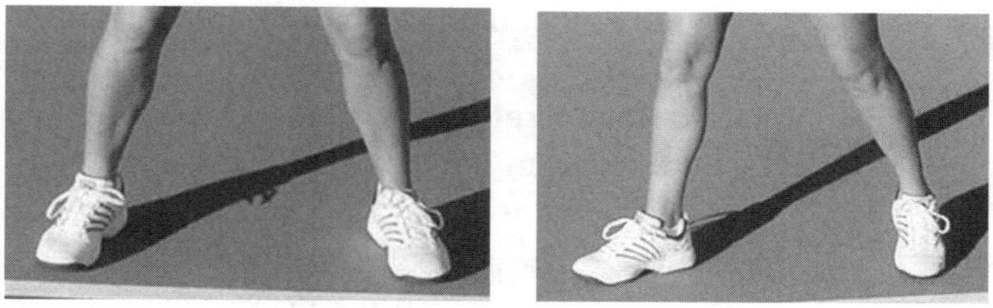

Figures 8 & 9
The "Jab" step to the player's right: from the ready position, (left) the right foot steps out and to the right.

While these two movements are sufficient for most players, there is one additional move that has been researched to produce more efficient lateral movement:

Drop Step or Gravity Step:

Here, the player actually brings the outer foot in, AWAY from the direction of desired travel. This movement causes the body's center of gravity to fall towards the direction of intended travel. For example, to move to my right, I will bring my right foot in towards my left foot and allow my center of gravity to fall to my right. This is immediately followed by the crossover step of the left foot, as in the first example. (Figures 10-12)

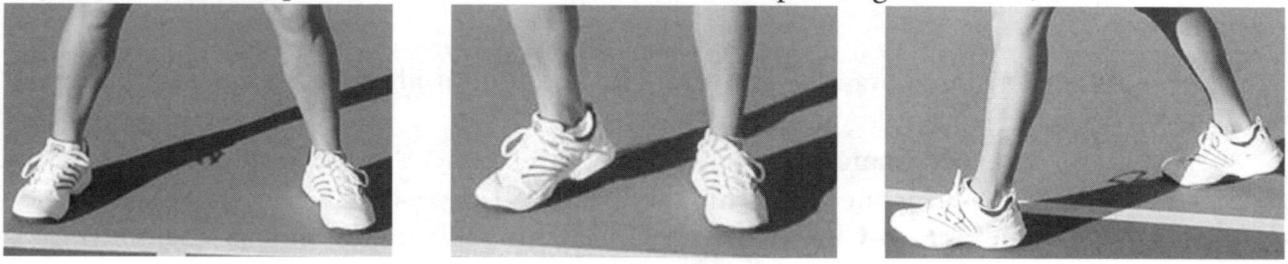

Figures 10, 11 & 12
Using the Drop Step to move to the player's right, the right foot comes in towards the left foot. (Figure 10 & 11) As the weight is transferred over this right foot, the left foot then steps across the body to the player's right. (Figure 12)

NOTE: Oftentimes, this movement is initiated by a simple bending of the outside knee, as opposed to actually bringing this foot in a step. You will see many top level players do both, depending on situations.

Both the Crossover Step and the Jab Step cause the body's center of gravity to move slightly away from the intended direction of travel. (This is because both steps' initial movements are done independent of the body's center of gravity.) The Drop Step, however, creates a favorable momentary imbalance in the player with their center of gravity moving towards the intended direction immediately following the Drop Step. (By the inside leg coming in, (Figure 11), the player's center of gravity is immediately moved outside this leg. This will cause the player to literally "fall" in the direction of intended travel!) Watch any pro match and you will see many examples of this Drop Step in action. Try each one yourself and see if you can feel the difference between each.

During the Shot

The vast majority of shots in a match should be hit with minimal linear movements occurring during the swing. Although highly skilled and experience players can create the proper balance and footwork while hitting on the run, most beginners and intermediate players notoriously find themselves running through shots due to faulty or absent split-steps or inadequate reactionary movements. Due to these preparatory mistakes, these players end up off balance when they do arrive at the ball. However, if a properly timed and executed split-step is instituted, most players should be able to arrive at most shots balanced and in control of their body.

Ideally, we want to be balanced and relatively calm during the swinging component of a shot. There are exceptions to this tactic. In addition to those shots so far out of reach that we have to run all the way to the point of contact, many skilled volleys will include a forward thrust of the body during the shot. This forward movement has little to do with the shot itself, however. It is more the result of a player attempting to cut off a shot earlier to give their opponent less time to cover the open court. Some shots actually will require a movement backward while hitting a ball. However, most shots in a rally will want to be hit under balance and control of the player. This will increase the hitting zone of most shots as well as provide a stable foundation between the body and the ground which most shots need for power and control. (Each shot will have its own specific footwork. In the following chapters on strokes, I will address each of these specific footwork needs.)

Today's modern groundstroke game incorporates three main footwork stances. These are:

- **Closed Stance:** This traditional position utilizes a crossover step at contact with the front leg and foot. (Figure 13)
- **Open Stance:** Used in today's power game, the open stance has the outside foot stepping out during the shot. (Figure 14)
- **Open-to-Closed Stance**: Usually hit while on the run, this combination step pattern starts with an open stance. The front foot will close at contact.
  This footwork pattern closes the lower half of the body while the upper half is opening during the stroke. This creates a whip-like body and is actually a very complex move. (Fig.15-16)

Advantages and Disadvantages

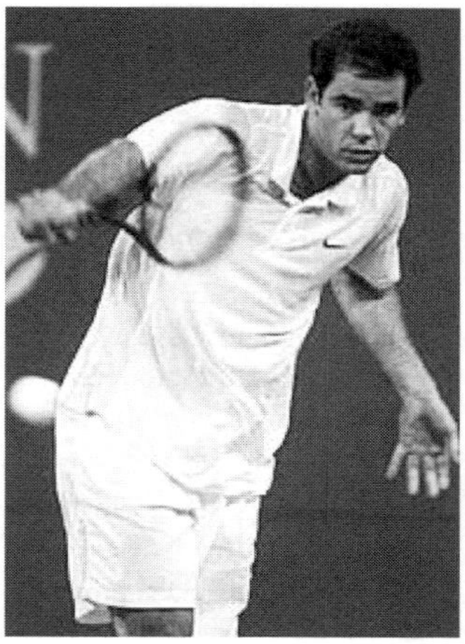

.Figure 13
Note the sideways positions held here in Pete Sampras' one-handed backhand, using a closed stance.

Closed Stance: (Figure 13) The action of stepping across the body sets up a good sideways turn and upper body rotation during the backswing. The position helps beginners learn how to turn sideways to the ball instead of facing the net and "pushing" the shot over. However, in terms of the mechanical advantage, the closed stance is actually counterproductive for players wanting to generate power. The reason for this is because the crossover step is what I call a "non-loading" step. That is, by tuning sideways the body does not possess any "potential energy". In fact, the body gains more potential energy AFTER the shot with a closed stance. The reason for this is simple: if players keep their back foot down during the shot (as they should), their body will coil up like a spring during the shot. In recoil, the player usually will swing their back leg around or step backward with their front, crossed over leg (as in a Break Step or a Pivot Step, which will be described later in this section). This action is reversed in an open stance stroke.

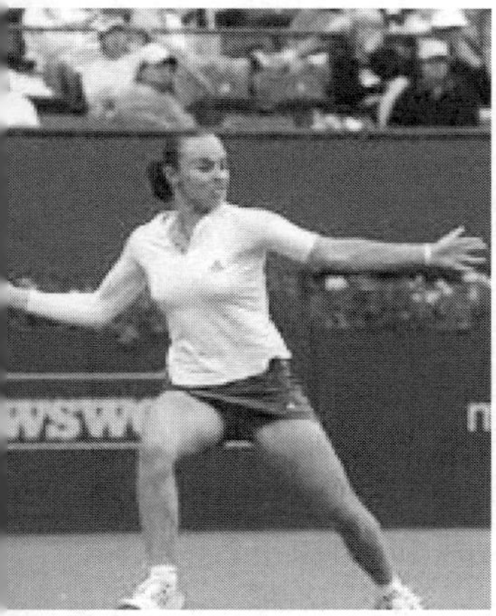

Figure 14
e, Martina Hingis sets up to ıer forehand with an open ıce. Note her sideways er body position compared er feet that are almost par- to the baseline.

Open Stance: (Figure 14) With the open stance players will coil their upper body so they are sideways to the ball. (This is virtually the exact same position as the Closed Stance position for the upper body.) However, their lower body is still facing the net. This coil between the upper and lower body creates torque that can be used as additional energy for hitting the ball. (As I will talk about body rotation or "angular momentum" later in this section, you will discover the tremendous power available through the coil and rotation of the body into the shot.) There is a release of energy and power through the release of this coiled position during the shot. Much like a spring that has been wound, the upper body literally springs open. When done correctly, this energy is passed on to the rack-et when hitting the ball.

Open to Closed Stance:

(Figure 15 & 16)

When a player is on the run, he often finds it difficult to get set and balanced and hit specifically either a closed or open stance stroke. Top players will often drive their front leg across their body, closing their stance in the middle of their swing. (See Figures 15 & 16, two pictures of Marat Safin.) Notice Safin is set

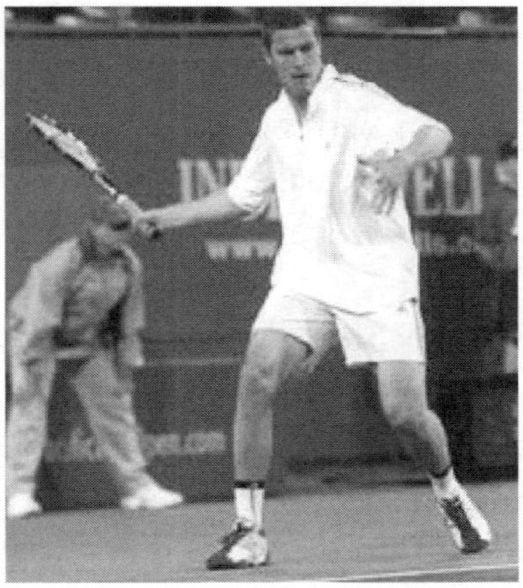

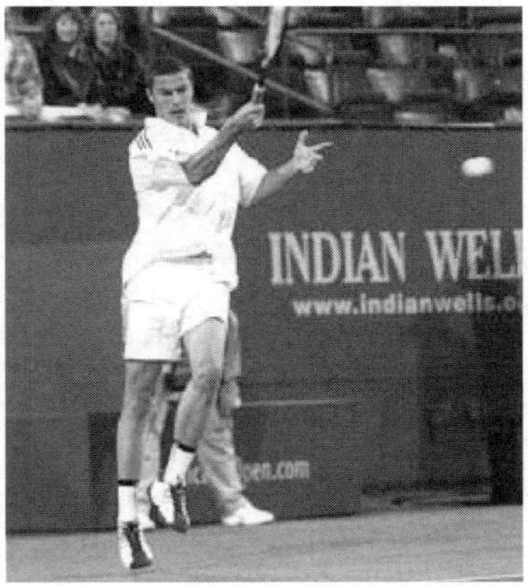

Figures 15 & 16
Marat Safin sets up to hit his forehand with an open stance. (left) During his swing (right), note his front leg steps in and across the body. (As in a Closed Stance position)

up for a typical open stance. However, due to his momentum he can't push off his outside foot and create what is called a "pivot step". (This will be discussed in just a moment.) Instead, he allows his left leg to whip across his body during the swing, which helps him remain balanced and does not open up his upper body too early during the swing. While this is actually a complex concept, it is not hard to accomplish and comes quite naturally for most students when they learn the Advanced Foundation for groundstrokes.

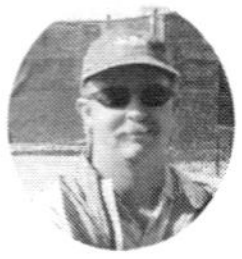

Author's Note - Hit and Hold

This exercise helps players learn to recognize where a shot ends and when recovery begins. Even when watching at the pro level, you can oftentimes observe the pros holding their follow-through for a brief moment following a shot. Hit and Hold means to hold your body still for no more than a half second or so. One learning advantage to this practice is that the player has a moment to evaluate the quality of the stroke instead of simply hurrying back to the ready position for the next shot. This evaluation moment also allows the player to note if they are balanced after the shot, the position of their racket on the follow-through, and a moment to "feel" what the shot felt like…a kind of muscle-storage practice. If the player hit a bad shot, by holding the follow-through for a moment they can usually identify what part of the stroke broke down. If they hit a great shot, they get to mentally replay the shot in their mind during that brief moment. If they are too busy trying to get ready for the next shot, much of this learning is lost. Also, even when players hit a great stroke, if they fail to hold the finish for a brief moment, the player loses the opportunity to let the good shot "sink in". Often a player will hit a great shot only to miss this opportunity to "savor" this great shot. The momentary hold following the shot will increase the player's ability to store the stroke mentally as well as physically.

Post Shot Recovery

Immediately following any shot, the body will require some element of recovery. This is necessary for two reasons: 1) the stroke itself may cause some imbalance immediately after the stroke; 2) the player will want to regain a neutral position to prepare for the next shot as quickly as possible.

This recovery footwork must be completely understood. Any action that is done at the wrong time can have serious consequences on the quality of the shot. If the shot itself is hit poorly (or erroneously) and it goes out or in the net, it won't matter much what your footwork includes after the hit! It is important to make sure that the shot is not compromised in favor of trying to get back in position.

There are several ways in which a player can incorporate recovery footwork in the course of a shot. However, as I just mentioned, players must be careful not to let the recovery steps impede the quality of the shot. Players can prevent this through understanding an important key position point: the "Hit and Hold" concept. (See insert above.)

RECOVER STEPS

There are two identifiable recovery steps players can use to help them gain better position following a shot.

- Brake Step: Used with a Closed Stance groundstroke
- Reverse Pivot: Used with an Open Stance groundstroke

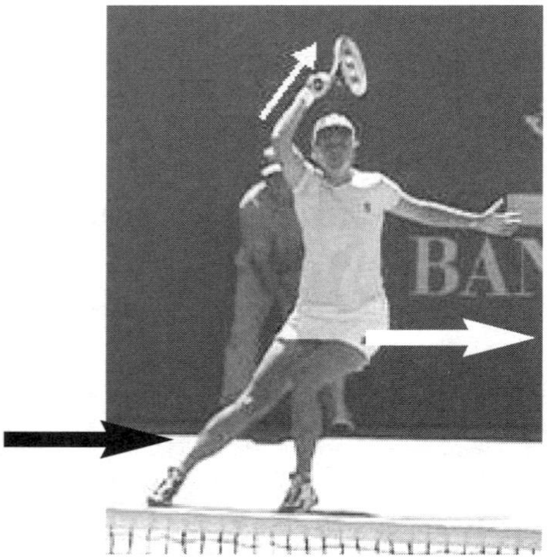

Figure 17 - Brake Step
Here, Lindsay Davenport pushes off her back, outside leg (right leg) in the course of her follow-through. This will allow her to return to a neutral court position as quickly as possible.

Brake Step: With most groundstrokes, players will be moving away from the center of the court to track and then hit the ball. In these cases, the player's body weight will also tend to be moving away from the center of the court during or just after the shot, (due to inertia of the body's movement). Obviously, the player will want to be able to recover back to the neutral or center part of his court as quickly as possible. The Brake Step is utilized with a Closed Stance hitting position. As the crossover step is actuated during the swing, the back leg will pause during contact, remaining on the ground in what I call a "toe drag" position. Immediately following the momentary pause of the back leg, this leg then swings around and plants itself on the court to the player's side. (See Figures 17 & 18) This foot then acts like a "brake" where the body can halt its movement away from the center of the court. The body can then push off this foot with substantial force to return to center of the court and a better ready position for the next shot.

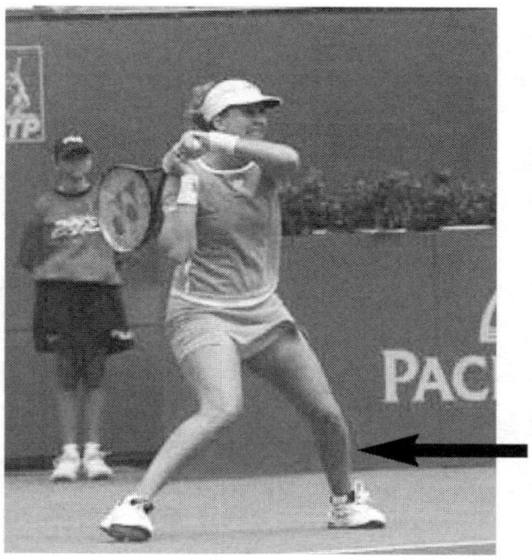

Figure 18
Monic Seles utilizes the brake step (with her outside left foot) here on her left-handed two-handed forehand.

Reverse Pivot: When a player hits an Open Stance groundstroke, the player tends to have more weight on the outside foot. Because of this, it is impossible to create a Brake Step as described above. However, the player can use this outside foot during the swing in what is called a "Pivot Step". As the body's momentum rotates during the swing, this foot pivots on the ground, usually around the ball of the foot. The opposite leg is then free to step backwards after the follow-through helping bring the body weight back towards the center of the court. (Figure 19) This Reverse Pivot can be also utilized on high bouncing balls hit deep into your court. The use of the Reverse Pivot actually increases a process called "Angular Momentum" (which will be discussed in a moment), and provides excellent racket head speed even as the player's body is moving backwards as contact is made.

BIOMECHANICS OF BODY ROTATION

Many instructors refer to "Rotation" as the act of turning their upper body into the shot at contact. While this is an action that is necessary for players in developing maximum torque and efficient racket head speed, it is also one of the most abused concepts in tennis. One of the biggest problems I see in ALL levels of players is the tendency to overturn prior to contact. I will address this issue in each stroke section in greater detail as it applies to each particular shot. However, there is a general, fundamental process about the rotation of a player's upper body that is undeniably critical in developing consistent advanced strokes.

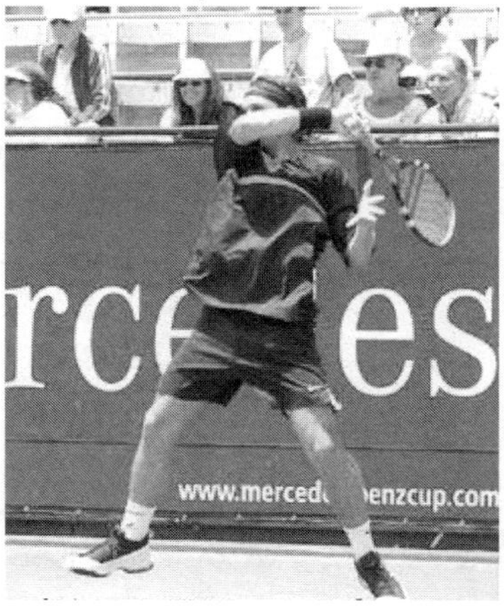

Figure 19
Carlos Moya has finished his forehand and stepped back with his left foot. This "Reverse Pivot Step" takes into account his weight moving backwards as he hit his forehand.

Tennis uses a principle in almost every stroke that I refer to as the "pendulum" principle. This simplistic concept is one of the fundamental "laws" to player development.

The pendulum concept refers to the action of the arm in swinging any club, racket, bat or other device. There are two vertical planes of motion in which a person can swing a racket. One plane is swinging the racket in a path that is perpendicular to the anterior plane of the body. This swing has the player facing square to the target and the arm motion in a straight line towards the target. (Tossing a ball underhand while facing the target is a good visual analogy.) The other swing-plane is parallel with the anterior plane of the body. This motion is created when the player stands sideways to the target with the arm swinging parallel with the chest. (This can be visualized by imagining a golfer swinging a golf club. They stand sideways to the target and generally make contact with the ball in this position.)

Beginners tend to favor the first pendulum action as witnessed by so many of them facing the net while making a swing. This perpendicular pendulum swing pattern creates a myriad of problems. In order to keep the arm and racket moving towards the target as in a tennis stroke, the action of the arm changes from a swinging pattern to a pushing pattern for most players. The racket is essentially pushed away from the body while the body remains open and parallel to the net. Players inevitably will bring the arm across the body during the swing, a natural reaction. This action brings the racket face out of the target line. Players tend to correct this problem by laying the racket head back and making even more of a pushing motion during contact. (This is how many "dinkers" end up hitting the ball!)

As I will describe in each chapter on hitting, the ideal biomechanical swing action occurs when the pendulum action of the arm is more parallel to the body plane. This requires the player to turn sideways for virtually every shot in tennis. This is why skilled players are seen hitting groundstrokes, volleys, overheads, and serves with their body essentially sideways at contact. While there are a few exceptions to this rule which I will explain later, when a player remains relatively sideways for the duration of the swing, through contact, the player will develop a much more advanced foundation for virtually every shot in tennis. As players develop, greater use of rotation comes into play, to the point that top players can be seen rotating almost 180 degrees during some forehand groundstrokes! However, most backhands, volleys, and slice strokes hit among skilled players maintain a much more defined sideways position through contact.

Power in tennis, as it relates to groundstrokes, serves and overheads, is primarily developed through the use of "Angular Momentum". Angular momentum is created when a player coils their body, which then allows for an uncoiling prior to contact. This uncoiling, done right, produces the majority of racket head speed when combined with proper arm movements.

Two of the most common footwork faults that contribute to over rotation in tennis are when the player either pulls the front foot away during contact, or the player steps out of the shot allowing the back leg to swing around prior to or during contact. Both of these problems change the orientation of the body to the swing, causing the body to open up. This over rotation generally results in players pushing the ball towards the intended direction instead of utilizing the more efficient stroke pattern associated with angular momentum. (See Author's Point.)

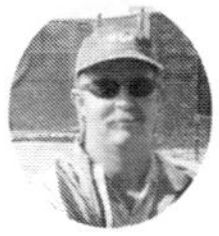

Author's Point

Many readers might recognize these two common footwork faults as the very desired movements described in the "Brake Step" and the "Pivot Steps" in the section prior to this. However the key concept is that these moves generally take place AFTER contact. It is when a player incorporates these footwork patterns prior to contact that creates problems in stroke development.

The biggest culprit in causing these undesirable leg movements is balance. When a player fails to get in the best balance and position to hit a ball, the center of gravity of the player falls outside the balance point of the player. This lack of balance will result in either of these leg movements I just described. The reason for this is simple: if the unbalanced player doesn't step out with one leg or the other, the player will fall down!

As I mentioned earlier in the section on footwork, a player can learn to prevent these undesirable movements by the "Hit and Hold principle. This practice helps players develop balance within most strokes.

Power—Angular Momentum versus Linear Movement

Even though the desired swing pattern places the player sideways for most shots in tennis, there is an element of body rotation that occurs in every swing. Advanced players tend to coil their upper body past this sideways position. This will allow the player to execute a powerful swing utilizing the gross motor movements of the larger muscle groups of the torso, hips and legs, prior to using the fine muscle movements of the arm without changing the desired swing pattern described above. Take a look at most shots hit by the pros. At contact, the players are, for the most part, standing sideways to the target. (A common exception to this is on some forehands that I will address in a moment.) As the racket reaches maximum acceleration at contact, the body will follow the swing more as a recovery phase, as opposed to a forced movement created by over rotation at contact. I have found that most players will indeed rotate at the correct time if they don't consciously try to rotate as they begin the contact phase of their swing.

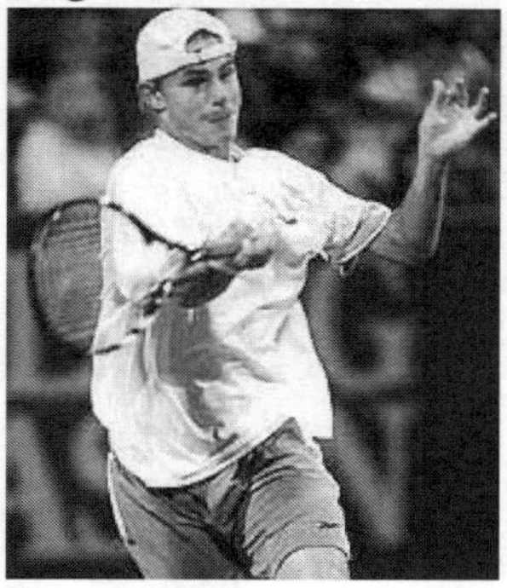
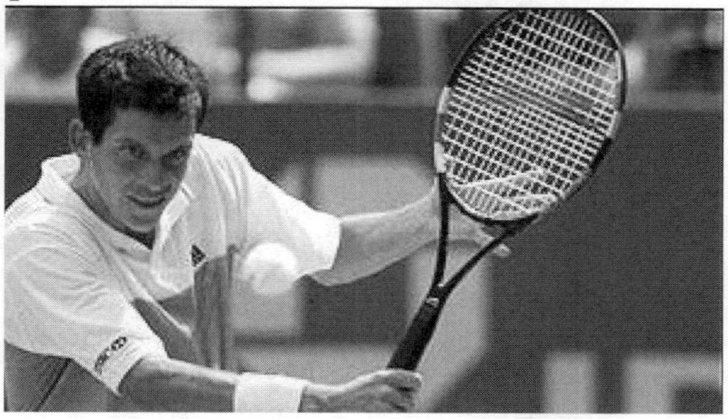
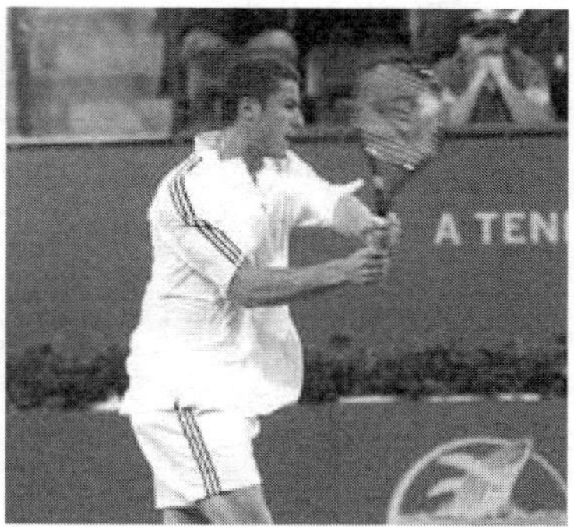

Figures 20, 21 & 22
Note the nearly sideways positions of each player during, prior and just after each of these shots.

There are exceptions to this sideways key position. Specifically, when players use a full Western grip for the forehand, the racket position at contact must be very far out in front of the player. Thus, those players using such a grip will tend to hit further rotated than our rule-of-thumb of staying mostly sideways at contact. (Figure 23)

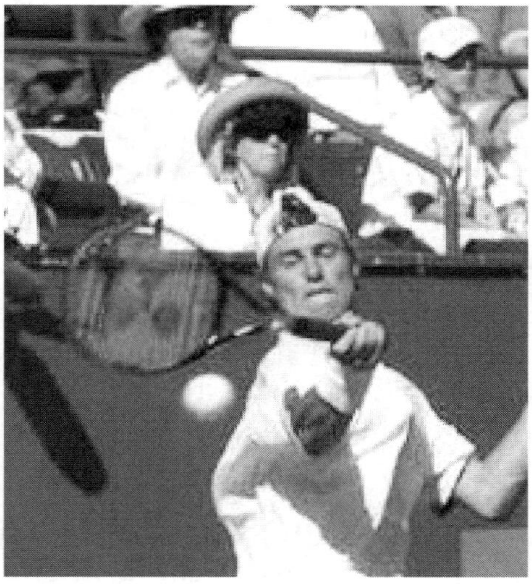

Figure 23
Lleyton Hewitt uses a full Western grip in executing his forehand. Notice that contact is more out in front of the player requiring him to open up his upper body further than players who use Eastern or semi-western grips.

The One-Quarter Turn Principle

Consider a proverbial lion tamer cracking a whip. To generate the rapid movement of the whip, the lion tamer actually slows his body down and lets the arm, forearm and, finally the wrist, accelerate the whip. This action is precisely what skilled tennis players do to generate high racket head speeds. The body, after the initial gross-motor movement, stops as the arm and racket speed up. Those players who swing the racket with the body find tremendous difficulty in developing racket head speed. Imagine strapping a racket to your waist and trying to rotate your body so the racket swings at the ball. As you can probably envision without even trying this, the swing would not be very fast! Look at this sequence of pictures below showing a forehand stroke.

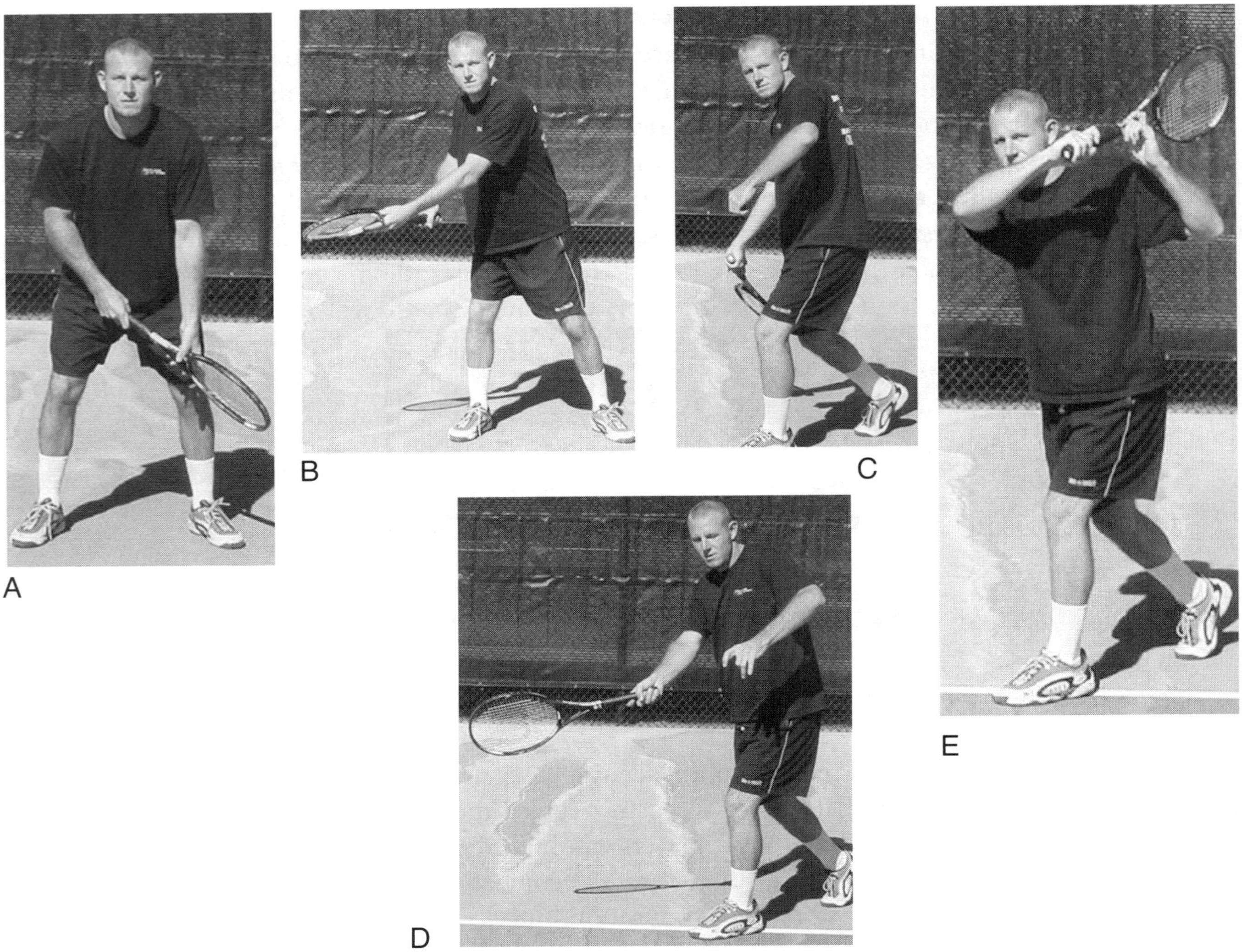

Note the one-quarter turn from ready position, (A) to backswing, (C). From the full backswing position, note the one-quarter turn back of the upper body at contact (D). Note that there is little or no movement of the upper body from contact (D) to follow-through (E)

Notice that the racket makes almost a full 360-degree arc around the body. However, the player only rotates one-quarter turn sideways on the back swing and a return of this one-quarter turn after the follow-through.

There are exceptions to this one-quarter turn principle. Many pros will over-rotate past this return point as a relaxation phase of a powerful swing. But even within these powerful swing patterns, you will find essentially the same basic foundation from backswing to contact point that is modeled here in this sequence. Perhaps more importantly, for players trying to learn and improve their strokes, over-rotating will generally produce questionable form and poor results instead of the imagined power they think will occur.

Linear Movements

Linear power involves a player moving in line with the target or other related direction. For example, a player who only steps into a shot without rotation of the body is moving linear in one direction towards the target. Or, another example is on the serve. If a player jumps upward during the service motion, this component of the serve would be considered linear as well. (Straight up.) Another example of linear swing patterns is the volley and the slice groundstroke, specifically the backhand slice. (Figure 24)

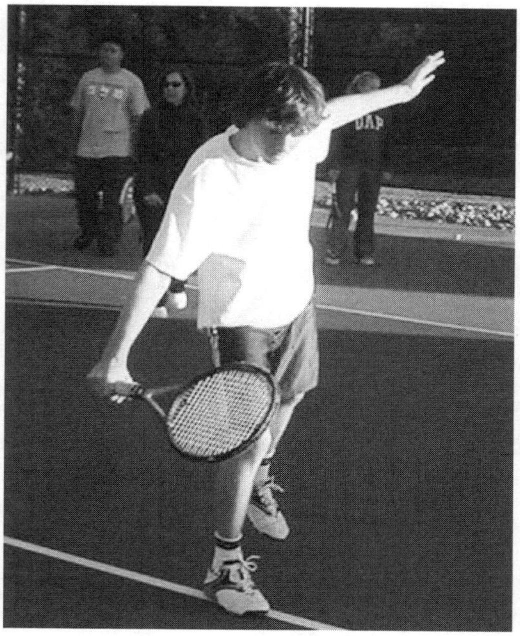

Figure 24
Notice the follow–through of a slice backhand is virtually in line with the target. This stroke pattern is "Linear" in terms of the stroke's direction

As you can probably distinguish, linear movements don't contribute a significant percentage of power to any shot. Imagine again strapping on a racket to your waist and only stepping into a ball to hit it, without using rotational movements as described above. Even if the racket were firmly attached to your body, the racket would only apply a small amount of force to the ball. (For most people the acceleration of the racket would be somewhere between 2 and 8 miles-per-hour!) So, if there is so little racket speed or acceleration associated with linear movement, is there a place for this type of movement in tennis? Yes.

When linear movements are applied correctly with angular motion, the results are significant. Stepping into the ball or moving forward into a shot can magnify the power -output of the angular swing pattern when used with the proper arm motions. In addition, the added linear movement can improve a player's position during a shot.

However, there are shots in tennis that utilize linear movements almost exclusively. They include mainly the volley and slice groundstroke. Angular or rotational movements on volleys and slice groundstrokes generally add not only complexity to the shots, but they provide unnecessary power that is not needed for both shots. (The one exception to this rule is on swinging topspin volleys. I will discuss this shot and how it differs from the more conventional blocking or short-stroke volley in Chapter 8 on volleys.) Because we are usually not looking for substantial power on volleys or slice groundstrokes, the power production of angular momentum is not justified. For example, perhaps 80 percent of the power required and generated on the volley comes from the moving ball itself! If a player at the net simply holds his racket firm and applies a slight linear movement either with the body or arm or both, there will be ample power for the volley to be effective.

Now that you understand the relationships between some of the physical and biomechanical laws of motion and movement, it is time to move on to the actual production of tennis strokes.

CHAPTER 8

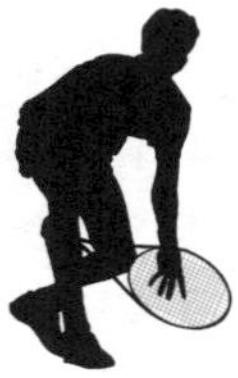

The Advanced Foundation– The Volley

Generally, there are two ways the volley has been taught throughout the history of tennis instruction. Most texts advocate the Eastern forehand and backhand grips for the novice player. The Eastern grips, the same used for hitting "conventional" topspin groundstrokes, are arguably easier for beginning players to "volley" a simple shot over the net. However, in assessing the need for player development most books recommend that players who want to progress past this basic volley capacity will need to make the change to the more "advanced" volley grip, the Continental.

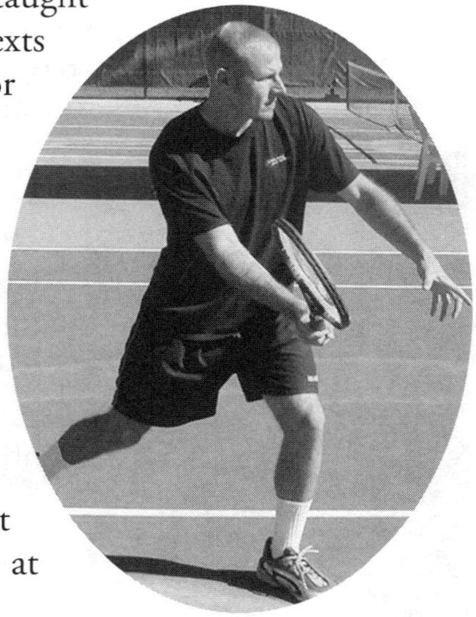

Figure 1
The Volley:
Progressive Player Foundation

As I have alluded in earlier parts of this book, such a transitional learning process is not only detrimental to the student, it is usually excruciatingly frustrating for most players. Those who discover that they do, indeed, need to make a significant change in their volley at some point will meet considerable physical and even emotional resistance!

I have found in my 29 years of tennis teaching experience that it is not necessary whatsoever to learn one method first only to have to switch at some time in a player's development. If a player applies the tools and methods described in this chapter, it will take most players no more time to learn the "advanced" Continental volley than it would to learn how to hit with the more elementary Eastern gripped volley. Save yourself a future of heartache and headache! Develop your volley with the Continental grip and never look back!

The Volley

It is no accident that I present the volley as the first chapter on hitting strategies. I start almost every on-court lesson with volleys. I also start all beginners with the volley. Starting with volleys has advantages for every level of player, some of which I mentioned in Chapter 6 on warm-up practices. However, if you are a beginner, or you teach or coach beginners, here are a couple of other reasons why it better to introduce players to the volley before moving on to ground strokes, serves, and strategy.

1. Players who learn groundstrokes first tend to have difficulty limiting their swing (both backswing and follow-through) when it comes time to learn the volley.
2. Because topspin is traditionally taught on groundstrokes, players who learn topspin first tend to hit with a similar topspin motion on volleys (instead of the slicing or blocking motion that I will be discussing later).
3. Typically, beginners find that blocking a ball out of the air is easier to judge than the bounce, speed, and spin of a groundstroke with a swinging racket.
4. It is easier to teach the Continental Grip if it is the first grip you are teaching. It is very difficult to teach any player the Continental Grip if they have first become comfortable with the Eastern forehand or other grips.

Footwork for the Volley

In the previous chapter I covered in detail the footwork associated with getting to a ball, hitting the ball, and recovering from each shot. The footwork for the volley can be executed correctly utilizing the same patterns discussed in Chapter 7. However, there are a few footwork concepts that must be clearly addressed in this chapter on the volley.

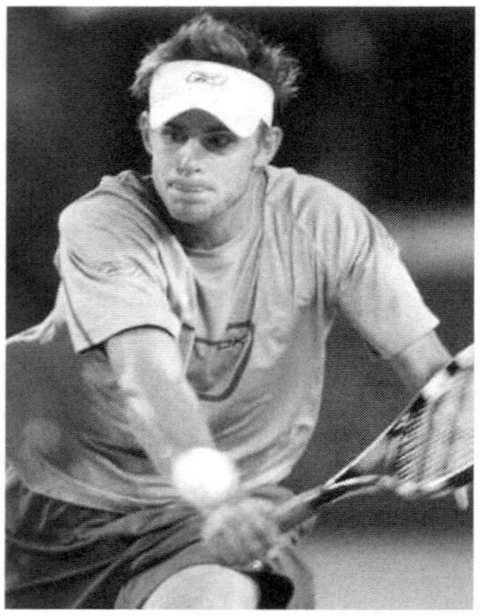

Figures 2 & 3
The backhand volley (above) and the forehand volley (below) are similar to each other on many levels

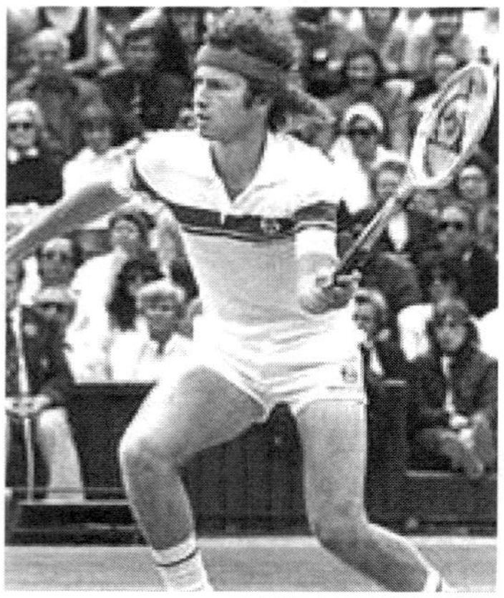

Perhaps more than any other shot in tennis, the volley is as close to a true "linear movement" stroke. That is, for consistent quality and success of each volley the player will want to reduce or eliminate the angular or rotational movements of the body during the shot. For many, the most common fault in this area is due to improper footwork during the volley.

The study of the footwork section in Chapter 7 and the application of the added concepts found throughout this chapter on the volley will provide every player with the footwork patterns necessary for executing superior volleys.

Forehand and Backhand Volleys

The volley is mechanically simple. A volley, when hit correctly, has a very short back swing and an abbreviated follow-through. The body is kept relatively still at the point of impact. With but a few exceptions, the forehand and backhand volleys are "mirrored" images of each other. (See Figures 2 and 3) That is, they should look essentially the same in terms of racket position at contact, racket orientation through the stroke, and other similarities. Because of these commonalities, I will be teaching both the forehand and backhand volleys simultaneously with defining differences expressed as needed. Let me break down the basic volley foundation in these sequential steps:

STEP 1. GRIP

Use the Continental grip for both the forehand and the backhand volley. (Figures 2 ,3 & 4) This grip is the choice of most pros on tour, most top college players, and most proficient club players... and it should be yours as well! There are several reasons why the continental grip is best suited for all players to learn from the start:

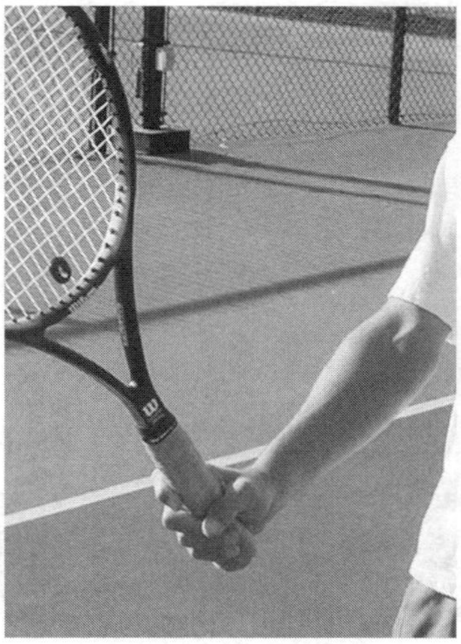

Figure 4
Continental grip in hitting forehand and backhand volleys.

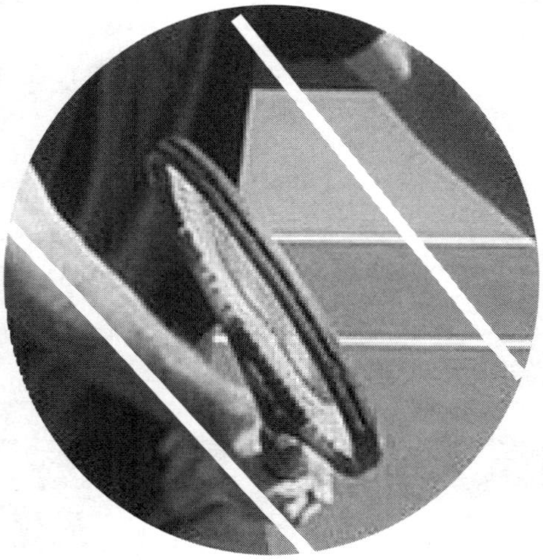

Figure 5
The continental grip on the forehand. Note that the racket lies almost parallel with the forearm.

• The Continental grip (Figure 4 & 5) is the perfect grip as it allows for the same action on both the forehand and backhand volleys. It is far better suited for low volleys than any other grip. The Continental grip might initially feel weak for most beginners because it does not put as much of the hand behind the racket during the shot (as the Eastern forehand and backhand grips do). However, since most volleys are hit with a slight cut or slicing action, the neutral racket face of the Continental is ideal for volleying the ball on both sides. For advanced players, when playing higher-level opponents, low volleys are common due to the advanced abilities of their opponents. This helps explain why virtually every pro, and top players in general, use the continental grip for most of their net play.

• As the name implies, the Continental grip is used for both the backhand and forehand volleys. Therefore, a great advantage to using this grip is the fact that players will not need a grip change between the two volleys. As players develop and play more challenging and competitive players, the advantage of not needing to make major grip adjustments during rallies is obvious. Quick exchanges at the net and rapid-fire passing shots require almost instantaneous reactions. The accuracy of obtaining a proper grip by having to make a grip change during such instances is certainly hindered. This is another reason we see almost all top players, especially those who play regularly at the net, utilizing the Continental grip.

• Players who try to utilize the Eastern grips for the volley usually need to overcome the distinct urge to hit their volley like a groundstroke. Typically, when using the same grips for groundstrokes as volleys, players tend to hit their volley with both a swing (like a groundstroke) as well as topspin. Topspin volleys are sometimes hit by pros and top players but only in certain circumstances. It is not advisable for beginners and intermediates to attempt the topspin volley until the fundamental volley with a continental grip is mastered. Even players who have worked hard to not hit topspin on their volley with these grips tend to revert back to this undesired swing pattern when the ball is hit at them with speed. Players almost always will repeat what is most ingrained in their swing pattern when they have little or no time to think or react.

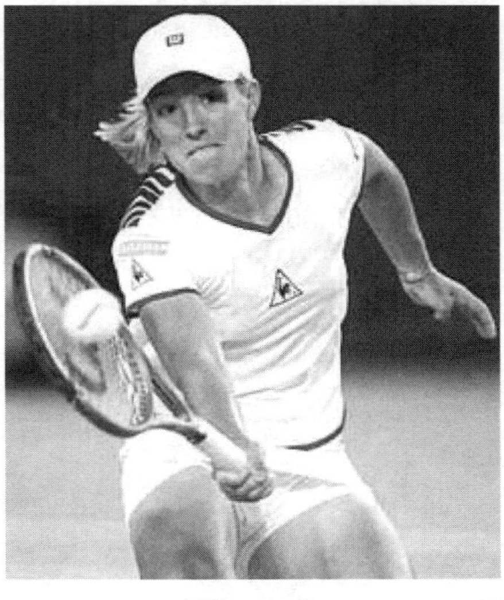

Figure 6
Here, Justine Henin-Hardenne demonstrates the parallel racket face to the forearm on the forehand volley at contact.

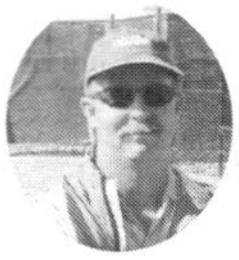

Author's Note

Most proficient players make subtle grip changes based on the Continental foundation. These changes are in response to recognized specific shots such as higher drives or balls that are slow moving. However, almost all top players utilize the Continental grip as described in this chapter.

• As most books recognize, the Continental grip is clearly the choice of advanced players. As we have stated many times in this book, it is incredibly difficult for players to make necessary changes in their strokes or grips as their play or skill develops. Thus, by learning the Eastern grips for the volley, players are sabotaging their ability to become advanced players.

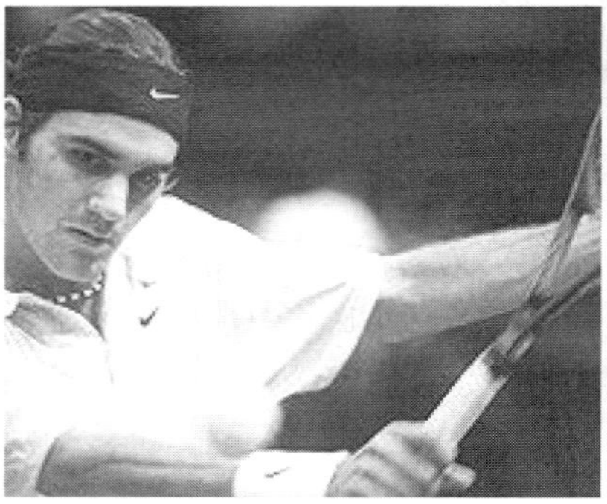

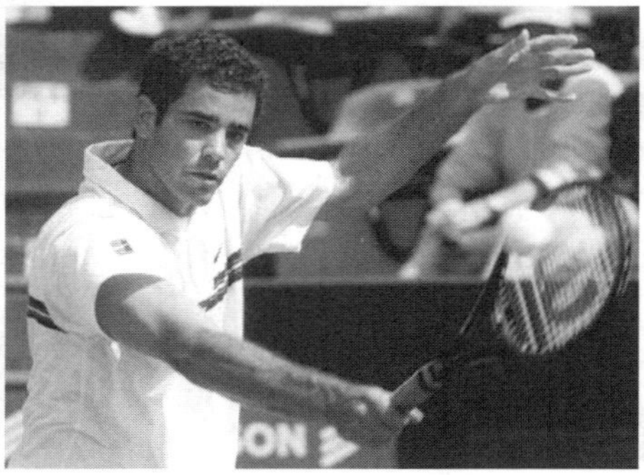

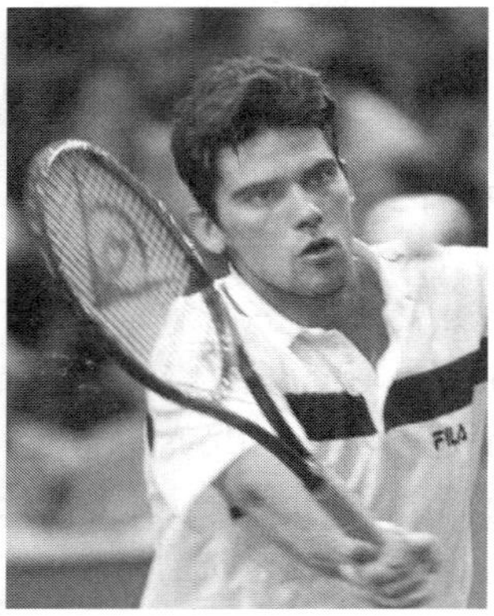

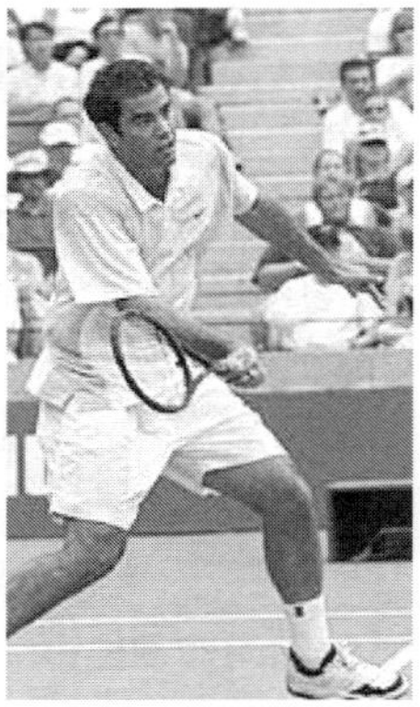

Comparison

Comparison - Note the similarities between the two backhand volley photos on the left and the two forehand volley pictures on the right. Notice that the grips, the arm positions, the off-arm's position, the racket face, the body position and the general positions of the feet are all similar in these examples. Skilled players almost without exception use universally accepted techniques to accomplish the volley.

How to "find" the Continental Grip

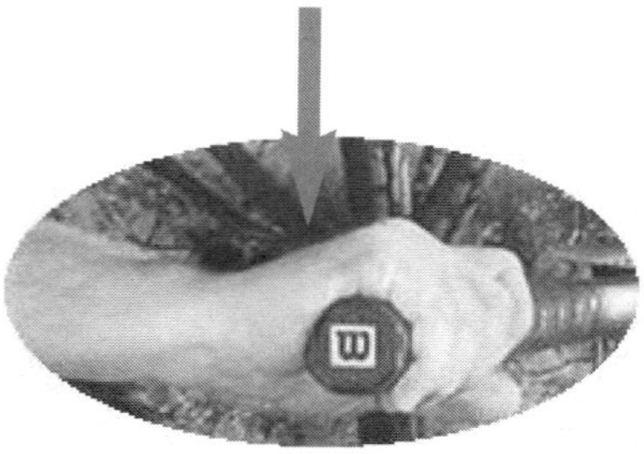

Figure 7
Look for that flat, back part of your hand.

For years I had been very disappointed in the way players were taught how to find the various tennis grips. The traditional way has always been to locate the base knuckle of the index finger and place it upon certain bevels on the grip. This has always been difficult for players for several reasons. First, the knuckles of players are often of different size and shape. Second, deciding just what part of the hand below the knuckle must be placed on the bevels of the racket's grip is quite ambiguous. Third, it is often difficult to identify exactly where the knuckle of the hand needs to be on the desired bevel of the grip. Thus, I designed a very easy and more accurate method of obtaining the basic grips and checking them quickly.

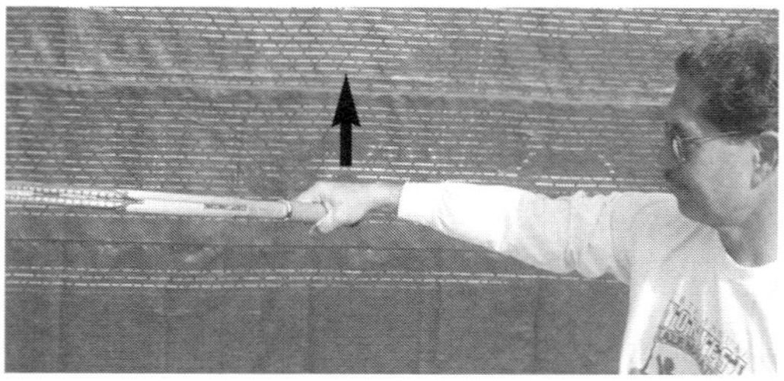

Figure 8
Eastern Forehand Grip. Note the flat part of the hand is facing the sky.

A. Hold the racket at shoulder height with a straight arm held out in front of the chest. The elbow should be straight. (Figure 8)

B. Hold the racket in the hand so the racket face is flat and parallel with the ground.

C. Hold the racket so that it is perpendicular to the arm.

D. While maintaining the racket face parallel with the ground, look at the back, flat part of your hand holding the racket. (See Fig7.)

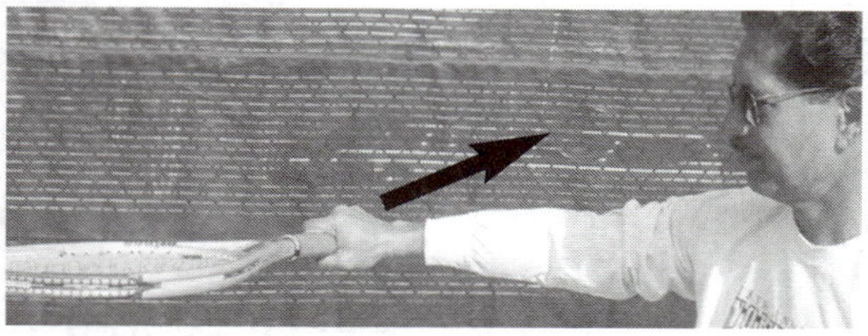

Figure 9
Continental Grip. Flat Part of hand is tilted towards the top of the player's head

• If the back of your hand is facing flat towards the sky, you are holding an Eastern Forehand grip. (See Figure 8)

• If the back of your hand is tilted back towards you, facing a point near the top of your head, you have a Continental Grip. (See Figure 7 & 9)

• If the back of your hand is tilted back even more, to the point that the flat part of your hand is facing your nose, you have an Eastern Backhand Grip. (See Figure 10)

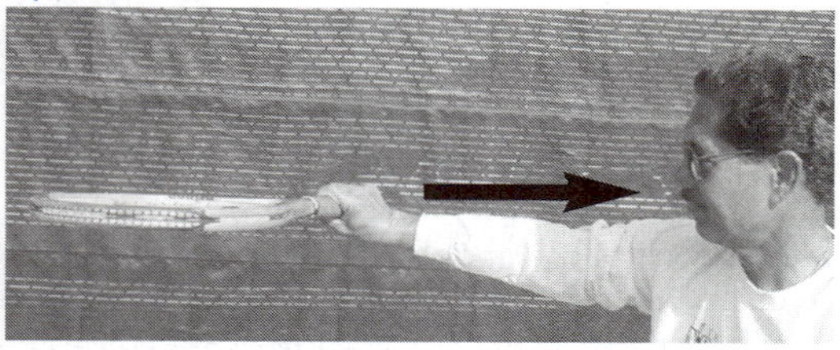

Figure 10
Eastern Backhand Grip. Note the flat part of hand tilts towards the player's nose.

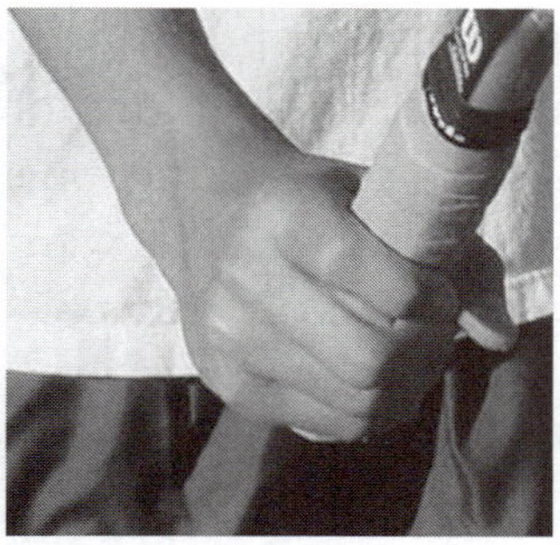

Continental Grip

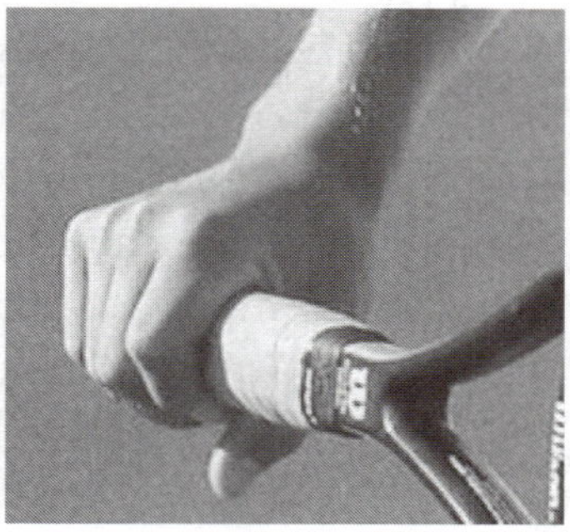

Eastern Backhand

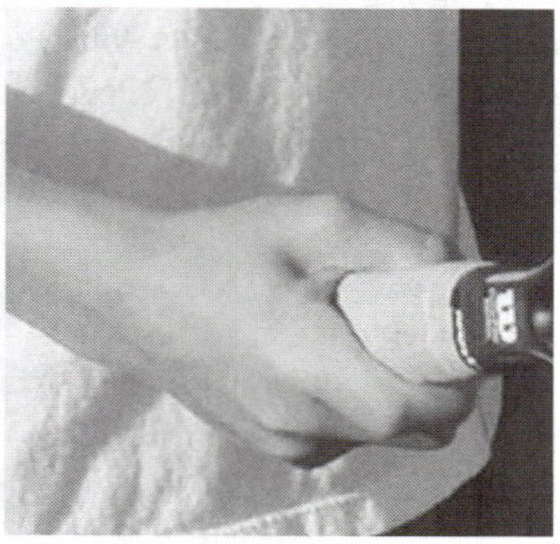

Eastern Forehand

HERE ARE THE THREE GRIPS FROM A DIFFERENT VIEW

Author's Note

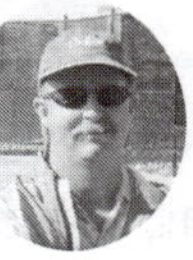

Years ago (and even today, among some teaching pros) the Eastern Forehand (Figure 11 & 12) and Backhand grips were the grips taught for the forehand and backhand volley. While it is true these two grips offer greater strength on the volley (due to the majority of the hand is behind the racket; see figure 11 & 12), the ability for players to advance their volleying abilities with these two grips is greatly handicapped. Because a beginner has the ability to hit "successful" volleys early in their lessons with the Eastern grips, pros sometimes favor the "instant gratification" that players get when using the grip. However, in choosing the Eastern grips for the volley, the player will become most frustrated when they discover the problems associated with their volley and want to change! In addition, the use of the Eastern grips creates a different stroke pattern than the stroke pattern used with the Continental grip. This additional problem compounds the difficulty in making the necessary change.

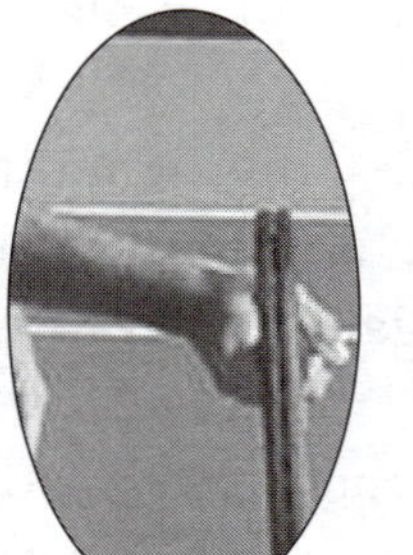

Figure 11
The Eastern forehand volley grip as seen from the side at the contact. This grip places more hand behind the racket. However, the racket must be held at a 90-degree angle in relation to the forearm. Compare this position with Figure 3.

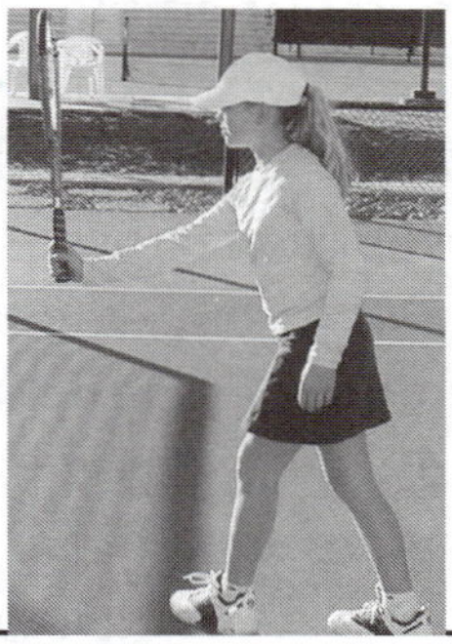

Figure 12
A very common problem when players use the Eastern Forehand grip: they tend to face the net and the on-coming ball like holding a stop sign. The only direction the racket can go from here is down!

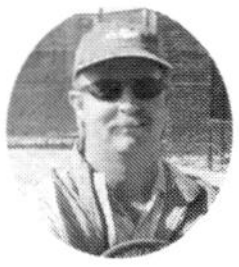

Author's Note -
Additional Notes on the Volley Grip

The basic Eastern Forehand and Backhand grips are generally recognized as "Topspin Grips". Due to the anatomical design of our hand and wrist, these grips tend to tilt the racket face forward as the arm moves towards the ball. As a result players in a quick exchange at the net, or when a ball is hit fairly hard to them, tend to close the racket face and end up hitting the ball downward and into the net. A player using either Eastern grip will have to consciously lay the wrist back to employ a flat or slice volley. With low volleys a player using Eastern Grips will have to twist the wrist at a difficult angle to get enough of the racket face tilted open to get the ball over the net.

Typically, one of the biggest problems in using the Eastern forehand grip for the forehand volley is the tendency to hold the racket up like a stop sign. (See Figure 12) This very rudimentary volley technique creates a situation that only allows the player to hit down on the ball. With the arm fully extended before contact, the player can only use the wrist to slap at the ball.

Another reason some pros teach the Eastern Grips is the belief that players won't have the strength to volley correctly with the Continental Grip. Yet, volleying the ball, when done with minimal back swing and follow-through requires only a small amount of strength. To emphasize this point, in demonstrations I often will employ only my thumb and index finger in holding the Continental grip to volley. With minimal effort (and proper form) you can volley the ball with a crisp, firm shot to the baseline utilizing only two fingers!

I have taught the Continental Grip to kids as young as 5 years old with 100% success! For those of you who teach tennis and think kids this young can't handle the Continental Grip, you are greatly mistaken! When you walk them through the progression of the stroke (as I will describe in this chapter), and employ the basic drills I will be prescribing, you will find that virtually every kid and adult can and will be hitting excellent volleys in no time at all! In fact, I have found in comparing notes with other pros who teach the Eastern grips to beginners, the actual learning time for players to hit with accuracy and consistency with the continental was essentially the same as those who learn with the Eastern grips. This discovery rules out the premise that the Eastern grips are faster for players to learn the volley. And, perhaps most importantly, by learning the Continental grip from the start, players will forego the need for change later as they progress!

In finding the continental grip, it is important that the racket is held parallel with the ground at shoulder height. When the arm is held straight (with the elbow straight) and the shaft of the racket is held at a 90-degree angle to the arm, the three grips described above will be quite accurate. This method is especially easy for young children to learn how to hold and check their grips. Other methods discussed in books and by teaching pros will contribute to your learning the grips. My method provides players who still have difficulty finding their grips with a different approach that might make more sense to them.

Tools for Mastering the Continental Grip

Because the Continental grip is usually not a natural grip in terms of comfort for most players when they are starting out, there are methods which players will want to employ to gain both comfort and control of the racket when using this grip. Players who first learned to volley using the Eastern forehand and Eastern backhand grips will need to "relearn" the grip (and the stroke) using the Continental. As I have stated, making a change in a stroke, especially a grip change, will be uncomfortable and frustrating. If you take these tools to heart and employ them as often as possible, you will make the change not only possible, but you will be successfully hitting progressively better volleys faster.

The practical part of these drills is that they are not only simple, but they don't require a court or a partner to execute them. Even though these tools are uncomplicated, the drills are critical learning processes essential to mastering advanced level volleys…so much so, that I employ them equally with my top nationally ranked players as well as beginners!

For beginners and especially those players trying to change to the Continental from the Eastern Grips, practice these drills several times each day for several minutes. About 10 minutes a day practicing these two drills will help most players gain a level of comfort and mastery of the Continental grip in a week or less.

It is critical to make sure you are using the Continental grip in each of these drills. Falling back to your Eastern grip will only hinder you from mastering the Continental grip and prevent you from hitting better volleys.

Tool #1 Down Bounces Continental

Down bounces incorporate the continental grip in a simulated forehand volley motion. The player will want to kneel down on one knee (right knee for right-handed players) and hold the racket so the hitting surface of the strings is facing flat towards the ground. Using the Continental grip, the arm is held out away from the body with the racket head bouncing the ball flat with a firm wrist. (See Figure 13) The initial goal for beginners is to hit 75 to 100 consecutive bounces. Young children will probably struggle a bit at first with this drill. However, if they practice it several times a day, they generally will be able to do at least 50 in a row within a few days. Practice holding the hitting arm firm and don't let the wrist "flop" the racket face like a teeter-totter. The entire arm moves in a subtle up and down motion; movement is generated at the shoulder instead of the elbow or wrist. Work to hit 150 consecutive bounces.

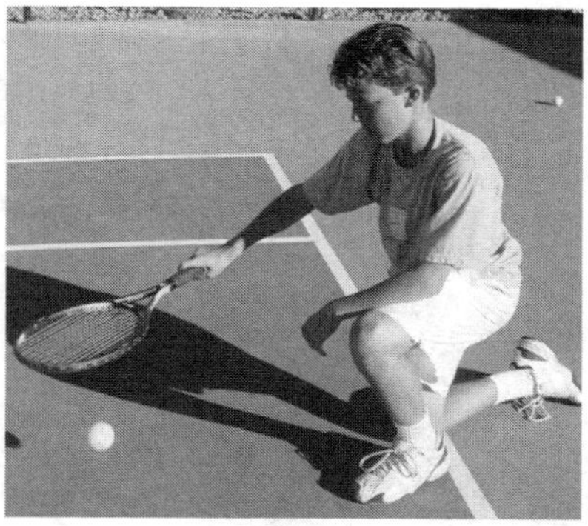

Figure 13
Down Bounces Tool
Keep your back straight and body relaxed. Maintain the Continental grip throughout.

NOTE: Even though we don't actually hit most volleys with a flat racket face as executed in this drill, the object is to allow the player to become comfortable with the Continental grip.

Value: This drill obviously strengthens a player's wrist and forearm while it develops an affinity for the Continental grip. This drill is also an excellent warm-up drill that uses a low impact stroke pattern to warm up the small muscles and tendons of the hand, wrist and forearm. It builds a player's hand-eye coordination and concentration while working the Continental grip in a repetitive movement. This short, overall movement simulates the forehand volley motion.

Secondary Drill: Tilt the racket face slightly so the racket brushes down the right side of the ball as you are bouncing it. This will cause the ball to have a slight spin and simulates the slicing motion of the volley. This is a bit harder to control because the ball spins off the ground. Yet, with practice you will be able to control the bounce without the ball getting away from you.

Tool #2 Up-Bounces Continental

This second tool is just like the first except the player bounces the ball up instead of down on the opposite side of the racket. Using the Continental grip the player stands and holds the hitting arm straight out in front, holding the elbow straight and rigid. The racket is held palm down at a ninety-degree angle to the arm with the racket face held parallel to the ground. (See Figure 14) With a very subtle movement of the arm, bounce the ball about 8 to 10 inches off the strings while maintaining the firmness of the wrist and keeping the elbow straight. Avoid bending the elbow at any time. Move your feet if the ball's position dictates a movement of the racket—as opposed to adjusting the racket's position by bending the elbow. Try to hit 50 to 100 consecutive bounces.

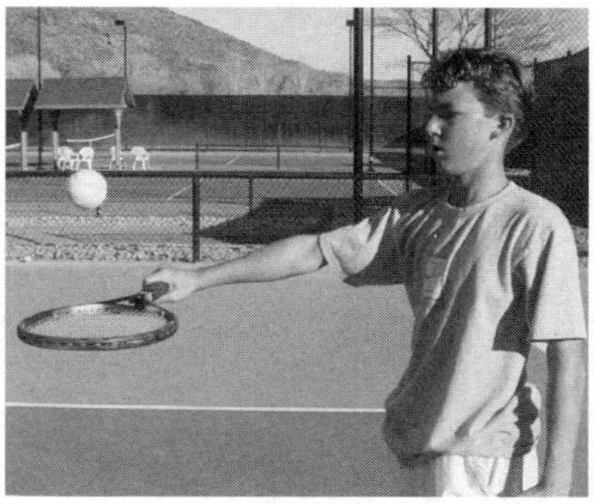

Figure 14
Here the Up-Bouncing drill with the continental mimics the arm position of the proper backhand volley. Note the similar arm and racket position to that of the backhand volley in Figure 17.

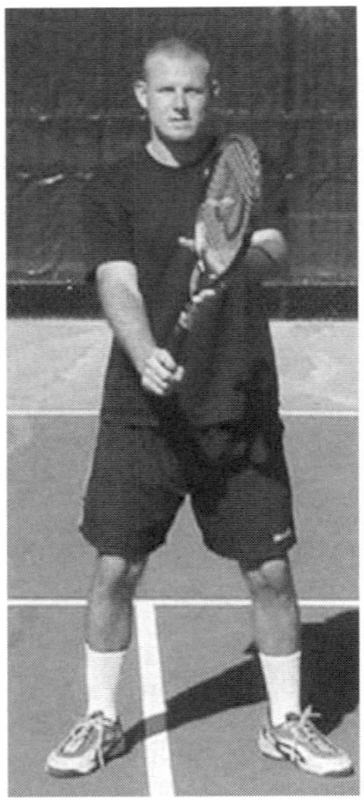

Figure 15
A comfortable, relaxed position at the net will allow for greater mobility and reaction speed to a volley.

Value: Like the down-bouncing tool, this is a good warm-up for the fingers, hand, and arm, helping prevent tennis elbow concurrent with wrist and finger injuries. Perhaps more importantly, this exercise is perfect for simulating the general backhand volley technique using the Continental grip. In addition, because the straight, firm elbow is critical for an efficient and consistent volley, this drill, when done correctly, focuses attention on this significant component.

STEP 2. READY POSITION

The ready position for the volley places the player's racket in the center of the body with the head of the racket held up. (Figure 15.) This position allows for easy access to either the forehand or backhand volley. By keeping the racket head up, you minimize the chance of the racket head dropping prior to or during the volley. Players who drop the racket head at the ready position will tend to be late in getting the racket up to the volley contact point. Cradle the racket at the throat with the off-hand. This will help the player turn the upper body as a unit on the backhand instead of taking the racket back with the arm.

The elbow of the dominant arm should be held close to the body, not sticking out like a chicken wing!

STEP 3. TURN

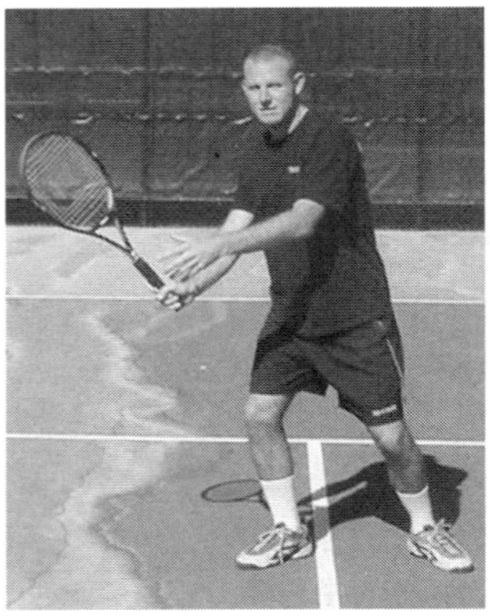

Figure 16
Note the similar shoulder turn for both the forehand and backhand volleys.

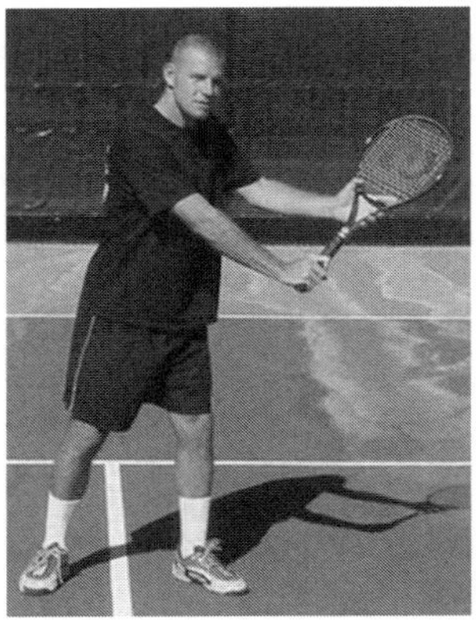

Figure 17
Use of the hand helps prevent the racket from being taken too far back

From a ready position: when you recognize that the ball coming to you is a forehand or backhand, first turn your shoulders sideways to the net. For right-handers turn your shoulders to the right for a forehand, (Figure 16), and to your left for a backhand, (Figure 17). Note that your left shoulder should be pointing to the net on forehand volleys and your right shoulder points to the net on backhands. (When learning proper volleys, this concept of pointing the shoulders to the targets is very helpful. However, on forehand volleys, because of the position of the shoulders, it is not as critical to turn the shoulders this far. Advanced players usually turn about 45 degrees on most forehand volleys.)

Don't take the racket back with your arm! By doing so, the racket will be taken back too far.

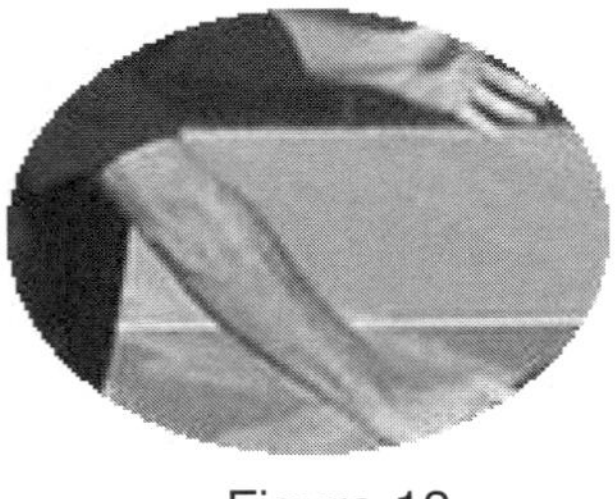

Figure 18
Keeping the dominant arm straight creates greater leverage and greater control for the backhand volley.

- *Notice that when you turn your shoulders, if you are hold ing your racket in the ready position, the face (or plane) of the racket naturally opens squarely to meet the ball. (Figures 16 & 17) Taking your arm back beyond this position will cause you to over-swing as well as impede your ability to make consistent contact with the correct racket angle. Use the off-hand in helping make the turn of your shoulders during the forehand and backhand volley. (See Figures 16 & 17)*

- *Keep the racket face open slightly. That is, tilt the racket so the hitting surface of the racket is pointed slightly up, over the net. (Don't over-open the face! This will cause you to float or pop up your volley.)*
- *On the backhand volley keep the dominant arm straight through the course of the volley. (Figures 17, 18 & 20) Avoid the natural tendency to bend the elbow of the dominant arm on the backhand volley.*

Explanation: By keeping the arm straight on the backhand volley the arm acts as a lever; the longer the lever, the stronger the force that can be applied by that lever. Also, by bending the elbow the player now has an extra joint to control in the course of the volley: the shoulder, the wrist and now the elbow. If a player conscientiously keeps the arm straight and firm, it won't take long for this move to become natural. This is one of the most important points for beginners and intermediates to keep in mind in developing an advanced backhand volley.

- *With forehands the elbow does not need to be kept straight. This is because the elbow can only bend in, not out, from a straight position. Thus, the bending of the elbow usually only adversely affects the backhand. In fact, with the forehand the elbow should be bent in slightly, bringing the racket closer to the body. If, indeed, the elbow were to remain straight during a forehand, the racket would be a considerable distance from the body making for difficult contact with the ball.*

- *Use the off-hand and arm to coordinate the shoulder turn, (see Figure 19). Many players tend to let this off-arm dangle at their side.*

STEP 4. CONTACT

As the ball approaches, attempt to meet the ball just slightly in front of your hip or front knee with the racket moving in a

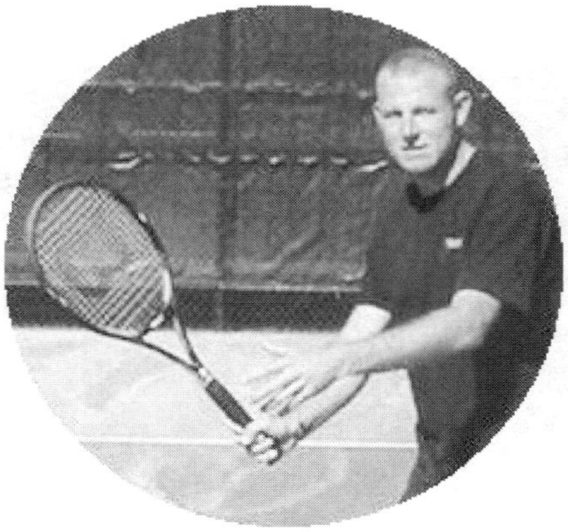

Figure 19
On the forehand turn, the left arm follows the right arm helping the shoulders make the turn. Some players leave out the non-dominant arm and end up only taking their racket back instead of simply turning the shoulders.

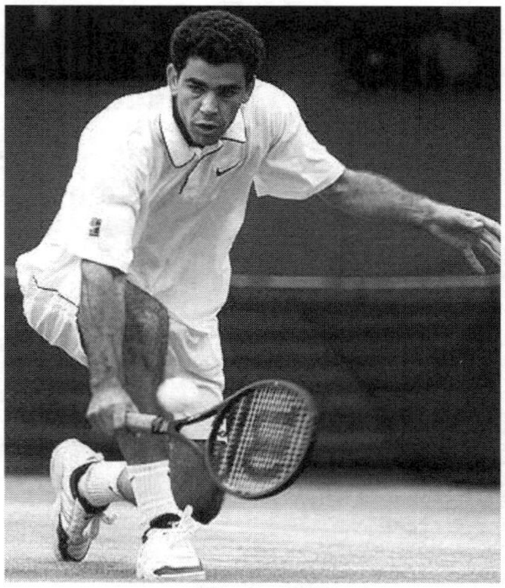

Figure 20
Note the straight lever-like dominant arm position on this backhand volley by Pete Sampras.

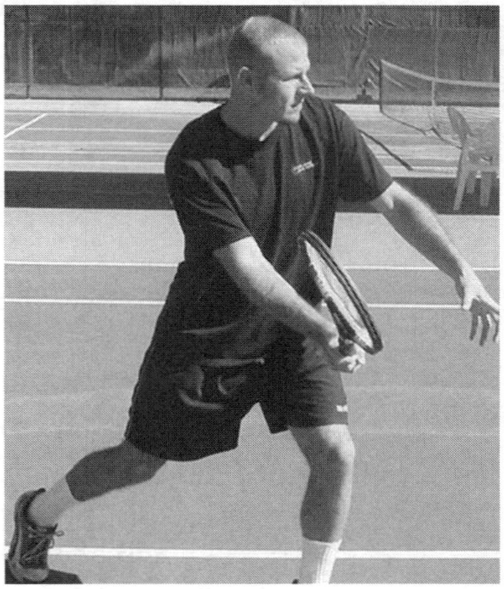

Figure 21
The contact point is just in front of your front Knee.

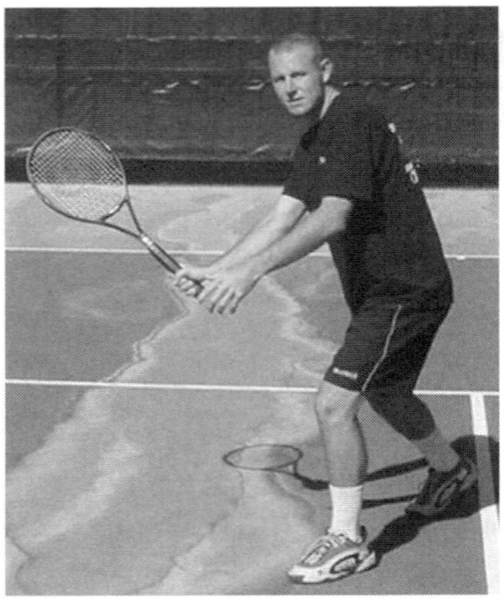

Figure 22
At contact, the racket head is held high, just as in the ready position. The shoulders remain sideways as well as the hips. This prevents the body from turning out of the volley and pulling the ball to the player's left.

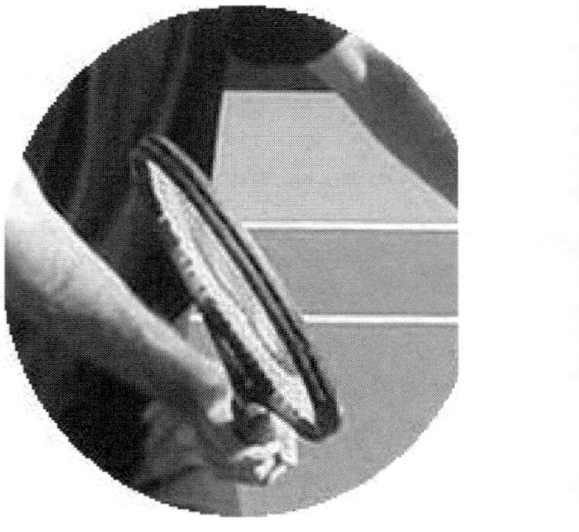

Figure 23
This is the open face of the forehand volley at contact.

downward and forward motion. (See Figures 21 - 25) I call this a "driving cut" since the racket moves down and through the ball in a very short stroke through the line of trajectory.

Explanation: The idea of moving the racket down through the ball with the racket face slightly open serves to accomplish several things:

a. The cutting action takes some pace off the ball (due to conversion of velocity to backspin), allowing the player to keep low shots—hit up and over the net—in the court. A flat racket face at the point of contact is very difficult to control. This concept is discussed further in a moment.

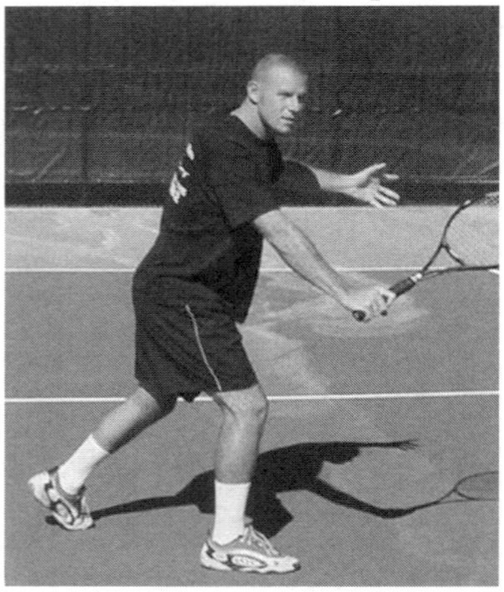

Figure 24
The proper contact point for the backhand volley

b. The act of cutting or slicing the ball helps the player prevent the racket from "flipping" over the ball. For many players it is hard to keep from using the wrist, and subsequently the racket moves at the ball in a "wristy" motion. We see this especially when a player is out of position making a desperation shot! The reality is, when a player is in trouble, the worst thing they can do is flick the racket at the ball using the wrist.

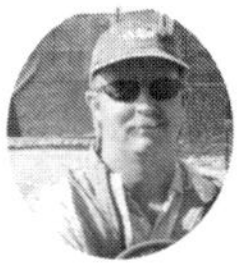

Author's Notes on
hitting a slice volley versus a flat volley

A ball hit with a perfectly flat racket-face will tend to rebound the racket at an angle towards the ground, dropping deceptiv lower off the racket face than players think. (See Diagram 1 n page.) To prove this point for yourself, hit a ball at a medium sp at a wall with the ball arching slightly downward as it hits the w (In most cases, this is usually what your opponent's shot will be do if you are going to volley. If your opponent's ball was on the rise wh you hit the volley, depending on the speed of the ball you are pro bly hitting an "out" ball!) Watch as the ball comes off the wall. rebound will angle down towards the ground quite quickly. A me um paced shot hit at a wall anywhere from 4 to 8 feet high will the ground off the rebound, landing anywhere from 3 to 10 feet fr the wall (depending how hard and how high you aim at the wa Now imagine standing at the net where you feel comfortable voll ing, (usually about 5 to 10 feet back). If you hit the ball with strings perfectly flat and with the racket blocking the ball usin minimal blocking stroke, the ball will land anywhere from the m dle of the net to the bottom of the net. (Remember the net is 3 f high at the center. If you are 10 feet behind it and hit the ball w this flat volley about waist-high, the ball will hit the ground appro mately two feet BEFORE the net!) Obviously, with increased vol speed we can get a ball to go higher and further. However, the ha er you hit the ball, the more likely the chance of an error in eit racket angle or contact point…both resulting in a lower percentage successful shots.

The spin of your opponent's shot will also affect the reflected an of the ball off your strings. An incoming shot with backspin w deflect downward off a flat racket face at a GREATER angle tha topspin ball. These principles often explain how a player standing erally right on top of the net will still find themselves hitting voll into the net!

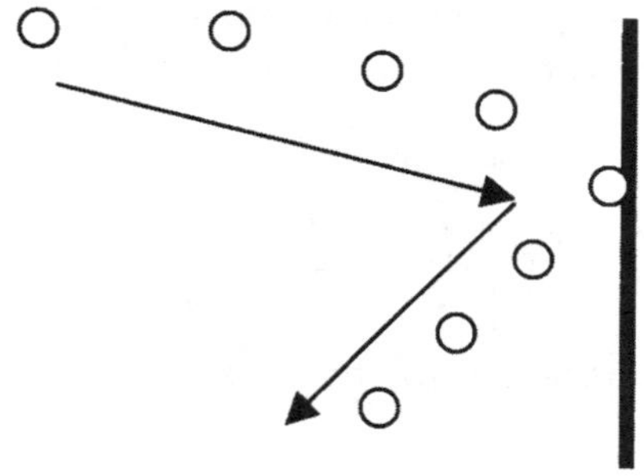

DIAGRAM 1
The angle of reflection of a ball off a flat surface is generally equal to the angle of incidence, (the angle the ball arrives towards contact). Gravity, as well as spin and speed of the ball, can increase the effect the angle of reflection has on the ball.

The chance of hitting the ball cleanly and in the desired direction is drastically reduced when this is attempted!

c. Ideally, cut down the BACK of the ball as you are driving forward and through it. Don't try to cut "under" the ball, as this will cause the ball to float up (unless you are attempting a "drop-volley" where slicing under the ball with finesse and touch will make the ball die on the other side of the net).

On low volleys it is doubly important to apply a slice to the ball. A hard hit ball, hit flat off your racket and angled up enough to clear the net, will usually land long due to the angle up that you had to hit the ball to clear the net and the speed of your flat ball. Players who don't have a slice on their volley tend to become "dinkers" at the net for this reason…they can't take the pace of the ball except by dinking the ball, usually with a floppy wrist and arm!

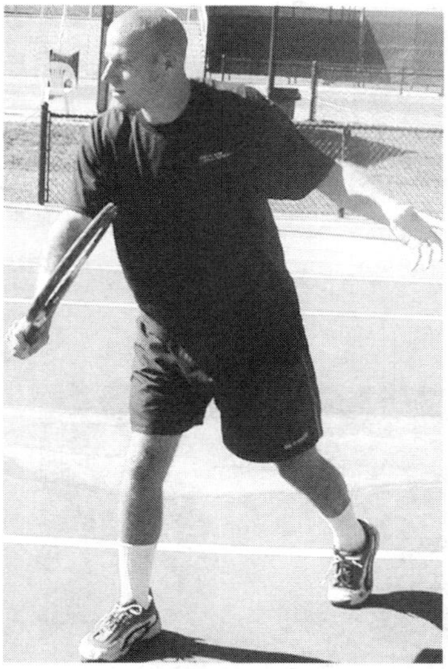

Figure 25
Similar to the forehand volley, the backhand volley is hit just in front of the front knee.

Another point made by some instructors is their claim that hitting a ball flat is easier to control and less complex than slicing the volley. I strongly disagree. A volley that is attempted to be hit with a perfectly flat racket face is dependent completely on the accuracy of that angle within two fields: a) is the racket angle correct in relation to the target? b) Does the player have control of the correct angle at contact? If the angle is off by even a minimal amount, the control of the shot will be far less accurate than using a slice volley technique. Certainly any volley method will be dependent on the accuracy of the player's racket head control. However, hitting a ball flat, even in the context of the problems discussed above, is certainly no more advantageous to a player than hitting with slice. The com-

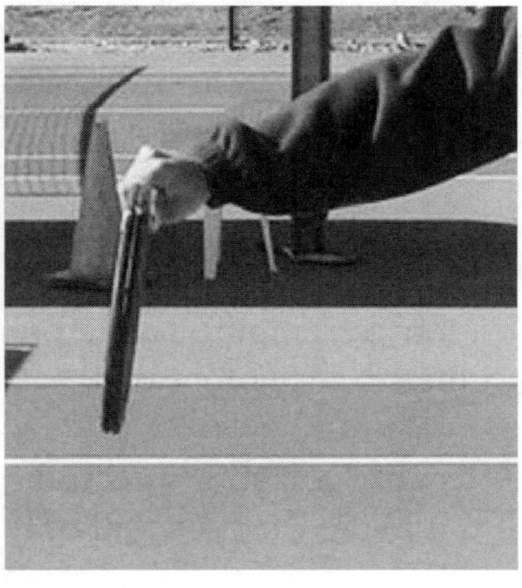

Figure 26
The Eastern backhand grip creates a flat racket face at contact. Notice the forearm at a 90 degree angle to the racket, similar to the Eastern forehand volley.

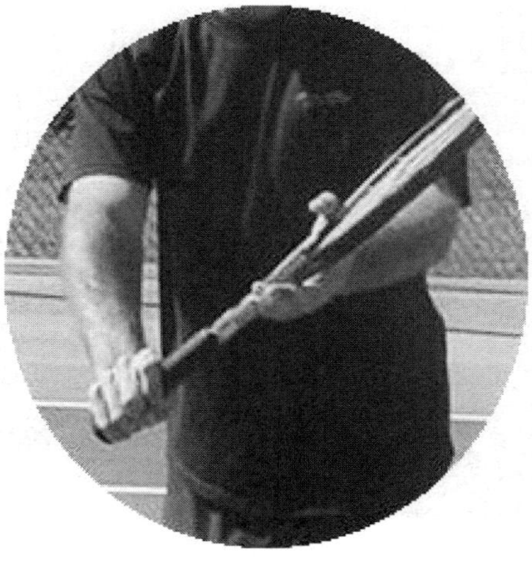

Figure 27
Here, the racket face on the turn for the backhand volley is set at the same angle it needs to be at contact.

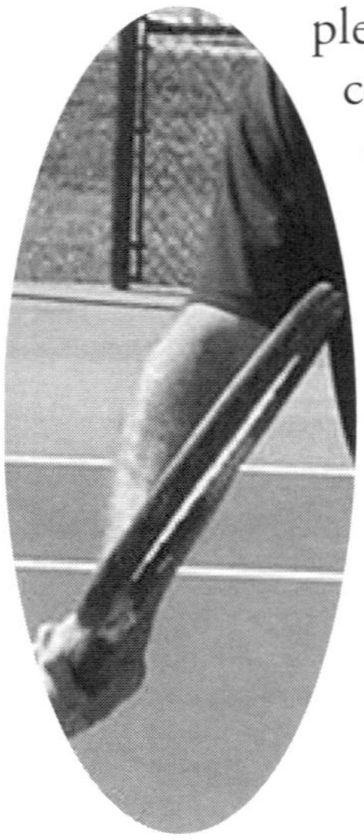

Figure 28

plexity of the slice volley, when executed within the methods described here, is no more complex than hitting the ball flat. In both cases, players will have to learn how to aim and control the racket.

KEEP THE PLANE THE SAME!

•*From start to finish the slightly open racket face stays in this position. (Figures 27 and 28.)*

•*The racket starts slightly above the path of the incoming ball and moves down, cutting the back of the ball in a blocking or punching motion. (I use both terms here as many people have different interpretations of both in how they apply to hitting a tennis ball.) I actually prefer the term "glide", as the short volley motion is smooth with minimal effort.*

•*After contact your racket should be slightly more in front of you from where you made contact, and the racket should still be the same position (in relation to the arm and wrist) as when you turned your shoulders initially. That is, the racket head should not drop during the course of the stroke, and, likewise, it should not rise up. The strings should still be facing the target.*

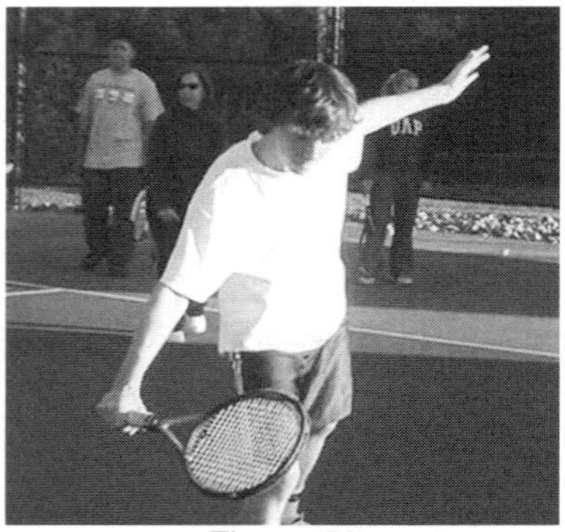

Figure 29
Note the arms spreading apart during the backhand slice or volley

Off-Arm Extension

A valuable learning tool in perfecting the backhand volley is the use of the non-dominant arm during contact. Skilled players will move this arm back dramatically during contact of a backhand volley or slice groundstroke. (Figure 29) This movement of the arm allows the player to maintain the desired sideways position during the course of the volley. You will see this exact same movement on slice approach shots on the backhand side as well.

Figure 30
The cross over step at contact

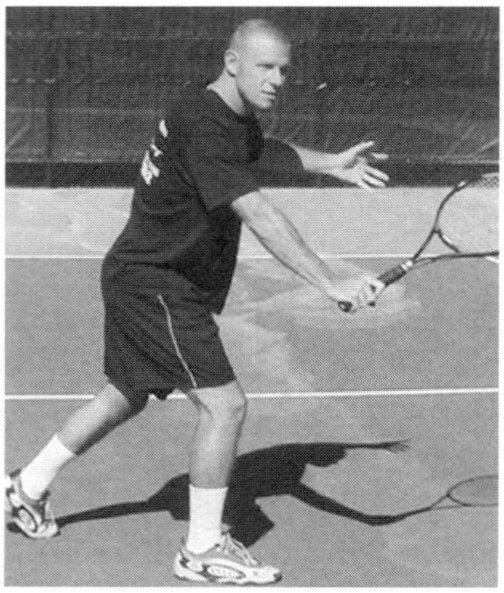

STEP 5. STEPPING INTO THE BALL

As you make contact, step with the right foot on backhands (Figure 30), the left foot on forehands (Figure 31). Step forward and slightly across your body. This will vary depending on whether the ball approaching you is coming into your body or well away from you where you will have to really reach as well as step. Often, you may have to step back with the opposite foot to create this proper sideways body position when a ball is hit right at you. Obviously, we don't want to step into a ball that is too close to us! By stepping back with the back foot, it creates the exact same body position as stepping across our bodies with the front foot. (I will cover more advanced footwork patterns later.)

• This step is timed differently for differently paced shots coming at you. In fact, in many cases, if the ball is moving fast, you will only

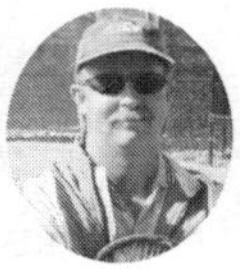

Author's Point

Many pros tell their students to hit the ball "well out in front of them." In theory and in practice this can be misleading. When players try to make contact too far out in front of their body, several problems occur:

1. The wrist must cock back considerably to get the racket face to tilt in proper position to hit the ball square to the target. This wrist-cock causes the player to "push" the racket forward away from the body instead of driving it with the arm across the body. (Compare Figures 25 and 26.)

2. With the racket way out in front, the player has literally nothing left with which to hit the ball. Notice in Figure 33 the arm is already forward. It can't move any more forward to apply force to the ball. This form results in the player "flicking" the wrist to make the forward movement. (Or they attempt to swing by rotating the shoulders or entire upper body...just as bad!)

3. With the racket so far in front of the body, the player can't see the hitting surface of his racket (except through the back of the strings!). (Figure 33) In fact, the frame of the racket usually hides a portion of the back of the strings as well. Even though the human eye can't pick up the actual contact of the ball with the strings (it is too fast for the eye to see), the eye does track the ball to the racket. When the object to which we are tracking the ball (the string surface) is out of view, it is very difficult, especially for beginners, to meet the moving ball cleanly and consistently. (See Figures 34, 35 & 36)

4. In the course of a volley the player usually has very little time to track the ball (compared to how much time we have to see and prepare for groundstrokes). By attempting to meet the ball far forward in front of the body, the player has even less time to track the ball especially within the last two feet or so, the area which is critical to hand-eye coordination.

5. Hitting the ball too far in front also limits the ability of the player to intentionally hit angle volleys. (Please see "Advanced Situation Volleys" later in this chapter.)

have time to turn your shoulders and block the ball. You won't have time to step into the shot. However, when time permits, by stepping in, your body's forward motion provides an added force to the ball resulting in more "punch" with no more added swing on your arm's part.

•Keep your back foot back. As with many other strokes, don't let the back leg "swing" around as you make contact. Likewise, don't pull your front foot away as you hit (as in leaning backwards). This improper move is very common among beginners and intermediate players.

Explanation: By swinging your back leg around as you are making contact (or, likewise, moving your front leg away), your hips will rotate towards the net usually prematurely. When the hips rotate, your body tends to over-rotate during the course of the volley. Usually, the shoulders will follow the hips, forcing your racket to "pull" the ball away from the target line. The result is that the player will automatically lay the wrist back to "push" the ball attempting to maintain the desired direction. Thus, by over-rotating the player changes the shot from a drive to an ineffective push.

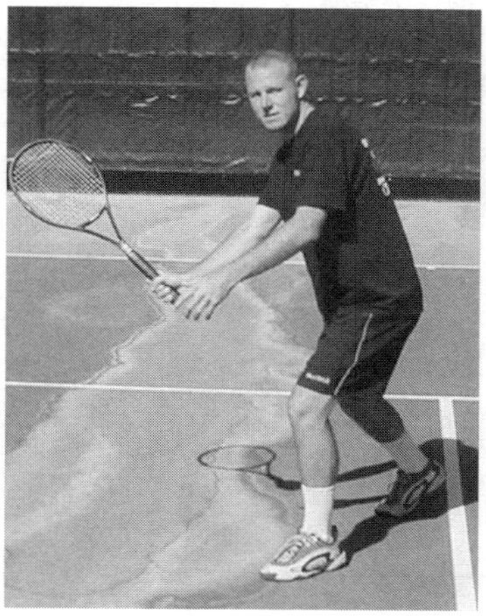

Figure 31
Notice the back leg stays back after contact The racket at the contact point is even with the front leg and the body sideway to the net.

• Ideally, you want to keep yourself as sideways as possible through the course of the volley. This will increase your ability to hit the same shot with accurate repetition.

• Your follow-through should be extremely short and compact.

• Your racket face should still be in an

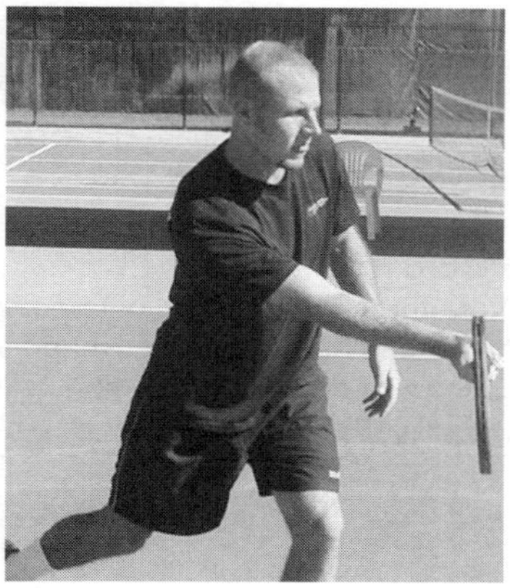

Figure 32
Notice the contact point (with Eastern forehand grip) forces the player to lay the wrist back.

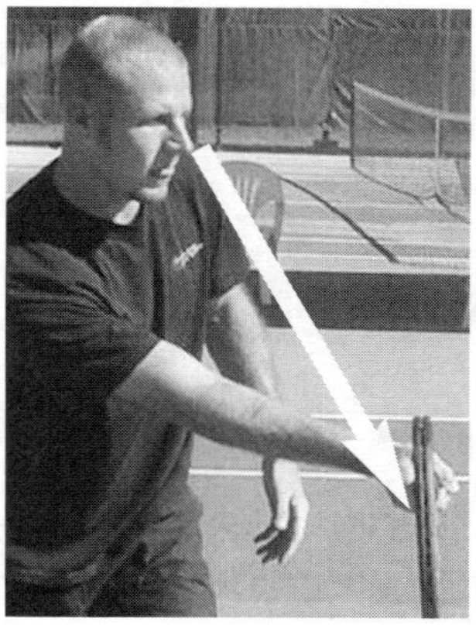

Figure 33
Compare how the eyes perceive the contact point here with an Eastern grip to that of the Continental in Fig. 34. Here the eyes are set behind the hitting surface.

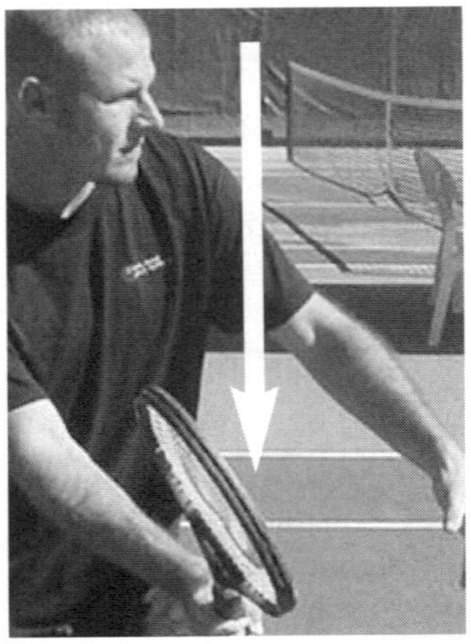

Figures 34 & 35
With the Continental grip, the eyes are set somewhat even with the hitting surface. Note Pete's Sampras forehand volley below.

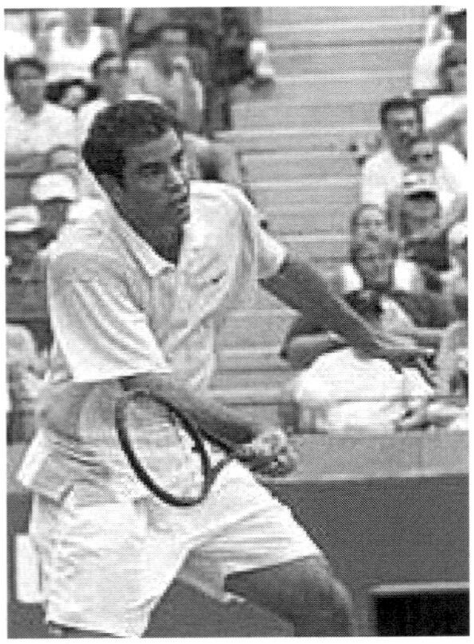

"open-face" position after contact. The racket should not turn over the ball or hit down on top of the ball. You can check yourself by holding the racket still just after the point of contact. By looking at your racket after contact, you can see if you have the racket still open or if you have used your wrist and turned the racket over the top of the ball. (If you do this, the racket face will be now pointed down at the ground…a good way to hit an easy volley into the bottom of the net!)

In directing a celebrity tennis event in 1999 I was teaching the volley to a small group of participants when one of the men complained to me that he couldn't get any power on his volley. Upon observation of his volley, I saw that the man was attempting to meet the ball with his arm already fully extended in front of him. (Similar to Figure 33.) Short of flicking his wrist he could not generate any substantial power on his volley.

His reason for this hitting position was, "My pro told me to hit the ball out in front of my body." Other players in the group voiced a similar directive that had came from their pros as well. After I described the limitations and problems related to this misconception, the gentleman attempted to hit the ball just to his side and slightly in front of his hip using the continental grip as I instructed. Within a half dozen hits he was hitting his volleys with far more pace and control.

"I'm cured," he exclaimed after hitting many successful volleys.

Some players may not hit as far out in front of their body as this man did. Inevitably, players who haven't been taught the differences as to where the contact point should be made (and those using Eastern grips) will attempt to make contact too far in front of them. In varying degrees, many of these players faced similar problems like the man I just described.

I want to emphasize, however, that we still make contact in front of us! It just does not need to be to the point where the racket is exhibiting the traits that I described above. This is one of those "classic" phrases that some pros use to help players NOT hit the ball late. However, be careful how you interpret it yourself.

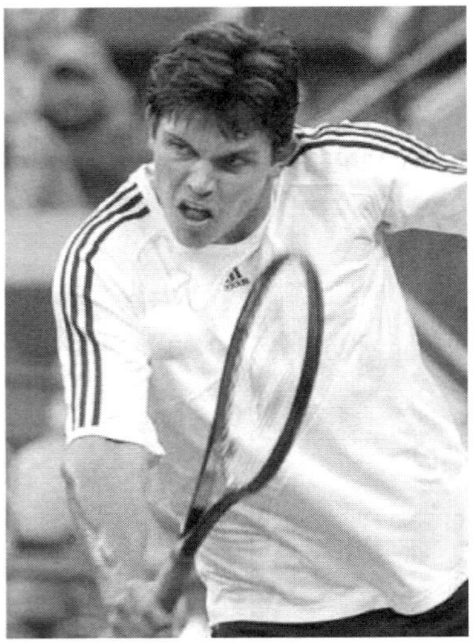

Figure 36
Note the contact point of the backhand volley by Taylor Dent is NOT out in front of his body but parallel with his side.

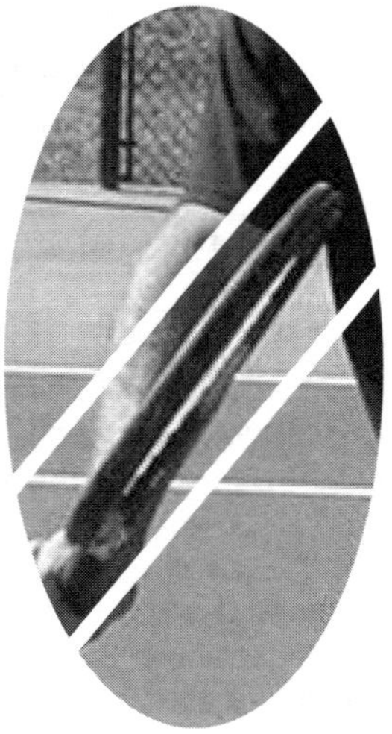

Figure 37
Note the racket lies almost parallel with the hitting arm on the backhand volley, (shown here), and the forehand volley. (Figure 38)

ADDITIONAL TIPS ON THE VOLLEY

- *Keep your racket head up and try to bend at the knees for low volleys as opposed to bending at the waist. A good tip is to keep your eyes as level with the ball as possible.*
- *Keep your racket head up as your arm moves the racket down and through the volley. Don't use your wrist or elbow to chop down on the ball.*
- *Try to get your eyes close to the ball on contact. Many players extend their arm too far away from their body and their eyes to control the shot. (Of course, you don't want to get too close to the ball either!)*
- *As a general rule of thumb, keep the racket parallel with the forearm. This principle will prevent the wrist from bending and produces a "picture perfect" volley! (See Figures 36, 37, & 38)*

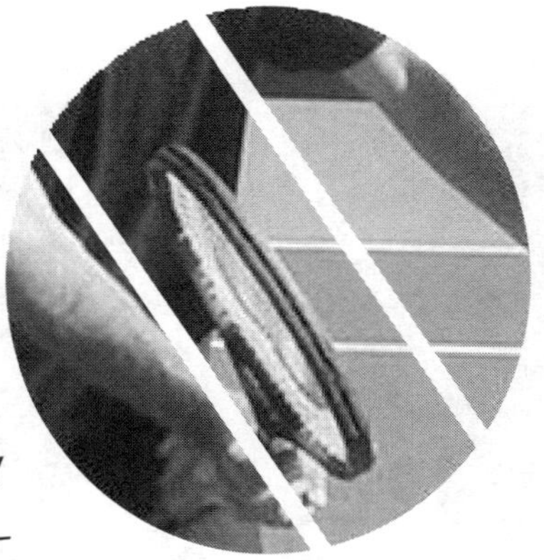

Figure 38
By keeping the racket parallel with the forearm, the arm and racket move as a unit. Note the similar arm and racket relationship as that of the backhand above.

Volley Summary

FOREHAND VOLLEY REVIEW

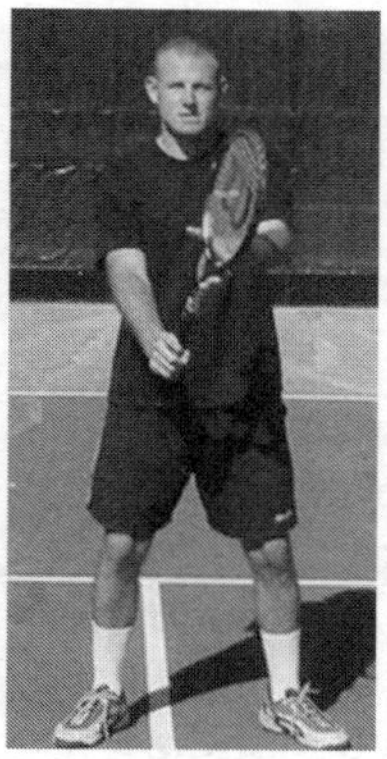

Figure A

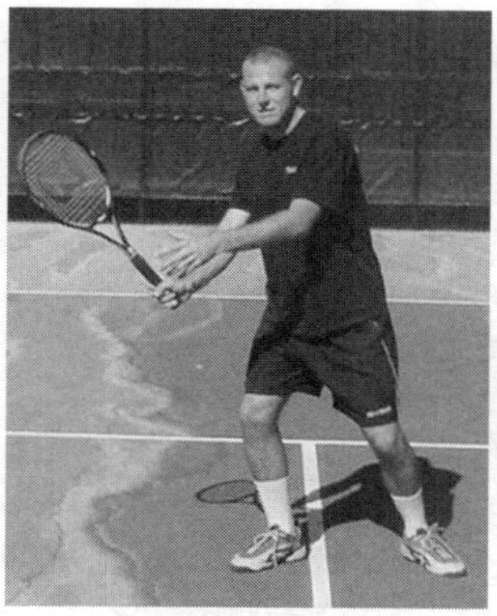

Figure B

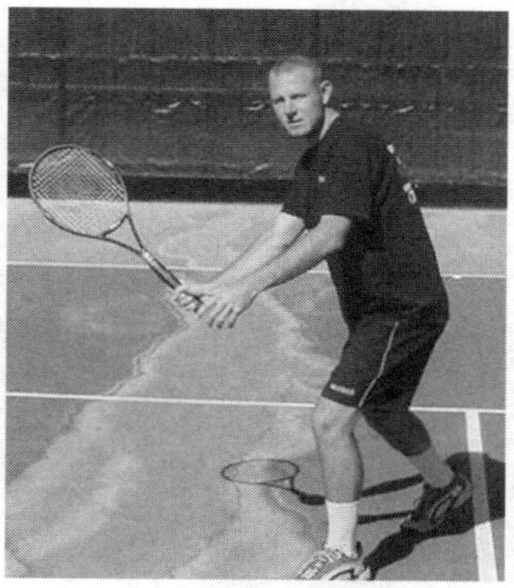

Figure C

FOREHAND VOLLEY REVIEW

Figure A: Ready Position
The player is able to turn to the right or left, depending on what shot has been hit by the opponent.

Figure B & D: The Turn
The upper body turns, taking the racket to the side. Notice the racket does not go back past the front knee

Figure C & E: Contact Point
The body remains sideways and the racket makes contact almost even with the front knee. Notice the step has occurred and it is across the body. From this point after contact, the player can hold this position to check balance and racket face.

Forehand—Side View

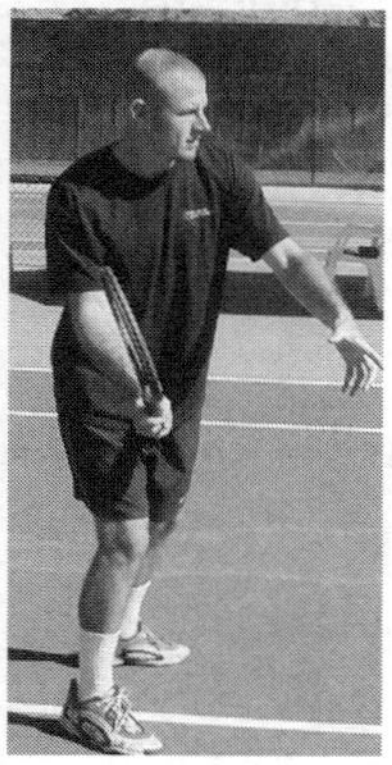

Figure D

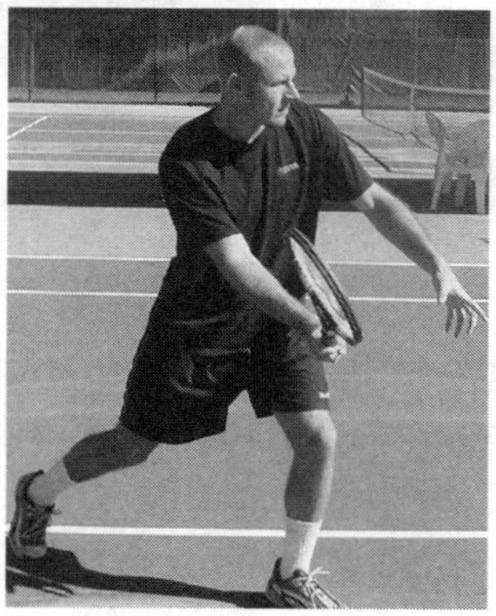

Figure E

SIDE VIEWS

Note the parallel position of the racket edge to the forearm. As the player turns the shoulders, the racket's face is towards the target. Contact is off the front knee with a downward, slicing motion. The body stays sideways after contact.

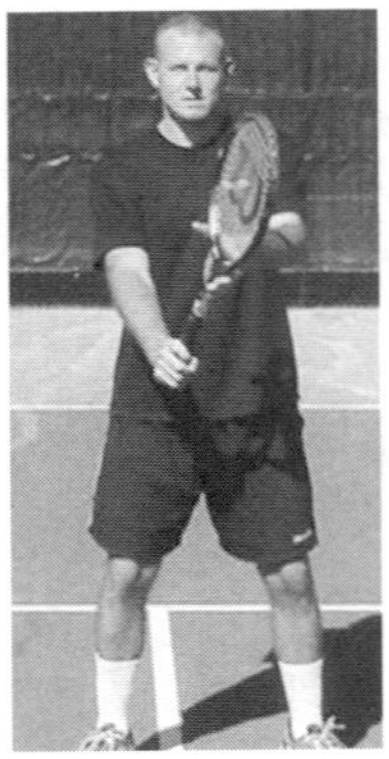
Figure A

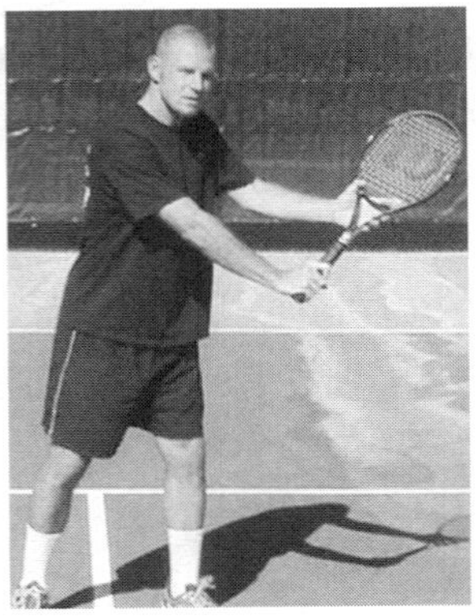
Figure B

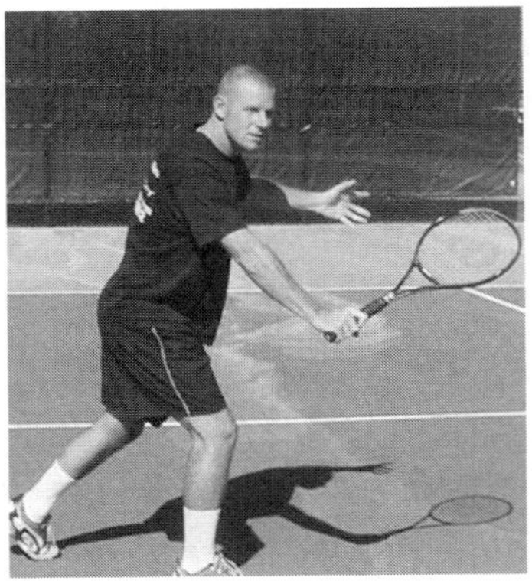
Figure C

BACKHAND VOLLEY REVIEW

Figure A: Ready Position
Notice the similar hand positions here as in Figure B, the Turn

Figure B & D: The Turn
The shoulders turn to take the rack back NOT THE ARM! The racket arm becomes straight with a locked elbow. The racket is still cradled with the left hand just as in the ready position.

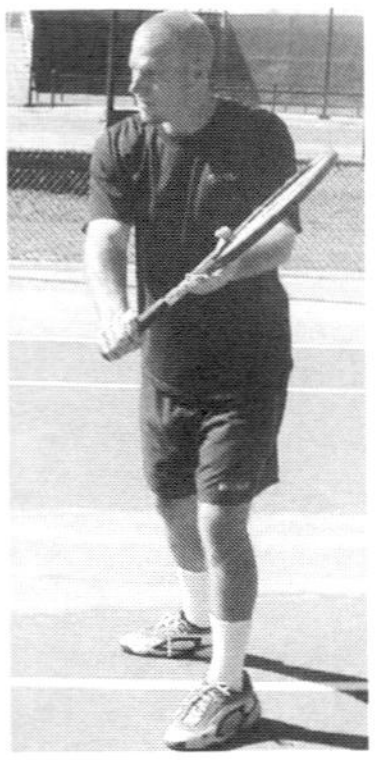
Figure D

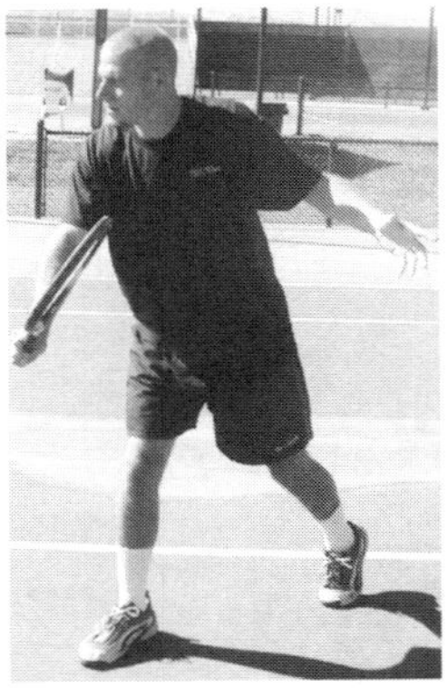
Figure E

BACKHAND VOLLEY REVIEW

Figure C & E: Contact Point
The step across the body with the right leg has occurred; the racket arm moves forward as a unit to meet the ball. The racket head is kept up and the arms spread apart to help maintain the sideways shoulder position through contact.

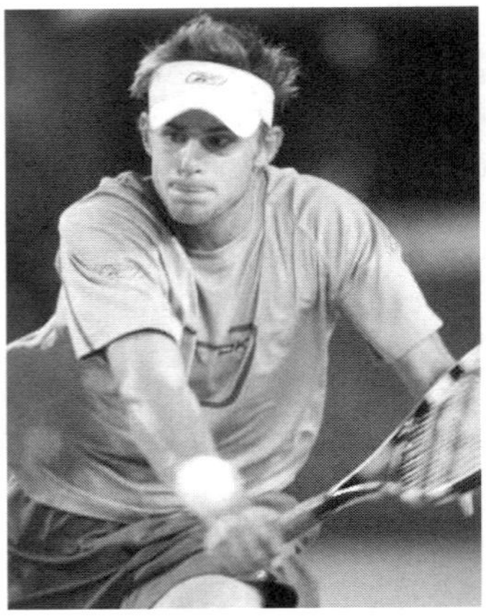

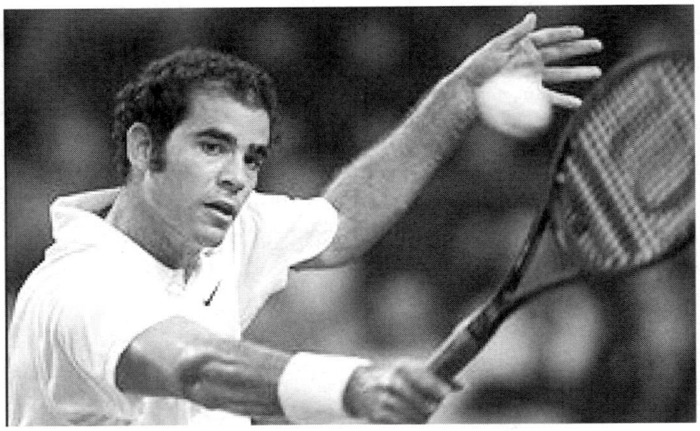

Figures 39 & 40
Note how parallel the arm and the racket plane are in each of these two pictures. Also note that the racket face is slightly open, beveled to meet the ball in a slice-like motion. Compare these two pictures with that of Figure D and E above.

Advanced Situation Volleys

Advanced volleys would include volleys hit while moving forward towards the net, or sideways as in poaching, or a combination of both movements. Also, deep volleys from behind the service-line are more difficult due to the distance the player has to track the ball and the fact most players tend to feel they need to swing harder at the ball when volleying from further back (which generally is not necessary!). Angle volleys are also considered advanced in that they require touch and timing; specifically, the Continental grip as described earlier is critical.

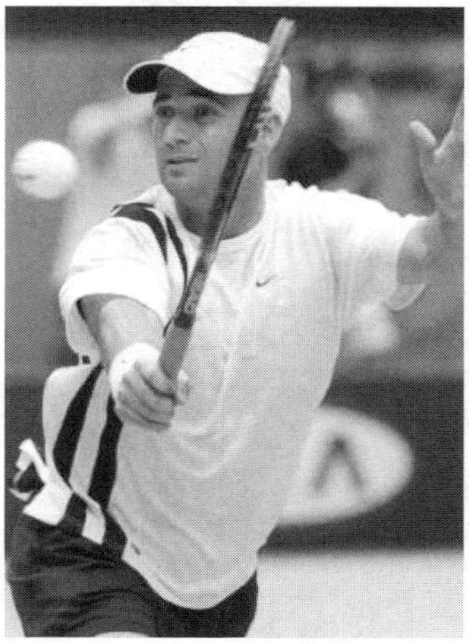

Figure 41
Note Andre Agassi's upper body is sideway to the on coming ball. Note also the correct step, straight right arm, Continental grip, and open racket face...all similar to the techniques used if he wasn't moving to the ball.

MOVING VOLLEYS

When you're moving towards a ball that you wish to volley, if possible try to pause your body's movement at the point of contact. Under some circumstances you may not have the opportunity to slow your forward momentum down enough in order to pause while making contact. In either case, it is important to keep your upper body (shoulders and torso) sideways through the point of contact. (See Figure 41) Keeping the back foot back on either the forehand or backhand volley usually will accomplish this. By pausing the feet at this moment, the arm can drive the ball more through the target line increasing the likelihood of the ball being directed at the intended target even if hit slightly early or late. If the foot steps through during this point of contact, the hips and shoulders tend to rotate towards the net causing the arm to be pulled across the body (as described in the basic volley form). The player in doing this will try to correct the swing by dropping the racket head back and pushing the racket towards the target. This produces a very weak and inefficient volley.

This idea of pausing is equally valuable when you are moving diagonally or sideways to the ball as in poaching. Keep in mind that the racket is attached to your arm which in turn is attached to your body. If your body is moving sideways to intercept a ball, then your racket is moving sideways as well! If you are still moving sideways as you are making contact, then the volley will become far more difficult due to the fact that your racket is also moving sideways! Advanced players have learned to judge and adjust to balls as they are moving sideways. As a result, they don't appear to pause at the point of contact. In reality, they generally do have a relative pause in their motion, usually seen as a very subtle hesitation with their upper body as they make contact while their legs continue to move through the shot.

Some noted instructors claim that when we pause, the ball will go downward into the net due to the feet stopping while the upper body tends to lean forward due to momentum. If a player is standing upright, he or she will indeed tend to bend forward at the waist in this scenario. However, for most players it is far easier to learn to hit volleys initially by maintaining body control through this pause than to allow the body to continue moving forward unchecked while attempting the volley. Thus, it is important for all players to maintain balance through proper footwork so the pause will be accomplished with minimal forward lean at contact. Also, for all beginners the pausing action teaches the proper footwork of not "walking through" the volley. Players who don't slow down at the volley usually over rotate and don't remain sideways through the contact point. They also usually can be seen missing some of the easiest volleys, over-running balls due to this lack of balance. Players who use the Eastern forehand and backhand grips tend to hit down on the ball with their upper body if they do stop abruptly. (See Figure 42) When players remain sideways on the volley as described throughout this chapter, such a lean at the waist seldom occurs. Only when players face the net do we see this downward lean.

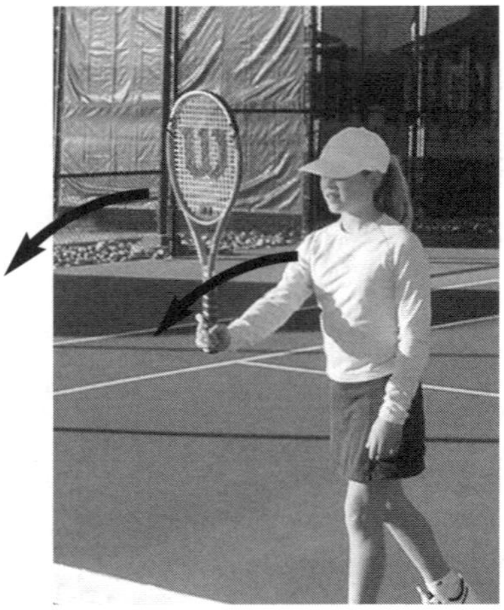

Figure 42
If a player uses an Eastern forehand grip and stops their foreward motion abruptly, they will hit the ball in the net.

THE CARIOCA STEP

When players are forced to accelerate to the ball with little or no time to pause, skilled players usually incorporate what is called a "carioca" step. This move is accomplished with the back leg actually moving slightly behind the front leg on volleys. (Figures 43 & 44) This carioca step serves a similar purpose as the off-arm: it helps the player remain sideways. If the player allowed the back leg to swing around as in another running step, the hips would rotate around defeating the goal of remaining sideways.

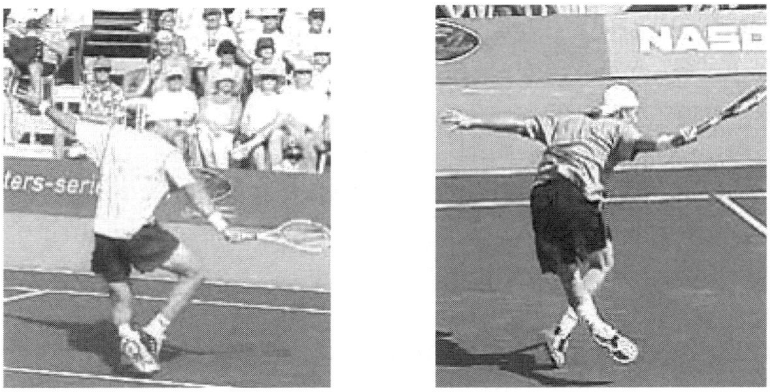

Figures 43 & 44 – The CARIOCA STEP
As players aggressively move forward to attack a backhand volley, the body must remain sideways. This is difficult to do while running forward. The back leg (left leg for righthanders) wants to swing around for another forward step. If this were to occur, the hips and body would rotate around during the stroke. As we have mentioned, it is imperative for the player to remain sideways for the volley so that the racket can continue towards the target as long as possible. Here, Patrick Rafter and Lleyton Hewitt have completed their volleys yet are still moving forward. Notice how they both remain sideways here, long after the ball has left the racket.

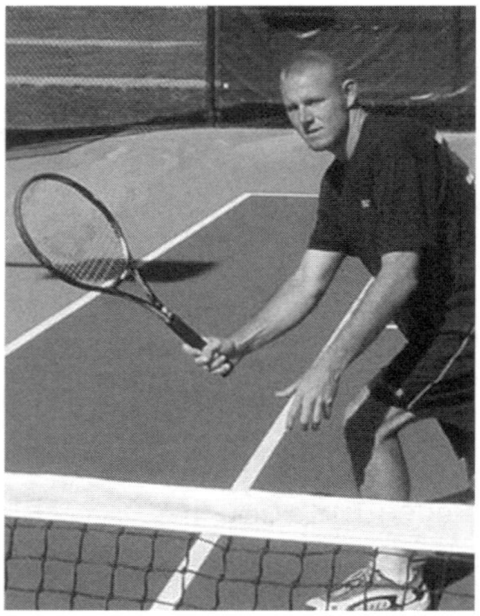

Figure 45
The forehand angle volley Notice the body turns away from the target. From the ready position, only a slight turn is necessary.

The carioca step allows the player to actually continue stepping forward. As the left leg moves in behind the right leg, weight is put on the left leg momentarily so the body can continue forward without rotating around. This is a critical part of hitting a successful volley while moving forward.

You will want to first learn to volley the ball correctly using the techniques discussed above. Once the volley foundation is built, it is far easier to move to more advanced levels of shot-making including using body momentum to move through the shot. You will be rewarded by a greater rate of improvement if you do.

ANGLE VOLLEYS

Angle volleys are, in my opinion, one of the most enjoyable shots to hit in tennis. When hit during a match they can be psychologically damaging to your opponents, perhaps more so than a killer overhead or put-away volley. The reason for this is that with an easy overhead or volley, your opponents are expecting the ball to be driven for a winner. Opponents tend to expect to lose the point on these shots. However, when you reach out and hit a low ball for an angle winner, it almost seems to stun your opponent. You can see their jaw drop and shoulders sag when surprised by this shot. It really can take the wind out of the sails of your opponent when done at the right time.

One of the most important points about the angle volley is the grip. Players who tend to favor the Eastern forehand and backhand grips usually have great difficulty executing effective angle volleys. This is because these grips cause the racket and the forearm to be nearly at right angles to each other. (See Figures 11, 12, 32, & 33.) This position makes it most difficult to execute any significant angle at the net.

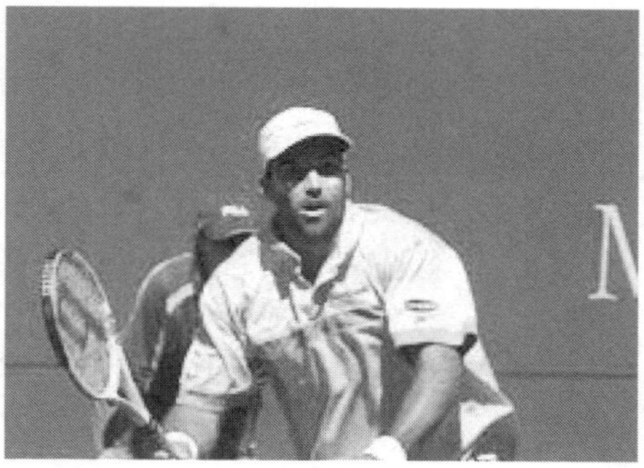

Figure 46
Note Patrick Rafter's early preparation for a forehand angle volley. The racket and upper body have established the proper turn.

The angle volley has some very important component parts to consider. However, perhaps more than any shot, players tend to convolute the angle volley when only the simplest moves are necessary. The first step is for the player to face slightly AWAY from the target. That is, you must turn your shoulders away from the angle in which you are hitting. (See Figure 45, 46, & 47) The reason for this is that if you face your target, you will have to take your racket back further than you need. This larger racket swing causes a loss in control, both in touch needed and in getting the racket back to the correct angle for the shot. In fact, if you are in the recommended volley ready position, you will notice that you only need to turn your shoulders to the side (so you face away from your target). In this position, the racket face is angled sharply to the side of your opponent's court with the racket facing towards the actual target! Making this simple move is all that is necessary in making an angled volley.

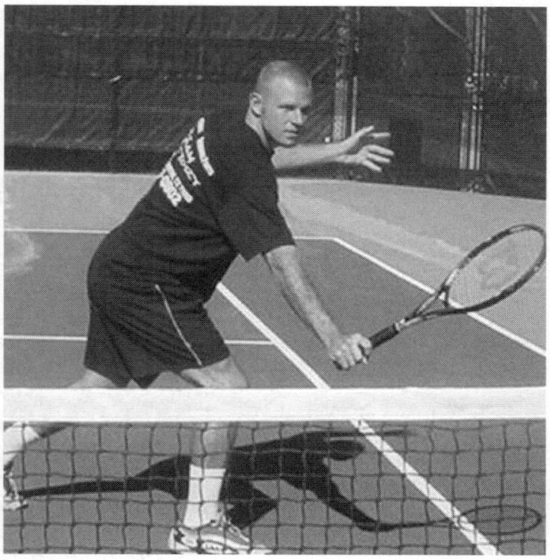

Figure 47 –The backhand angle volley.
Similar to the forehand, the player turns away from the target and uses the racket face as a mirror to "reflect" the ball. Absolutely no backswing is used in the angle volley.

I like to use the analogy of a beam of light and a mirror when talking about angle volleys. The idea is that the ball in flight towards your racket is the beam of light; your racket face (plane) is the mirror. Use your racket strings as a mirror to reflect the beam of light (the ball) to a desired point on the court. If you were going to reflect a beam of light with a mirror to a given point, you wouldn't move the mirror once the proper angle had been achieved. This same principle is applied in how to approach hitting an angle volley. Once the racket is in position to meet the ball, the angle of the racket not only remains the same prior to contact, but it doesn't change during or after contact.

Also, angle volleys should be hit with touch. Some players like to swing at their angle volleys thinking this is more effective. In reality, this is the farthest thing from what you want to do! Hitting angle volleys hard increases the likelihood of hitting the ball too far, causing the ball to go wide. Also, if you hit the ball from a higher angle, such as hitting from a couple of feet above the net tape, the harder you hit, the higher the ball will bounce, usually giving your opponent more time to run down the volley.

As a general rule, angle volleys should not be hit when the ball is hit from a point higher than your shoulders, especially balls that are coming soft from a high trajectory.

There are a couple obvious reasons why this is not advantageous. First, balls hit from a higher point on your side of the net will logically bounce higher when they land on your opponent's side of the court. Second, if you get to a high ball near the net, you really should go for the "kill" put-away since it is a relatively sure winner. (There is nothing worse than having a sure put-away, only to miss it by trying to hit a "fancy" drop angle shot!)

There is another reason you should not hit an angle volley from a slow, high ball that is dropping from a high possible contact point: it is extremely difficult to hit a ball that is falling almost vertically with a racket that is angled nearly vertically. The timing is very difficult. It is much easier to let the ball drop (one of those exceptions to the rule!), and hit it from a much lower position allowing the racket to hit more under the ball as you're angling it off to the side of your opponent's court. Generally, if I feel I need to hit an angle shot from this position, I try to make contact with the ball and my racket about level with the top of the net. Here are some reasons I might recommend the attempt of letting a ball drop from a high position to this lower point:

- *I didn't feel I could move up to the ball with enough time to have a good opportunity for a hard-hit winner*
- *Opponent(s) are standing far back near the baseline anticipating the smash*
- *I am intentionally trying to wear my opponent out by having them try to run down a short drop or angled shot.*

When to hit the angle volley

Many players don't know the best time to attempt the angle volley. Let me say that it should be used much more in doubles than in singles. The reason for this is that:

a) You have more court width (doubles alleys);
b) You have more opportunity to hit from the side of your own court, opening up the possibility of hitting the angle volley with a greater degree of angle;
c) If the angle volley isn't hit well, in doubles you have a partner to cover the open part of your court.

In singles you leave yourself vulnerable if your angle shot isn't a winner. In singles the drop-volley down-the-line is the better shot. It cuts down the amount of open court your drop-shot might leave you if it isn't perfect.

DROP VOLLEY

The Drop Volley, a volley that is hit to intentionally die close to the net on your opponent's side of the net, is one of the hardest volleys to hit with accuracy and control. The drop volley works on the same principle as a drop shot hit from a ball that has bounced first. The difficulty in hitting the drop volley is creating the right amount of softness and backspin on the shot to get the ball over the net, yet die on your opponent's side of the court. Technically, the drop volley is hit the same way as we have described hitting the volley in this chapter. The only difference is that the ball is hit with a more open racket face and the arm actually gives with the shot, minimizing the force applied to the ball. Practice the shot by opening up the racket face and hitting the bottom side of the ball at the contact point. Your first few shots undoubtedly will go too high. But as you develop your volley skills, your ability to hit the drop volley will also improve.

TOPSPIN VOLLEY

Decades ago the topspin volley was seldom, if ever, seen among the pros. What was once considered a low-percentage shot is now used and taught to advanced players of all ages. One of the reasons, I feel, that the topspin volley has evolved over the past 15 or 20 years is the insistence of players to play and practice only a baseline game. This trend of top players to bang out groundstrokes created, out of necessity, the topspin volley. These players did not spend the time to fashion effective volleys or volley strategies in their game. Hence, when a baseliner was forced to the net, their response was to hit the ball the only way they were comfortable…with topspin! Recently, even players with solid volleys utilize the swinging topspin volley in certain situations.

In reality, the topspin volley is simply a topspin groundstroke taken out of the air before the ball can bounce. The difficulty in producing the shot with reliability is the issue of racket head control when swinging through a ball that is not necessarily slowing down as much as a ball that has bounced first. This truly is an advanced shot in the sense that the timing of hitting the ball with a full swinging motion is critical. Players who have developed solid topspin groundstrokes can begin to experiment with hitting and practicing this shot. However, those whose groundstrokes are suspect will fare much better by hitting the fundamentally sound block or cut volley from anywhere on the court a volley is encountered. I highly recommend that all players first develop sound volley skills, as described in this chapter, before deciding to experiment with the topspin volley.

The best time to hit the topspin volley is when the ball is higher in the air and somewhat of a floater. This gives a player the needed time to calibrate the swing rhythm and set up for the shot. Certainly, a hard hit ball will create difficulty in timing the swing and contact point to keep the topspin volley in the court. Most players utilize the swinging volley from behind the service line. Usually when players have a high volley inside the service line, the most efficient and effective shot is a normal drive volley to the open court. But, behind the service line, in order to create an offensive volley, a player will want to have more pace than can be generated by a normal block or punch volley. Thus the topspin volley can provide this added power.

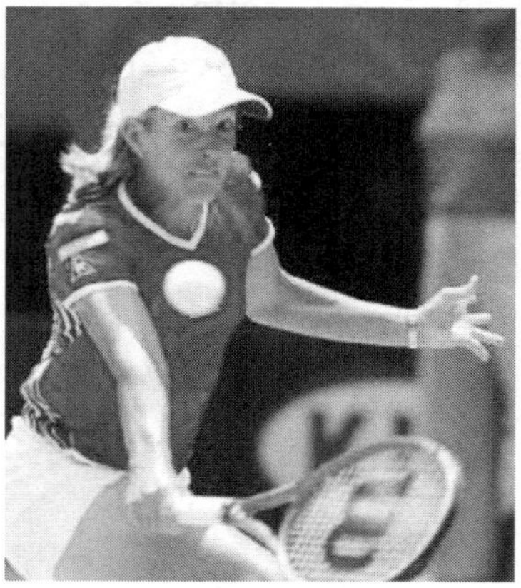

Figure 48
Notice the relatively similar racket orientation to the arm and body on both the higher volley (See Figs 39 & 40) and the low ones, seen here in Figures. 48 & 49.

LOW VOLLEYS

One of the most intimidating volleys, especially for beginners and intermediate players, is hitting a low volley out of the air. A combination of factors contributes to this fear. Eastern forehand and backhand grips are notoriously poorly suited for low volleys. The wrist must be cocked at a difficult angle and most players simply can't negotiate the

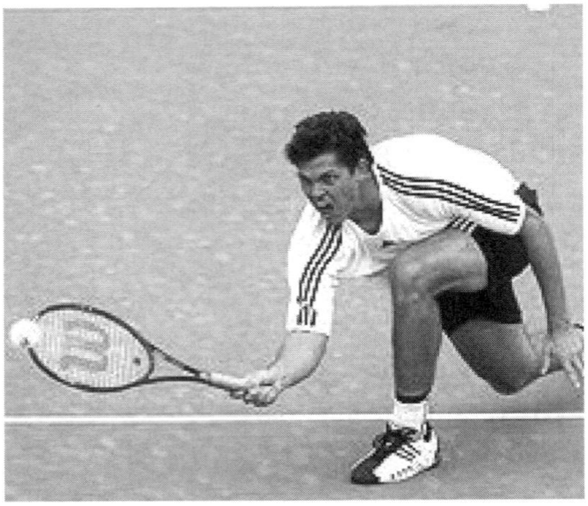

Figure 49
By bending the knees, the player can lower his center of gravity and keep the racket in the proper position.

racket head open enough to get the ball up over the net. Also, beginners tend to drop their racket head on low volleys instead of bending the knees. This lazy move creates difficulty in hitting a consistent volley.

The low volley must be attempted while keeping the racket head up and the hitting arm straight. (See Figure 48) This position allows for the leverage of the arm to be utilized while slicing the low volley. If the racket head drops, the player tends to flick the racket at the ball in an attempt to get the racket to lift the ball.

In an effort to maintain this racket formation, the player must bend the knees. There is no substitution for getting low. Players who don't bend their knees tend to bend down at the waist. This will put the player out of balance in addition to putting strain on their back. (See Figure 49)

HALF-VOLLEY

The half-volley is, in my opinion, a misnomer. The actual method of hitting a half-volley correctly more resembles a short, groundstroke-like motion than a correct volley motion. In this light, the half-volley could be named the "half-groundstroke" instead. Regardless of what the shot is named, players must understand the principles of how a correct half-volley should be hit.

The half-volley is a ball that is hit immediately after it bounces, usually near the feet. Because contact is made while the ball is rising quickly from the court, the motion of hitting the ball differs from both the volley and the groundstroke. However, the half-volley takes from both strokes in correct form.

Unless you are able to create more time in hitting the half-volley (usually by quickly backing up before striking the ball), it is not recommended that the slicing or cutting action of the volley as described in this chapter be used. Because the ball rebounds off the court at an angle almost parallel to the angle of an open racket face as used in hitting a normal volley, cutting the ball will usually result in a miss-hit or a pop-up half-volley.

Diagram 2

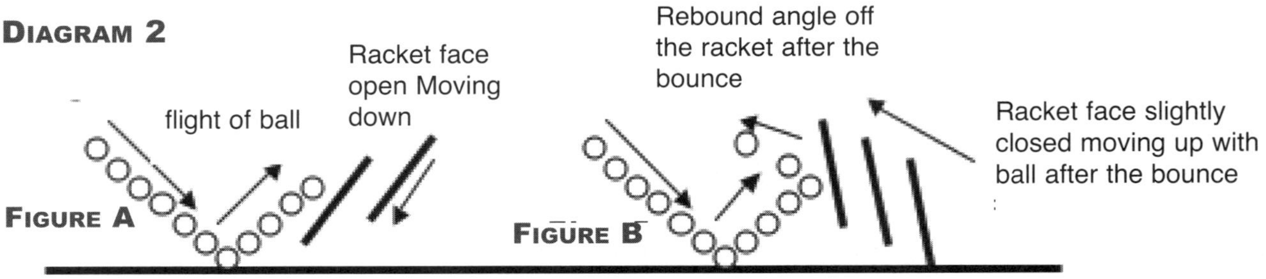

As you can see by this diagram, an open racket face (Figure A), moving down and forward, moves almost parallel with the path of the ball after it bounces. The racket held at this angle could produce miss-hit shots. Usually the ball catches either the bottom outer edge or the inside top edge of the racket, depending on the timing. In Figure B the racket face is closed slightly and moves up as the ball bounces from the court. You can see how the ball will meet the racket face more squarely in this pattern of movement. The key to directing the ball with control is to move the racket up and through the ball with minimal changes in the plane of the racket. This requires the shot to be hit with a firm wrist and a very short motion. Through practice, players get a feel for the half-volley in terms of how much motion and racket face angle is needed.

As you can see, the half-volley mimics the volley in the short motion of the stroke. It also mimics the topspin groundstroke in the low-to-high motion of the racket. It is this action of the slightly closed racket face moving up through the half-volley that imparts clean topspin on the ball. This helps the ball drop quickly on your opponent's side of the court which, in turn, helps keep your opponents from driving the ball down your throat!

Many players are confused as to what grip they should use on the half-volley. Since the stroke is an upward topspin stroke that resembles a shortened groundstroke, many think their standard topspin grip should be used. While the logic in using this grip is rational, it has a very important drawback. Because a player is moving in to the net and is in a position to volley the ball should it come high enough and fast enough, players should use their continental grip for the half-volley. The reason for this is position. The closer toward the net you end up, the more likely you will encounter a volley. By holding a topspin grip as if anticipating the topspin half-volley, you will have difficulty hitting a volley when a well-hit ball is hit in the air to you. If you encounter a slower moving ball that is dropping and you can back up or set up for the topspin, then, by all means, change your grip to your topspin groundstroke grip. In this situation, because the ball is moving slower (giving you time to both set up your position with your feet as well as establish a topspin stroke), you obviously have time to change your grip. But, when coming to the net most shots will be moving too fast to maintain a topspin grip, and there will only be a split second to change to the continental grip.

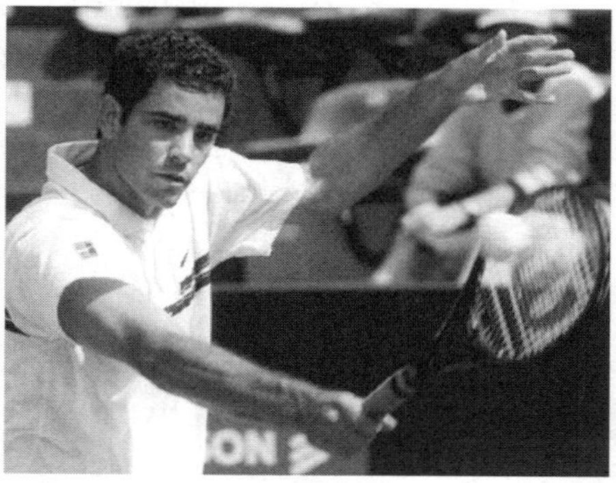

Figure 50
Note the racket head held above the wrist on higher volleys.

HIGH VOLLEYS

The high volley is one of the most difficult volleys to execute cleanly and with consistency. One of the problems most players find is that the higher the volley is in relation to your body, the more the arm tends to swing in an arc. This arc causes the racket to swing down more on the ball when the ball is hit slightly early, or when hit late the racket will tend to hit the ball too high. This same principle also makes the player hit the ball long when striking the ball late. Because the arm is connected to the shoulder, the arm, along with the racket, acts as an upside down pendulum. Please see Diagram 3.

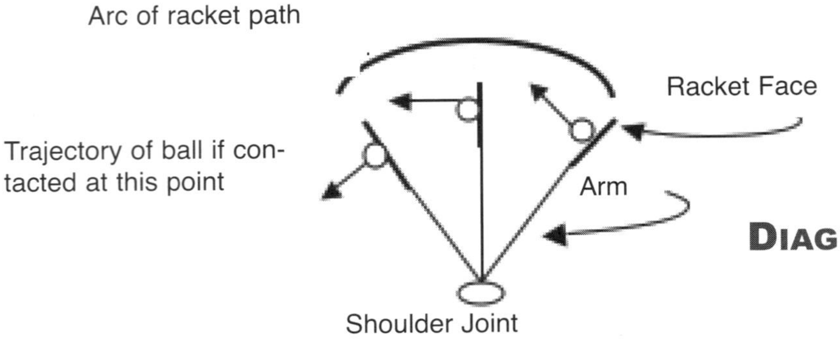

Diagram 3

Diagram 3
The "Reverse Pendulum"

On high volleys the arm and racket act like an upside down pendulum, swinging around the shoulder joint. This action results in the racket face – and resultant trajectory of the ball – to change throughout the swing.

As you can see from Diagram 3 if the arm and racket move parallel with each other, the contact point and resultant trajectory of the ball changes constantly. We often refer to this movement as a "windmill" swing due to the arm arching around the shoulder like the blades of a windmill. In order to hit your high volleys correctly and accurately, you will need to avoid this common stroke problem.

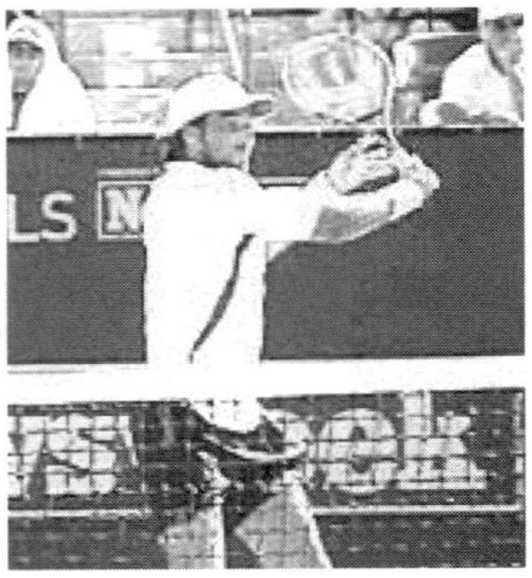

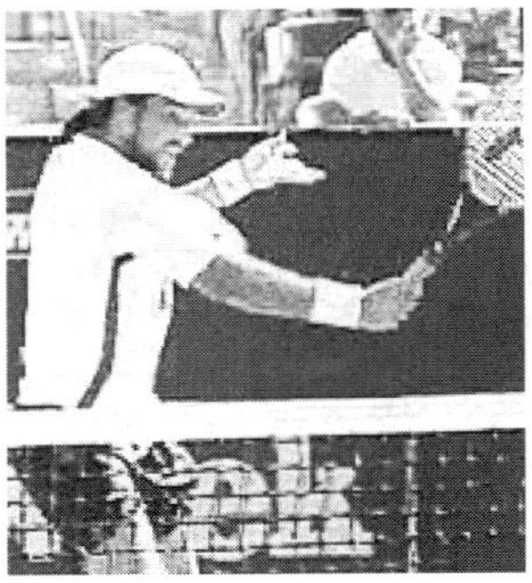

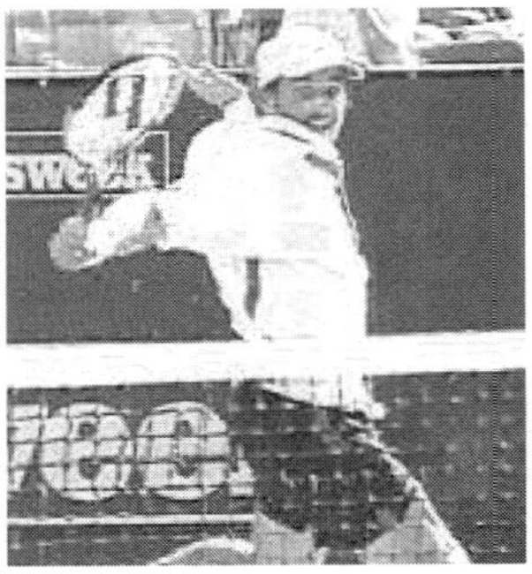

Figures 51, 52 & 53
On this shoulder-high volley, Patrick Rafter starts his racket back high with a short backswing. Contact point is parallel with the front shoulder with a slight open racket face. On the follow-through Rafter remains sideways as his racket clearly slices downward and through the target line

There are two ways to hit a high volley within the bounds of our advanced foundation. You will want to learn both techniques, as there will be times each is applicable in match situations.

High Volley Method 1: High Volley hit as a Volley

When presented with a high volley a conservative approach to hitting the volley is to keep the plane of the racket the same as long as possible through the contact zone. (See Figures 51, 52, & 53) This requires the racket to drive through the ball in more of a linear motion as opposed to a rotational swinging motion as shown in Diagram 3. Some advanced players will make subtle changes in their grip (usually toward somewhat of an Eastern forehand grip on certain forehand volleys), as this does put more hand behind the racket. Because the motion on higher volleys does require more strength than lower balls due to the higher position of the racket to the shoulder, the Eastern grips can help provide greater power on higher balls. However, it is imperative that the player makes sure that the racket still stays slightly open through the volley. Because of the tendency to hit down on higher balls, players inevitably hit more of these shots into the net than they might on lower balls. Also, generally, higher balls that are hit as volleys are usually arching downward more than waist-high or low volleys. (Obviously, if the high volley is not dropping and instead going straight or upward with some velocity, it probably is going out!) Players who try to hit the ball flat, instead of the slight cutting action described in this chapter will find their shots rebounding off their flat racket faces at a greater angle down than they usually expect. (Refer to Diagram 1) This is why tennis great Arthur Ashe said in his book, Arthur Ashe on Tennis, that ALL VOLLEYS, NO MATTER HOW HIGH OR LOW THE BALL IS, SHOULD BE HIT WITH UNDERSPIN. I will add an addendum to this phrase: while learning, unless you plan to intentionally hit a volley with topspin, all volleys should be hit with some aspect of underspin.

High Volley Method 2: High Volley hit as an Overhead

If the incoming ball is high enough to be hit head-high or higher, the same technique used to hit an overhead can be incorporated with a more offensive result. If a player intends to hit this shot, there are two very important points to address in addition to the basic overhead technique:

a. Make sure to bend the knees to make the high volley essentially become an overhead. Players often will swing standing upright with contact much lower than a traditional overhead's contact. This will result in the player having to lay the racket face way back to prevent hitting the ball literally down into the ground. Typically, these players will end up hitting the ball too long due to the result of the racket face being laid back and not being able to release the racket head through the course of the swing.

b. Shorten the overhead swing. Due to the fact that high volleys present less time for preparation, players will quickly discover a loss of control when attempting to hit the high volley as a full-speed overhead. It is highly recommended that the player turn sideways just as they would for their regular overhead from a higher lob-type shot. However, during the turn players should not only get their racket back quickly, but it should be taken back in a shorter radius than when hitting the full overhead. The contact of the ball and the follow-through should also be abbreviated to help prevent the player from over rotating and over swinging. Overall, the arm swings very little. The racket and forearm simply pronate at the ball while keeping the elbow high. Like the serve and overhead, if the elbow drops before contact, the player will have a hard time getting the racket head ahead of the hand in time to still hit the ball from a high enough point and still angle the ball down in to the opponent's court.

Hitting the high volley as an overhead requires much greater timing of the stroke and a sense of discipline in not letting the ball drop too far and over swinging. However, the overhead, when hit correctly from this position, is a far more effective shot than simply taking the shot as a volley.

Commentary on the Volley

It is of fascinating interest to me that so many books contradict not only themselves, but they contradict what I consider to be common sense. So much so, I feel that I should point out a few of these irregularities so you won't be confused if you happen to come across them in your pursuit of tennis knowledge.

COMMENTS ON THE EASTERN VOLLEY GRIP

Arthur Ashe made these statements about the Grip in his book Arthur Ashe on Tennis: "Unless you are purposely trying to hit with underspin, [with the Eastern grip] you will impart a little topspin to the ball, whether you like it or not, even if you think you're hitting it flat."

As I have already mentioned, Ashe also instructs, "All volleys, no matter how high or low the ball is, should be hit with underspin." While Ashe was not necessarily known for his tennis teaching, he is right on target with these statements.

A contradiction comes into play when we look at how he and others teach the basic volley technique. Ashe talks about the Eastern forehand and backhand grips as "a good basic grip to learn even if you want to switch to something else later. You are going to meet the ball squarely right from the start."

If a beginner is going to want to learn to hit volleys with underspin as they should, why should anyone be taught to hit volleys with an Eastern grip that naturally promotes a topspin result? While I agree that the Eastern grip is usually the more comfortable grip for beginners (only because the continental is unfamiliar to most!), this teaching strategy fails to acknowledge the clear contradiction of what actually happens when players employ the Eastern grips on their volleys.

A noted tennis researcher who was popular in the 1970's, believes beginners and pros alike should use their regular Eastern grips when they volley. He oftentimes refers to his "research" showing how his "experiments" demonstrate there is sufficient time to switch grips between the Eastern forehand and backhand grips. I would agree that this is true for beginner and intermediate players who may not see as much net play or encounter as many hard hit balls coming at them as the more advanced players often do. However, the issue of having sufficient time to switch between these two grips is definitely NOT true for skilled players playing other skilled players! Consider higher levels of doubles play. These rallies often include all four players at the net during many volley exchanges. Players who insist on playing with the Eastern grips get caught time and time again doing the "windshield wiper" move…a move that is basically hitting volleys on both sides of their body with the same Eastern forehand grip and hitting the ball on the same side of the racket. If you want to see spastic looking volleys, watch many of these players who use the Eastern grips in a quick volley exchange! And, perhaps more importantly, if these Eastern grips prohibit continued progression towards skilled play, why spend one second using them?

Some instructors promote using the Eastern grips in hitting volleys flat, insisting that a flat ball is easier to hit with control. As I have mentioned in this chapter and shown in Diagram 1, any incoming ball that has a downward trajectory will rebound off a flat surface at a downward angle of reflection. Combine this explanation with Ashe's statements about the Eastern grips producing topspin, and you have a clear answer why so many beginners and intermediates alike can stand literally only a couple of feet from the net and still bury even high balls into the bottom of the net on their volley! In addition, some of these instructors insist that the Continental grip forces you to be much more coordinated and talented. I have taught over 3000 players, many of them as young as 5 years old.

With few exceptions, all of them mastered the basic volley using the Continental grip in essentially the same amount of time as other did who were being taught to volley with the Eastern grips. The difference between my students and these others is that my students will never have to change the way they volley as they get better! And if you follow the methods in this book, NEITHER WILL YOU!

But, perhaps more importantly, consider the required preciseness of hitting a ball flat. If the player is attempting to hit a volley perfectly flat towards a target, and the angle of the racket is off, tilted down at even a miniscule amount, the ball will most likely be hit into the net. (Again consider what Ashe said about the Eastern grip's natural tendency to hit topspin!) A player who opens the racket face and applies a slight slice on the ball will be much more likely to get the ball up and over the net with consistency due to the many inherent and accommodating conditions that are met when hitting a volley with a slice.

Consider too, that most shots hit as passing shots are hit at net players with topspin. The slice action promotes the use of the "Spin Advantage" I discussed in Chapter 7. It becomes much easier to control a ball with slice, especially on topspin shots hit at us while we are at the net.

And consider in singles or doubles the preciseness of any grip change when you are coming to the net, making a split-step, and having to move with the split-second reaction speed required in retrieving a passing shot. I would hate to rely on trying to grasp correctly any Eastern backhand or forehand grip during the reactionary moment of a hard hit ball in singles or in doubles. And despite what a few teaching pros might believe, the reality is that there are virtually no pros or even top club, college, or high school players who elect to use the true Eastern grips on their volleys. (One exception would be for those who are hitting intentional topspin volleys as described earlier in this chapter.)

Sequence of Learning

HERE IS YOUR "CHECKLIST" FOR LEARNING THE VOLLEY CORRECTLY.

1. *Grip: Clearly understand the continental grip for both the forehand and backhand volley.*
2. *Ready Position: Remember the racket head should be held high and the elbow held close to the body.*

3. *Turn: The shoulders turn sideways to the net. (More sideways on the backhand than the forehand.) Minimal backswing with the arm.*
4. *Racket face: beveled slightly open and held slightly higher than where contact will be.*
5. *Arm Position: On the backhand, the hitting arm is held firm and straight on the backswing. The forehand, the arm can be bent and held closer to your body by keeping the elbow closer to the body.*
6. *Contact: Just off your front knee. Don't try to reach for the ball, especially on the backhand. Don't compromise the correct arm and racket positions by reaching. Keep your eyes level with the ball if possible.*
7. *Footwork: Start with a closed stance by stepping across your body with the front leg. If necessary, step back with the back leg if the ball is coming into your body more. This will create the correct sideways position for contact.*
8. *Post Contact: Hold your follow-through for a moment after contact. Check to see if your racket face is still facing towards the target and has remained slightly open. Also, check that the racket head is still held up and has not dropped at the wrist.*

ADVANCED VOLLEY CHECKLIST

While there is technically no difference between the way you first learn to volley and what we would call an "Advanced Volley," there are some things that can be done once the player has mastered the initial learning sequence above.

1. *Limited footwork: Once the proper body-turn and arm positions are mastered, players can eliminate the step and closed stance. As long as the upper body turns, the player can simplify the footwork if the shot dictates.*
2. *Relaxed follow-through: When a player gains firm control of the racket past contact, the player can relax their stroke and not necessarily hold the racket still after contact. This means the player may have a follow-through longer than recommended in the learning stages. This post-contact swing is a relaxation phase that prevents the player from being too tight.*
3. *More slice or less slice: Once the player can effectively hit a firm slice volley, options can build upon this stroke. Adding more slice can help keep a ball very low after the bounce on your opponents side. Hitting the ball flatter can add pace to the ball.*
4. *More movement through the volley: When a player has mastered the volley, the body can move with greater force through the shot.*

> *After the split-step, the player can move with greater emphasis through the ball giving the shot greater pace. This will help players keep from letting the ball drop more than if they simply let the ball come to them.*

This sums up the basic volley form and function. Throughout this book, I will refer to elements I have discussed in this

CHAPTER 9

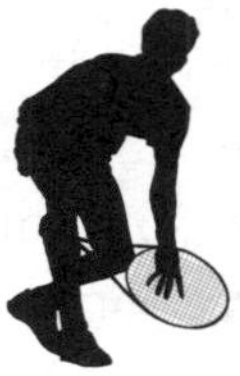

The Backhand Groundstroke

The Advanced Foundation: The Topspin and Slice Backhand

Introduction

For many recreational tennis players the prospect of hitting a backhand groundstroke can induce a sense of fear unequaled to anything short of asking your girlfriend's father for his daughter's hand in marriage! The backhand has often been associated with weakness in most players' games initiating an entire strategy among many opponents:

"Hit it to his backhand and attack."

"Just keep it to her backhand and you're in the next round."

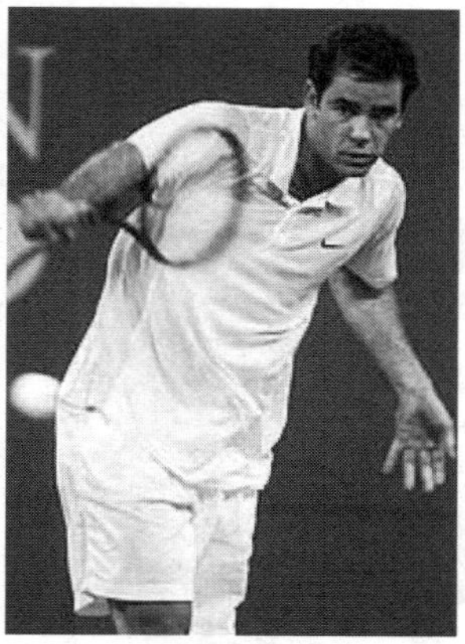

Figure 1
The one-handed backhand is still around!

This generality exists due to several factors. The first factor being that the proper form for hitting a backhand is not initially comfortable for most players. Players who don't receive adequate instruction (or don't apply the same!) often find themselves flailing at their backhands with a complete lack of feel and form required to execute an accurate and reliable stroke. Thus, anxiety and fear creep in every time the ball is hit to the backhand side of the court! Sweat forms on the forehead and the palms of a player's hand, not due to exertion necessarily, but often due to the stress and fear of simply hitting a backhand! Players will often run around their backhand to hit the forehand instead...even if it exerts twice the energy!

What creates this fear is that for most players (those who have not developed the proper backhand technique) find hitting the ball on the backhand side incredibly difficult. This difficulty can result in a tremendous lack of confidence, and a lack of confidence often leads to some very ugly and unproductive backhands! However, players who work towards the development of proper and skilled backhands usually find that their backhand does not have to be a handicap!

Two Backhands

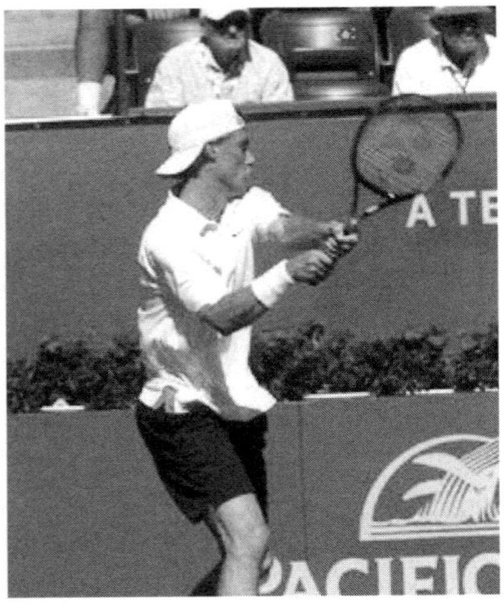

Figure 2
The two-handed backhand has gained dominance in men and women's professional tennis over the past two decades.

I think most people know there are two general methods in which a player can execute a topspin backhand groundstroke: a one-handed backhand (Figure 1) and a two-handed backhand (Figure 2). The question for you might be which one should you use?

The problem for nearly all players beginning to address this question is that the one-handed backhand "feels" easier to hit than the two-hander. The reason for this is that the one-handed backhand offers a sense of freedom of movement similar to the one-handed forehand. In addition to this simplified explanation, the two-handed backhand requires much greater emphasis on proper footwork. Usually when a one-handed backhand player is introduced to the two-handed backhand, the player feels a sense of limited reach and inability to get in a comfortable and balanced position to hit the ball cleanly. Many of these players quickly abandon any further exploration of the shot and revert back to the one-handed backhand... as flawed as it may be!

However, this seemingly limiting component of the two-handed stroke is one of the reasons why the two-handed backhand is indeed the best stroke to learn first! The two-handed backhand literally forces a player to get in proper position. Because players can hit the one-handed backhand from a variety of positions (most of which are not associated with proper form or consistent reliability), it is difficult for players to develop the discipline needed for proper footwork development and a stable swing pattern. In addition, the two-handed stroke generally helps players develop topspin faster than the one-hander. Also, the two-handed backhand helps the player develop proper body coil and rotation during the stroke.

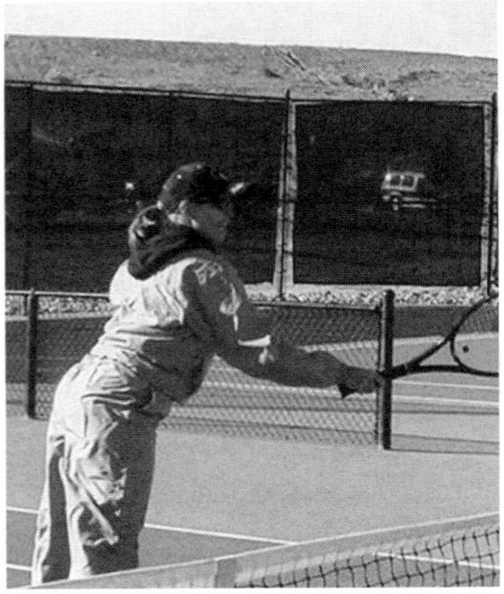

Figure 3
If players continue to play with inferior form, they will never acquire the techniques necessary for advancement

If you currently utilize a one-handed backhand, one that you know is inadequate, it is never too late to learn the two-handed stroke...even if you have been playing for years. This is not to say that a one-handed backhand can not be properly learned and executed successfully. Later in this section I will offer the procedures for hitting the one-handed stroke giving you power to make this decision for yourself. However, it is my recommendation for all players to learn the two-handed backhand first. After given ample time for improvement, a two-handed player usually finds it easier to change to a single hand backhand than the other way around. (This is exactly what tennis-great Pete Sampras did!) Even for intermediate and advanced players, learning the two-handed backhand can open your eyes to understanding the favorable backhand mechanics, allowing many of you to discover a completely new and exciting way to hit your current backhand better!

If you are an intermediate or advanced player, several ideas presented in these sections will offer you additional tips to improve your existing stroke as well as open your eyes to ways that can fine-tune your backhand into becoming a weapon.

History of the Two-Handed Backhand

While some of you will want to get right to the instruction of the backhand, it is both interesting and revealing to examine the historical changes in the backhand. This examination is for those of you who wish to understand both the physical properties of the stroke as well as the psychological components that have led to these changes. Thus, I offer a short history of the backhand.

ONE GRIP...AND THAT'S ALL!

Back when the strategy of tennis was predominately a net-attacking game, players of historical significance mainly played using the Continental grip for their backhands (and usually their forehands, serves and volleys as well!). Their one-handed backhands consisted mainly of flat drives and smooth slices, and for the first 100 years or so, few players deviated from this norm.

Those who did stray from convention disproved naysayers and experts alike over time. Australian Vivian McGrath possessed a two-handed backhand in the 1930s and went on to not only be the youngest male tennis player ever selected to the Australian Davis Cup team, but to hand losses to several of the world's top players during his career. Other two-handed backhand players who became champions in this early period of the 1930's and 1940's included two other Australians, John Bromwich and Geoff Brown. Renowned Aussie Davis Cup Captain Harry Hopman foresaw the future when it was reported in 1951 in Sporting Life: "...I believe that we have not seen the last of the two-handed players."

And, of course, Mr. Hopman was so right!

The rise of the use of two-hands on the backhand can be arguably traced to the desired use of greater topspin. If this is accurate, we can ultimately look back to the development of Rod Laver's heavy topspin groundstrokes as a precursor of the two-handed backhand. Even as Laver hit a one-handed backhand, his formidable use of topspin on both sides inspired the use of such spin in the subsequent strokes of those who followed. And this led to the discovery that, for a great majority of players, producing topspin on the backhand was far easier with two hands. Not only is the use of two hands on the backhand easier to execute appropriate form for most players, but beginners develop significantly more effective backhands earlier in their development through the learning of the two-handed backhand as a whole.

I find it amazing that tennis strokes prior to the early 1970's seldom consisted of any two-handed methods. Considering other "swing" sports such as golf, hockey, cricket, and baseball which used two hands, tennis seemed to shy away from what we would consider a logical swing choice based on the fact that these other sports utilized them almost exclusively.

Interestingly, legendary champion Jack Kramer wrote in 1949: "The use of two hands not only weakens your strokes but robs you of confidence and gives your opponent a psychological advantage." Paul Fein, in his book "Tennis Confidential", reported that after Bjorn Borg won the 1974 French Open, reporters would frequently ask him when he was going to start using a one-handed backhand. Consider, too, that from 1884 to 1996 only one woman player using a two-handed backhand ever won a Wimbledon singles title (Chris Evert). How much dominance has the two-handed backhand established on the women's tour since then? Since 1997, not one women's Wimbledon title has been won by a single-handed backhand!

Beginning in the early 1970's the traditional look of the backhand, first among pros and later among up-and-coming juniors, was about to be revolutionized. Beginning with the "big three", Bjorn Borg, Jimmy Connors and Chris Evert, the two-handed backhand finally gained the needed respect that would firmly establish the shot not only as legitimate, but also as a weapon for many. Soon, teaching pros around the world began introducing the shot to players of all ages and within 30 years the transformation would be significant!

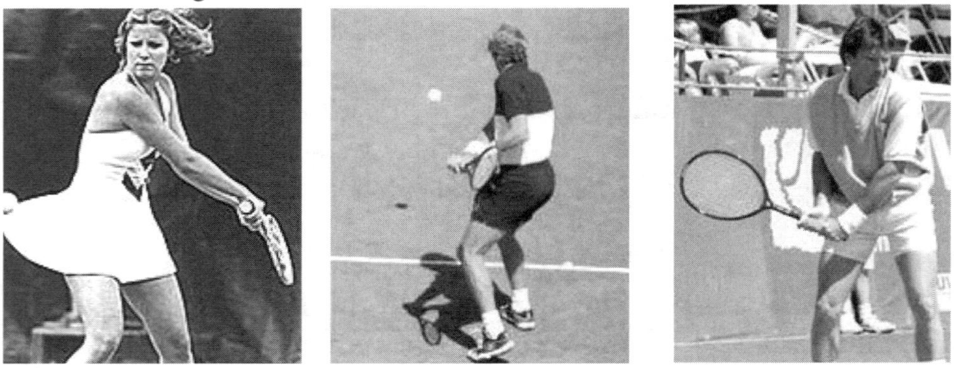

BACKHAND PIONEERS

Chris Evert, Bjorn Borg and Jimmy Connors not only showed that the two-handed backhand was a weapon, they dominated tennis for over a decade.

Ironically (and logically), even as Evert, Borg and Connors dominated tennis for years, few other significant two-handed players would emerge among the pro ranks for some 20 years! I add logically because prior to these three becoming champions, few pros were teaching the shot. It would take the right combination of pros recognizing the value of the shot, then learning how to teach the shot, and finally teaching enough talented junior players the shot—before players began to emerge from junior tournaments to the professional circuit.

Today around 70 percent of the top 100 men use a two-handed backhand. Over 90 percent of the top 100 women use the shot. Considering that prior to 1968, not one pro in the top 50 used a two-handed backhand, these statistics reveal a remarkable revolution of the shot. Perhaps no other sport has witnessed such a radical and nearly complete transformation in the technical aspect of its sport than this.

While the two-handed backhand continues to grow in popularity among almost all skilled players, there are still champions among the best in the world today who use a one-handed backhand. Justine Henin-Hardenne of Belgium, Amelie Mauresmo of France, Gustavo Kuerten of Brazil, and 2003 Wimbledon winner and runner up, the Swiss player Roger Federer and Australian Mark Philippoussis are among current top-20 world-ranked players on the men's and women's professional tours favoring the one-handed backhand.

The question for many students in learning to play tennis might be which backhand is "right" for them? The better question, however, should be "Which backhand will lead to progressive improvement?" In my experience, for the great majority of players (looking to excel in tennis), there is one answer to this question: the two-handed backhand. This statement is not to assume that all players will end up progressing with a two-handed backhand. However, players who first learn a two-handed backhand develop necessary skills related to faster and more proper backhand development than players who attempt to first learn the one-handed backhand. Interestingly, among all my 3000-plus students, (where all have been taught the two-handed backhand as their foundation backhand stroke), most can hit a very skilled one-handed backhand when they so desire.

In fact, some end up developing the one-handed backhand as their sole backhand technique. (Much like Pete Sampras, many players who start out with two-handed backhands can make a relatively smooth transition to a one-handed backhand with comparably less frustration than going from a single handed backhand initially.) In most cases, the transition from two hands to one on the backhand is much easier to accomplish than taking a one-handed backhand and then trying to learn a two-handed backhand.

Because I believe the two-handed backhand should be taught first, I will discuss the techniques associated with the two-handed backhand first. For those who wish to understand or develop a skilled one-handed backhand, these techniques will follow the two-handed sections.

The Two-handed Backhand Topspin Groundstroke

One of the elements that helps players learn the two-handed backhand correctly is the inherent use of Key Position Points that the two handed stroke provides during the course of the swing. If these key position points are met, a "proper" two-handed backhand is almost self-working! With only a few exceptions the two-handed backhand is clearly the most similar stroke among the pros. Watch for the similarities of the stroke among all the pros, men and women. You will quickly recognize these key position points in most of them once you have studied them here.

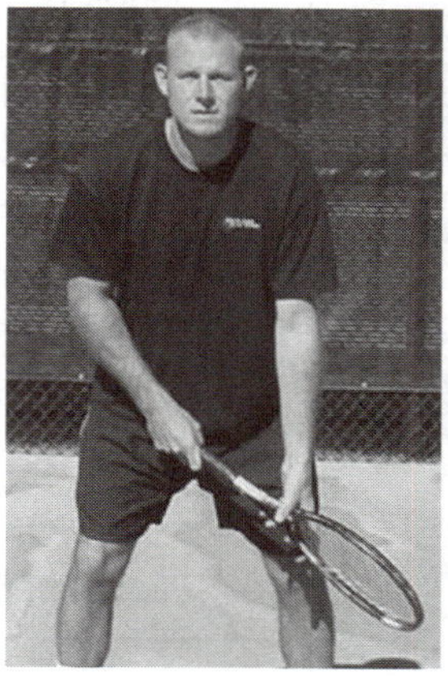

Figure 4
Here Scott has a neutral Continental grip, racket pointed down, and slightly flavoring his backhand side.

READY POSITION

Unlike the volley, which has most shots hit with the racket moving down and forward from high to low in the course of the short stroke, the topspin groundstroke is hit with the racket moving from low to high with the strings brushing up the back of the ball. This difference alone should signify a difference in ready position between the two strokes. Because the racket must get below the ball at some point during the topspin groundstroke, the player can shorten the distance that the racket is taken back during the backswing by lowering the racket head during the ready position. (Figure 4) Depending on the type of backswing used by a player (loop, semi-loop or straight back), the ideal height of the racket during the ready position can vary between players. Many players on tour today point their racket head down towards the ground in their ready position…an unimaginable position a decade or so ago! I will mention this ready position again when I address the backswing later in this section.

One issue in the ready position that can be debated is the position of the off-hand. Some players prefer to position the non-dominant hand at the throat of the racket. From this position the hand can slide down the shaft of the racket during the back swing. (Fig. 4) Lindsay Davenport is an example of a professional using this method. On the other hand, many players will elect to hold the hands together in the backhand position while waiting for the ball. This obviously minimizes the time needed to grasp the proper grip for the two-handed backhand. (See Fig. 5) Refer back to Chpt. 7 for more on the Ready Position.

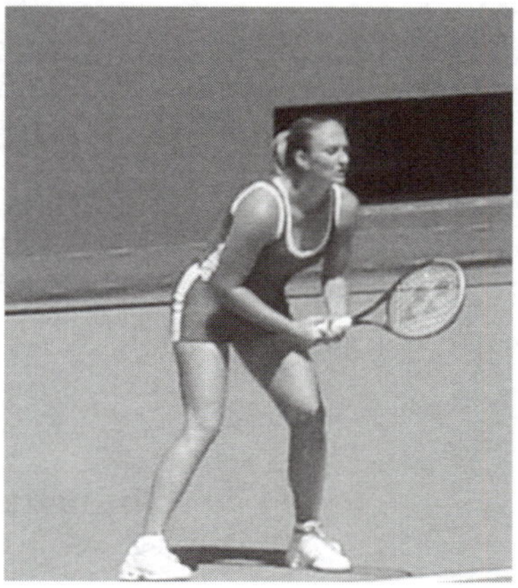

Figure 5
Mary Pierce anticipates the serve with his racket held in the "two-handed backhand' position.
Photo by David Smith

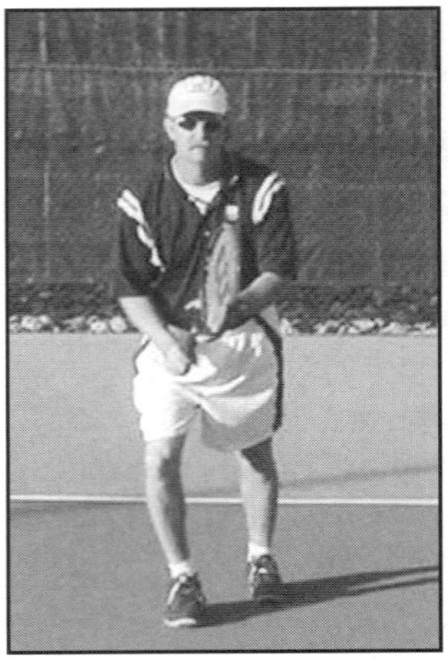

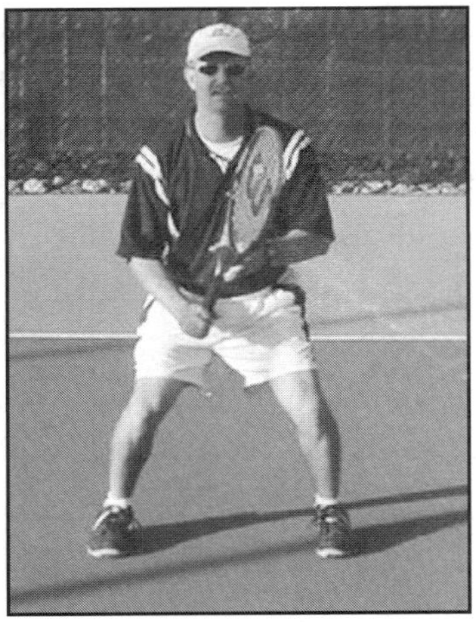

Figure 6 & 7 - "The Split Step"
As the player moves to any position on the court, (in figure 6, the player is approaching the net), just as your opponent hits the ball, you come to a momentary pause, or "split step".

SPLIT-STEP

The most important part of any ready position is the balance of the player just prior to their opponent's contact of their shot. One of the biggest mistakes players make during any point is the lack of a split-step, maintaining the subsequent balance necessary to make a controlled move to the next shot. Next time you watch a match on television, note this move by every player during every point. I have already discussed the split-step in depth in Chapter 7. However, it is such an important part of every shot in tennis that a timely review here in this chapter can be helpful.

Basically, the split-step is accomplished by the player pausing any directional movement with a slight split-step of the feet. (See Figures 6 & 7) This momentarily places the player's center of gravity over both feet and in a position ready to move in any direction deemed necessary by their opponent's shot. Highly accomplished players make this move with extraordinary subtleness and smoothness. However, you will still see this split-step accomplished by watching both feet bounce to this position just prior to their recognition of their opponent's shot followed almost simultaneously by their movement to where the ball will need to be hit. A split-step should be executed prior to every ball hit to you. No matter where you are on the court, it will be crucial to be in a balanced position prior to the recognition of where you will need to be to hit your opponent's next shot.

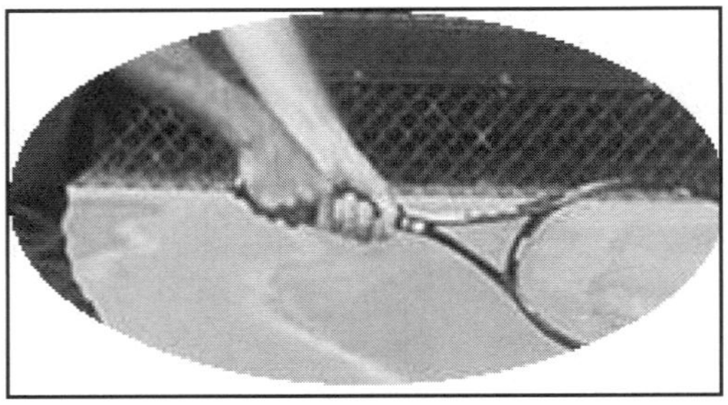

Figure 8
The right hand is continental, the left hand is an Eastern Forehand grip. It is easy to see why the two-handed backhand is often referred to as a "left-handed forehand"!

Grip

(Refer to Chapter 8 on Volleys for additional Grip Information)

The most dominant grips used by top players using a two-handed backhand is a Continental grip on the dominant hand (right hand for right-handed players) and an Eastern forehand grip on the other hand. (See Figure 8) The dominant hand is held at the bottom of the racket handle with the non-dominant hand gripped comfortably just above. (The hands should be touching but not overlapping.) Most two-handed backhands are technically stroked with the same general pattern as a "left-handed forehand" (again for right-handers). There are a few exceptions. Tennis great Jim Courier hit his two-handed backhand with almost the exact same form as most one-handed backhand players hit. (Figure 9) The grip necessary for his type of backhand is an eastern backhand grip for the dominant hand and almost a semi-western grip for the upper hand. Since this grip is somewhat unique to only a few players, most top players today follow the continental/eastern forehand grip combination.

Because the two-handed backhand stroke closely resembles a left-handed forehand, there are a couple of drills I highly recommend to all two-handed backhanders. These drills will help all players become more proficient at hitting the two-handed backhand.

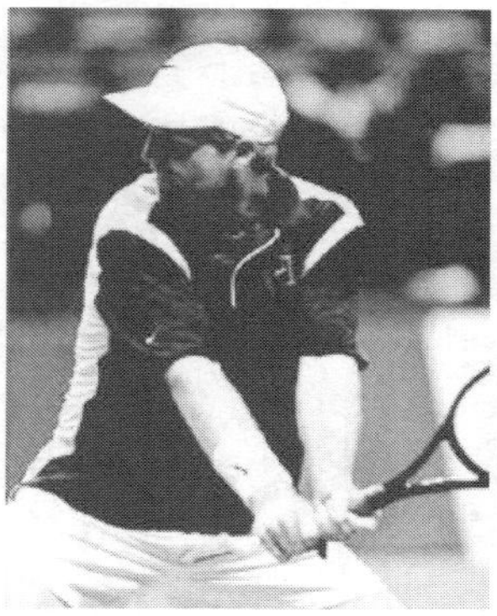

Figure 9
Jim Courier used an Eastern backhand grip on his dominant hand, similar to that used by players hitting a one-handed backhand.

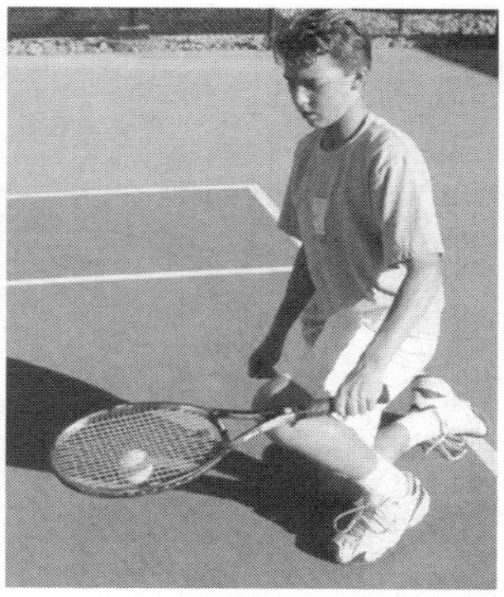

Figure 10
Here, A.J., a right-handed player, is bouncing the ball left-handed with the Eastern forehand grip. This will condition the "off hand" to be more coordinated and skilled for the two-handed backhand.

DRILL #1: BOUNCING DRILL CONTINENTAL

This drill is described in the Volley section.

DRILL #2: LEFT HAND (OR OFF HAND) EASTERN FOREHAND BOUNCES

This is the same drill as #1 except the player uses his or her off hand (left hand for right-handers) and uses an Eastern forehand grip instead of the Continental. Because the two-handed backhand is dominated by the combined use of both the right and left hands, it is equally important that the player train both hands in developing strength and coordination. (See Figure 10)

For right-handers, kneel down on your left or right knee and bounce the ball on your left side or in front of you. Using the Eastern forehand grip the player should attempt to bounce the ball at least 50 or 100 times consecutively. If you have never done this, it will be initially difficult to bounce 10 in a row, let alone 50! However, within a few days of practice you will improve quite quickly. Keep the wrist firm and use the arm instead of a floppy wrist to bounce the ball.

The added coordination you gain from this drill will translate into more precision and skill when you hit your two-handed backhand.

The Two-Handed Backhand Stroke

BACKSWING

After the split-step when the player recognizes the ball will be hit with a backhand, the next move is essential. The shoulders must turn and the arms take the racket back. (Figure 11) For beginners I recommend a "straight back" swing. That is, the racket stays low with the arms straight and the rackethead pointed down towards the ground. (Figure 12) This position is the most efficient in terms of getting into position to hit topspin. Obviously, when the player deems it time to swing at the ball, from this position the racket only needs to

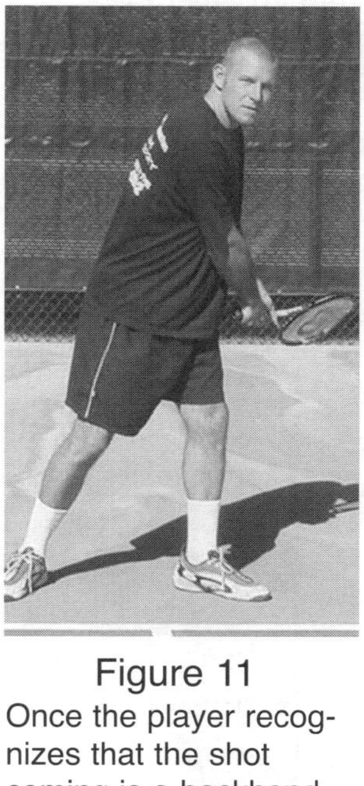

Figure 11
Once the player recognizes that the shot coming is a backhand, the shoulders turn, facilitating the backswing. Note the right shoulder points towards the incoming ball.

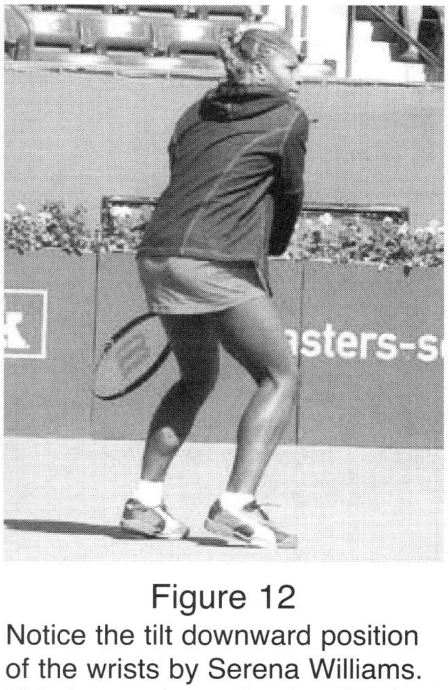

Figure 12
Notice the tilt downward position of the wrists by Serena Williams. This keeps the racket head below the ball prior to contact. The amount of brush upward on the ball will dictate the amount of topspin the player will apply.

come up to the point of contact (unlike the loop back swing where the racket will start above the ball prior to "looping" down below the ball before contact). When a player needs to move to the ball, it is wise to be moving with the racket back in the backswing position. This will allow the player to simply swing forward at the ball when they arrive. Many players will run to the ball only to find themselves having to suddenly take the racket back AND swing at the ball all at once. This is why many beginners and intermediate players feel rushed every time they have to hit a ball! (And why they often find themselves hitting the ball late!) Advanced players have learned to move and get their racket back in position in plenty of time, for most shots. (Which is another reason they are advanced players!) As players do advance, many will incorporate a half-loop, half backswing position instead of the full, straight-back backswing mentioned. This technique does provide greater rhythm and utilizes the slightly more efficient movements associated with the loop. However, I have seen most players have difficulty with racket head control and development of a stable swing pattern when this procedure is attempted first. On the other hand, those players who learn a straight back swing pattern first, almost always are able to evolve their swing into some aspect of a loop without losing control. Obviously, if many of the world's top-ranked players incorporate a straight back swing pattern (among them are #1 and #2 current world-ranked women Serena and Venus Williams!), we can assume that there are few, if any, limitations to this stroke, even at the highest levels! (See Author's Note below.)

During the backswing the wrists should lock the racket in this pointed-down position. The wrists will remain in this position through contact. (See Figures 11, 12, 13 & 14)

Also, during the backswing players will want to flex their knees once they have moved into position to hit the ball. By bending the knees prior to contact, players can move their weight up and forward during contact, adding greater body inertia and force to the stroke. This is not going to make a huge difference in racket speed. However, for advanced players, this small percentage will make a difference in their effort to have an edge over other advanced players.

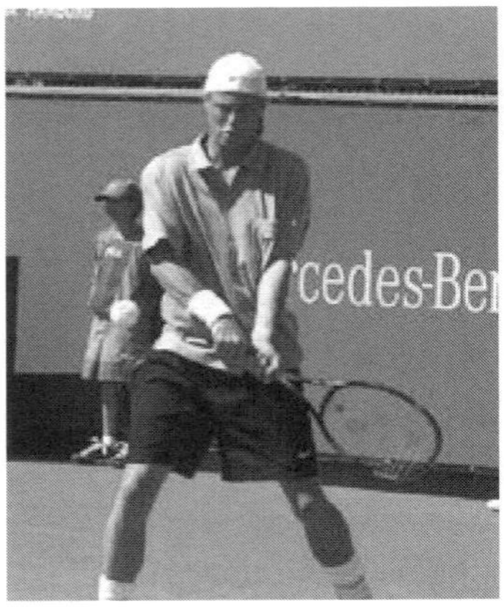

Figure 13
Here, Lleyton Hewitt has his racket head is pointed down. This is the perfect preparation position for the topspin backhand.

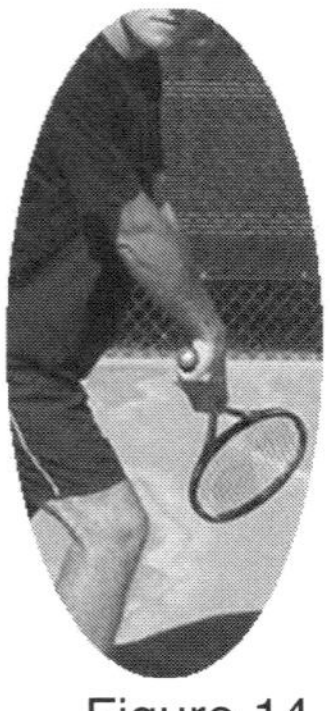

Figure 14
Here, the racket head is pointed down and the racket face is also slightly closed.

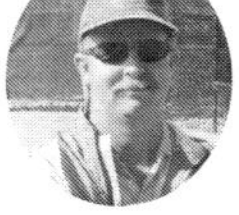

Author's Note

Since most advanced players develop some aspect of the loop swing almost automatically (as their stroke becomes more defined), I generally teach the straight back pattern as the player's foundation. I have found that beginners, who are taught the loop prior to learning how to control their racket head on the backswing, tend to have difficulty deciphering where their racket head is prior to contact. This lack of control limits a beginner's ability to hit topspin properly or consistently.

Loop Swings

Most advanced players create a semi-loop or a full loop backswing. These swings utilize gravity in creating a more continuous swing once the racket starts its backswing. The full loop is created with the racket head taken back high, usually above the shoulders. A semi-loop swing starts the racket back just above the waist. However, the timing of using either loop swing is far more critical due to the racket literally having to change direction in one continuous motion.

The course of the loop swing takes the racket head back

above the waist or above the shoulders (in a full loop backswing). (See Figure 15) As the player continues the swing, the racket head drops down below the ensuing contact point and then is brought back up in one motion to hit the ball. For the most part, this stroke is continuous. However, often players will pause at the backswing, holding the racket at the high point of the loop progression. The downward motion and subsequent brushing up of the ball then are done as one sequence.

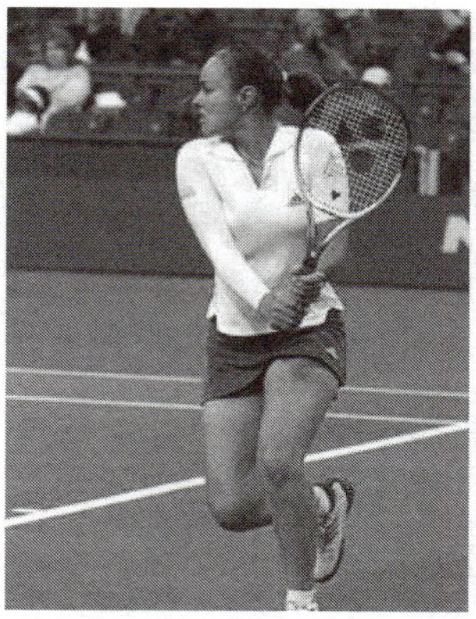

Figure 15
Martina Hingis prepares to hit her backhand with a significant loop backswing. Note the high racket head position at her shoulder's

Often, a common problem associated with players learning the loop swing too early in their development is an inability to get the racket head down below the ball prior to contact. This results in the player hitting the ball too flat or with underspin instead of the desired topspin.

Generally, players will develop a natural loop in their swing as they progress. Players can add the loop component easily if they learned the "straight-back" backswing first.

KEY POSITION POINT #1

The hands drop down near the left hip at this backswing point. (Figures 13 & 15) For added emphasis on learning how to hit topspin, the player can bend their knees and actually have the racket head nearly touching the ground on the backswing. (By actually touching the ground, this can give the player a physical attribute to which to associate the backswing.) Many players have difficulty locating their racket once it is taken back on the backswing. Former baseball or softball players are notorious for bringing the racket up high on the backswing since the movement is so closely associated with taking the bat back in baseball. + squash players!

KEY POSITION POINT #2

The wrists tilt downward allowing the racket head to drop well below the contact point. (See Figures 12, 13 & 14) The more the racket head is pointed down below the wrists, the more topspin is available to the player, (as long as the head of the racket doesn't rise up prior to the start of the forward motion of the stroke).

A very important point during the backswing is that the racket face (the hitting side of the strings) is NOT facing up. (See Figure 14) If the racket face is open at this point, the player will either have to roll the face of the racket closed during the contact phase or end up hitting the ball sky high. As a general rule of thumb, the angle of the racket face should be pointed down at an angle between 5 and 15 degrees. Generally, players who want to hit a lot of topspin on their backhand will add the greater amount of tilt downward of the racket face during the backswing. The more the racket is tilted down, the more the vertical path the racket will need to take in hitting the ball.

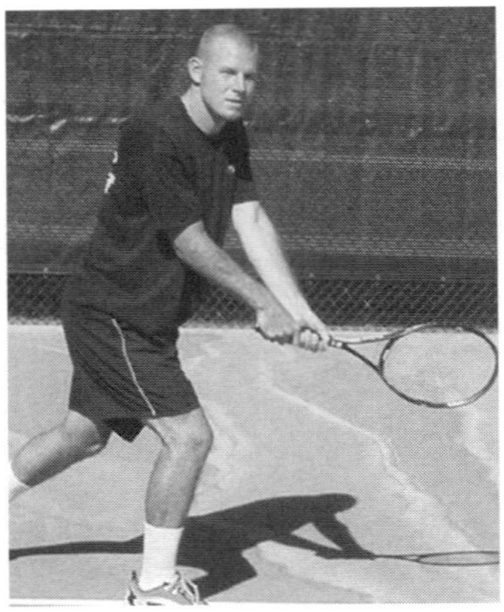

Figure 16
Closed Stance Backhand. For right-handed players, the right foot will step into the shot, across the body.

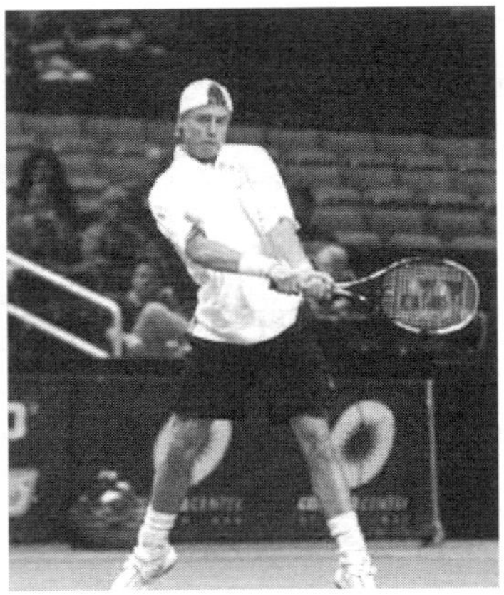

Figure 17
An "Open Stance" backhand. The upper body must coil and turn sideways to the on-coming ball.

CONTACT

After a player has gotten the racket back and has properly moved to the ball, he will now swing the racket upward and forward to contact the ball. With the two-handed backhand, this is almost self-working. From the low backswing position the arms move together towards the point of contact. The wrists remain locked in the same position as they were during the backswing.

Just prior to contact, the right foot will step forward and slightly across the body. This "Closed Stance" position helps prevent the player from opening the hips and shoulders too early. (See Figure 16)

Advanced Notes: A move now being made by a number of advanced players is a backhand being hit with an "Open Stance" position at contact. Research has shown that more power can be generated if this open stance is used properly. The key to a proper use of the open stance is a complete upper body turn. (See Figure 17) If the shoulders don't turn all the way (perpendicular to the net or more), the player will either pull the ball too far to the right or the player will end up pushing the ball out away from his or her body towards the target in a very ineffective move.

NOTES ON OPEN STANCE GROUNDSTROKES

An open stance groundstroke does create greater torque for the body to use during the course of a swing. (Greater torque can produce greater power.) However, because we seldom ever hit a ball as hard as we can, the question I pose to players is, "If this move for beginner players does not produce accurate strokes, will more power be an advantage or disadvantage?" Obviously, more power used on inaccurate strokes will produce far more errors. Players who learn the more conventional closed stance backhand (and forehand for that matter) will be able to transition easily to the open stance stroke if this is desired. This is because the closed stance provides a better method of learning how the shoulders and upper body turn in preparation for the shot.

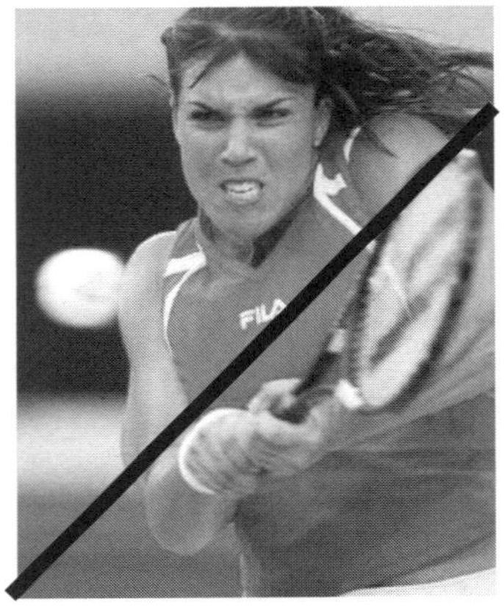

Figure 18
The dominant arm (right arm here) remains close to the body at contact. Note the similar line from elbow to racket tip.

KEY POSITION POINT #3

For right-handed players, the right elbow will stay fairly close to the body at contact. The right elbow bends as the racket moves up to strike the ball. (See Figures 16 - 21) The left arm can stay relatively straight (Figure 16 & 17) or be bent (Figure 18, 19, 20, & 21) at contact. This combination of the elbow close to the body and the left arm driving through the ball creates a proper racket plane of motion for topspin. If the racket head remains below the ball prior to contact, utilizing this Key Position Point will insure topspin on your backhand..

Parallel Plane

In most two-handed swing patterns there is an identifiable Key Position Point where the forearm runs parallel with the mid-line of the racket. This is true for low, mid, and high balls.

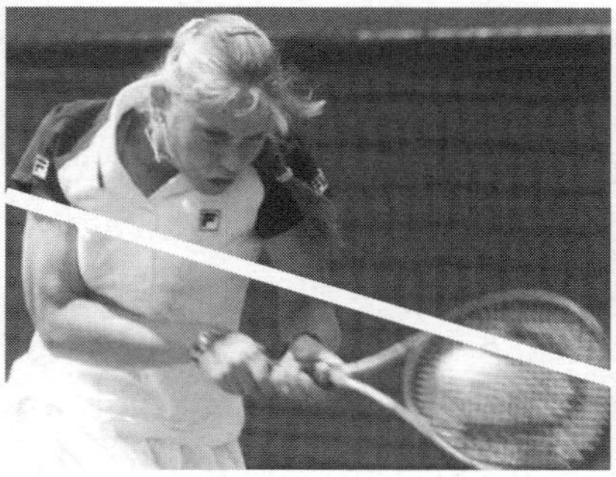

Figure 19

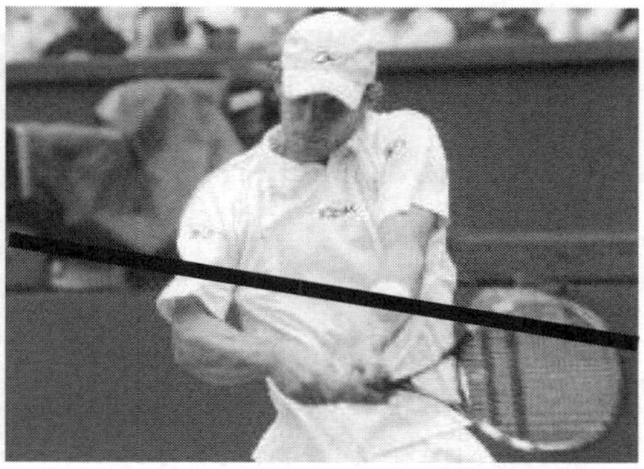

Figure 20

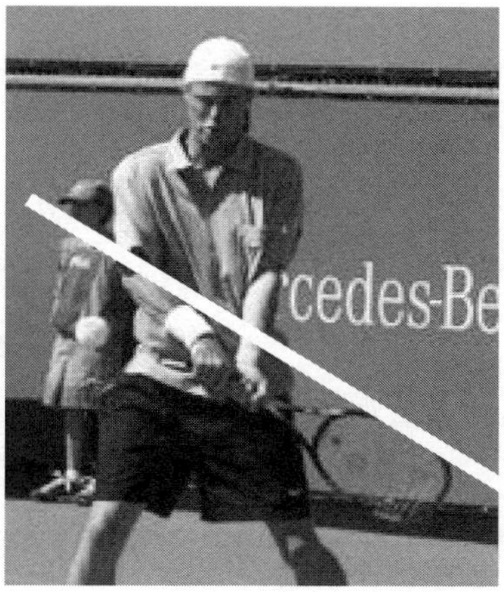

Figure 21
As most all skilled two-handed players near contact, the position of the racket is held in a virtual straight line from the dominant elbow drawn to the tip of the racket.

KEY POSITION POINT #4

With the two handed backhand, there is a commonality among skilled player where there is nearly a straight line extending from the elbow to the tip of the racket as the racket moves through the contact phase. (See Figures 19 - 21.) This position allows for the non-dominant hand to work as if it were hitting as a one-handed forehand. The tilt of the wrist of the dominant hand, (and the use of a continental grip), allows for this position to be achieved.

Follow-through

As the arms move through the contact point, the left arm will pull the racket up over the right forearm. Because the right elbow is the pivot point for the swing, the left arm (along with the right forearm and hand) acts as the force needed to hit the ball. (Figure 22) It is important for the player NOT to break the wrist and forearm position through the contact point. Players sometimes "flick" the left hand over the right hand causing the racket face to change position at contact point. This "rolling" the racket over the ball is very inaccurate.

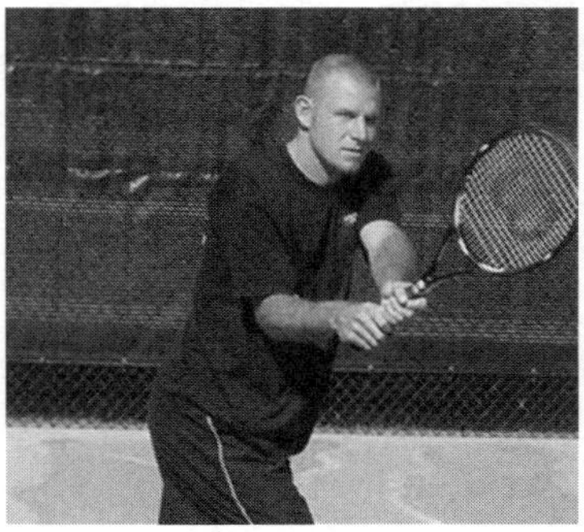

Figure 22
Note the pivot point of the stroke around the dominant arm's elbow. The left hand helps drive the racket up and through the ball.

$E=MC^2$

PHYSICS NOTE

This relationship of the arms and racket create a third-class lever. The object of a third-class lever is to create speed of the applied force. The strings of the racket apply the force of the hands and arms (and body as we will discuss in a moment) to the ball.

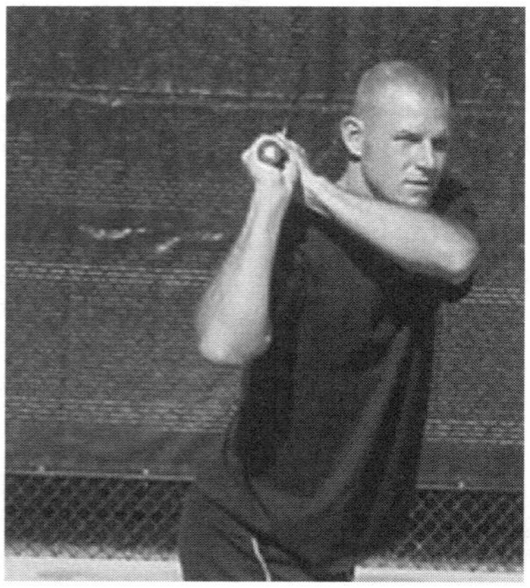

Figure 23
During the follow-through, the racket continues up and over the right shoulder.

After the ball has left the strings, the arms continue in a relaxation phase of the stroke. The left arm continues up and the right elbow usually will lift up away from the side of the body. (Figure 23)

Two of the biggest mistakes players make in attempting the two-handed backhand is (1) they pull the dominant elbow across the body during contact, or, (2) they lead with the right elbow pulling the racket through contact with the right arm. Both of these actions contribute to poor form and little, if any, topspin.

KEY POSITION POINT #5

The left arm continues up during the relaxation phase to the point where the biceps of the left arm come up to the chin of the player.

A great tool for teaching little kids is to say, "kiss your biceps" (on their non-dominant arm) on the follow-through. This gives the kids an exact point where their arm must finish on the follow-through. (See Figures 23 & 24)

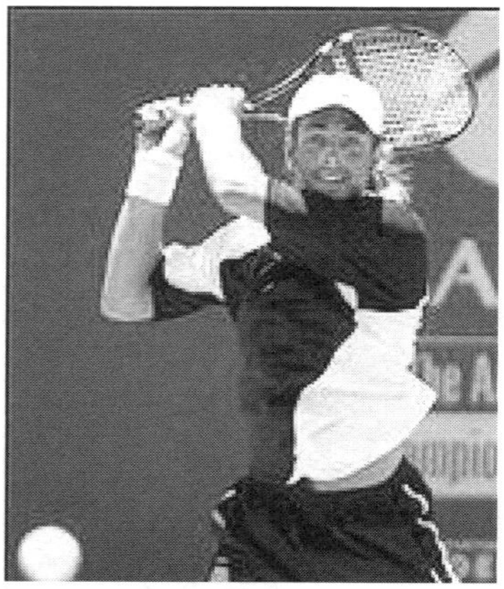

Figure 24
Note that the finish of the backhand brings the non-dominant arm's bicep directly to the chin of the player. "Kiss the bicep" tool is an excellent way to have players understand where their arm needs to be after contact.

Footwork Blunders

The most notorious fault for players when executing groundstrokes (forehand or backhand) is allowing their legs to swing around, opening up their body. This error is caused when either the back foot sweeps around the body during contact or the front foot pulls back. As you can see, either move will open up the hips and the shoulders early. This results in the player pulling the shot to the right on the backhand. The player's body usually recognizes this result subconsciously, and the player ends up pushing the ball back towards the target in an abbreviated swing. Doing this enough times, the player begins to develop this pushing type stroke as their main backhand and fails to produce strokes that can improve and be effective.

To help train the player's body in preventing this over-rotation due to the back leg swinging around, it is very helpful to "drag the toe" for a moment after contact.

Another fundamental flaw created by this opening up of the body

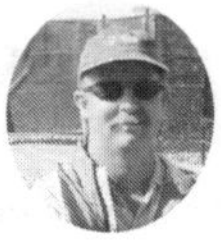

Author's Note
Brake Step after Tog-Drag

As I will mention later, skilled players will swing the back leg around after contact in what is called a "Brake Step." However, it is important to establish completion of the main contact portion of the swing prior to this back leg swinging out. This is accomplished by dragging the toe momentarily at contact. (See Figure 25) After contact and toe-drag, the player can release this back leg and make a break step. (See Figure 26)

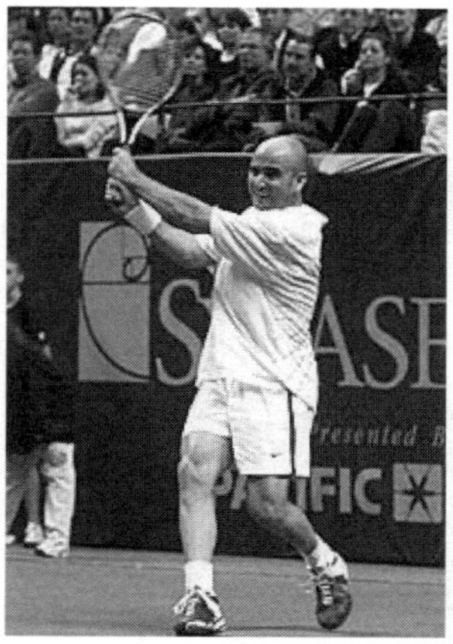

Figure 25
Note the back foot "Toe Drag" at contact anad during follow-through.

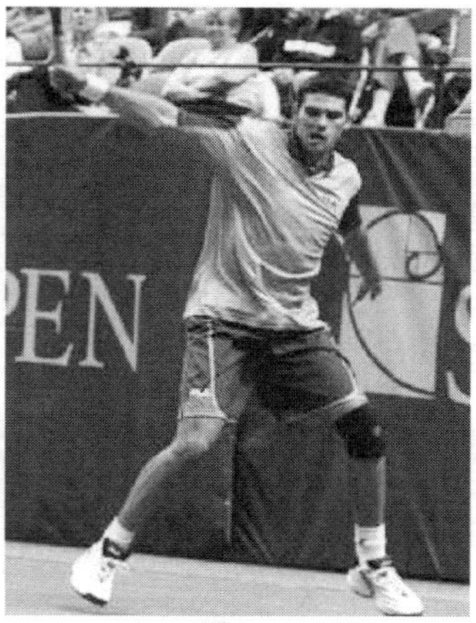

Figure 26
Here, Mark Philippoussis releases his back left leg after contact has been made on his one-handed backhand

during the swing is that the player actually uses the speed of the body turning as their racket speed. That is, the racket moves through the stroke at approximately the same speed as the body is turning. This produces an incredibly slow swing. (While some instances a player may utilize this swing pattern for a difficult shot, for control, players who develop this stroke pattern as their normal swing seldom progress groundstrokes to their optimal potential.)

The exception to this procedure is when a player, usually skilled, keeps their upper body closed while either hitting an open stance stroke or executing what we call a "reverse pivot". This move swings out the lower body, usually as a fast recovery step to get back in position for the next shot. However, the timing of this footwork pattern is done just after contact, not before.

Body Rotation

I have purposely left the issue of body rotation for the end of this section. There are several reasons for this. First of all, the body rotation (the act of turning the shoulders or upper body during the course of the swing) is basically self-working if a player executes the stroke as described in this chapter. The position of the two-handed backhand sets up the shoulders correctly when the racket is taken back. When the player executes the swing to hit the ball, the body rotation through to contact is usually correct. A player need not emphasize the rotation back. Typically, when a player consciously tries to utilize the proper body rotation, they tend to do it much too early. Also, body rotation produces only a small percentage of rackethead speed even when correctly applied. It is the combined movements of the body, legs, and arms that provide the quality of stroke speed. Players who sacrifice stroke form in the name of additional body rotation end up defeating the proper stroke intention.

Body rotation refers to the "kinetic chain" of larger muscle groups working in harmony with smaller muscle groups in the course of an athletic move. As you have noticed, I did mention during the backswing instruction that the shoulders and upper body do turn sideways (with the right shoulder pointing usually towards the net or on-coming ball). The act of the arms working in the correct sequence mentioned will institute the correct body rotation for most players.

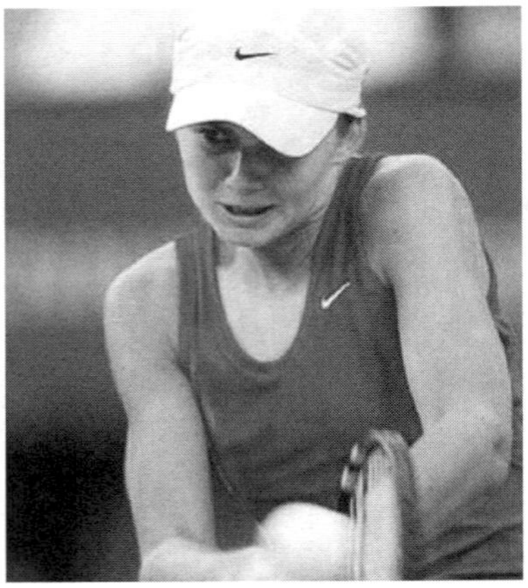

Figure 28
Here, Daniela Hantuckhova is making contact yet her body rotation is still sideways facing the camera.

One-Quarter Turn Principle

Beginning players tend to over-rotate, especially at contact and follow-through, when first learning to hit the two-handed backhand. Generally speaking, the maximum preparation turn and recoil from that turn is ninety degrees or one-quarter turn. Observe the vast majority of top players and you will notice that although the racket moves almost (and sometimes greater than) 360 degrees around the body, the actual turn of the body is one quarter. That is to say, the shoulders start by facing the net, followed by the body (or shoulders) turning sideways prior to contact. (Figures 27 & 28)

At contact, players will generally slow down this rotation back to the net, which speeds up the arms through the swing path. Like cracking a whip, the slowing down of the large muscle groups allows for the arms to speed up. After contact is made, the inertia of the swing will bring the shoulders and hips further around.

At conclusion of the follow-through, the body finishes facing the net. Occasionally, you will observe the pros recoil greater than their starting point. This exaggerated over-rotation is usually a result of a greater force applied to the ball. The body's natural inertia carries them past this one-quarter return. However, it is important to notice that at contact the body seldom is over-rotated as we see so often in beginner and intermediate players.

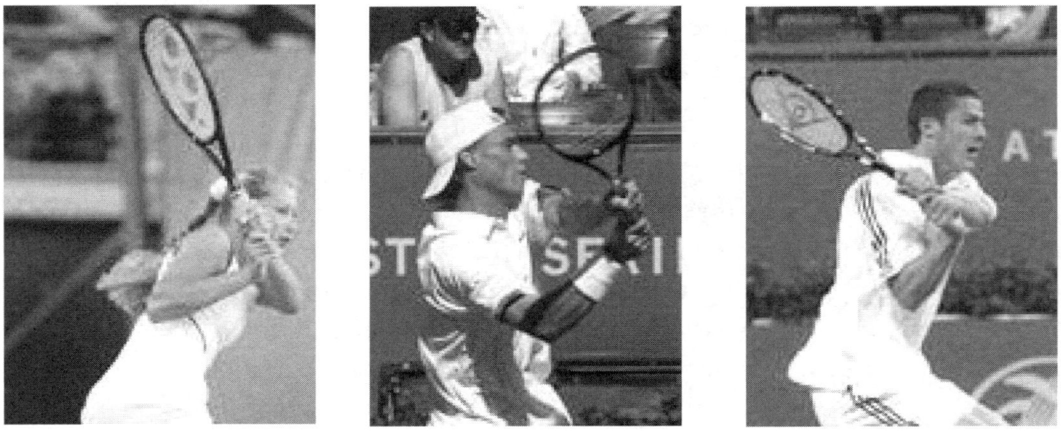

Figures 29, 30, & 31
Note these three pictures demonstrate the body's position after contact has been made. The hips remain almost perpendicular to the net while the racket has pulled the upper body around, back to our starting position (of facing the net.) While each player's position is decidedly different due to where the ball is, note the similarities of the hips, shoulders, and racket.

Two-Handed Backhand Sequence Review

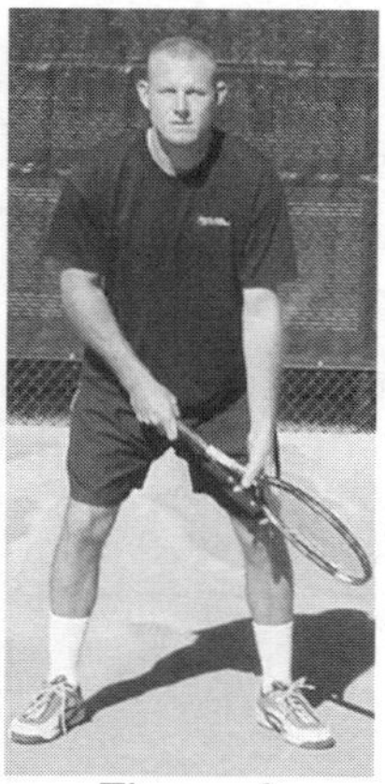
Figure A

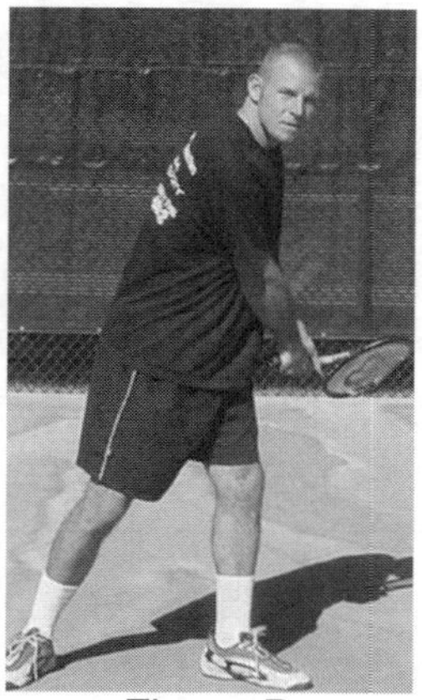
Figure B

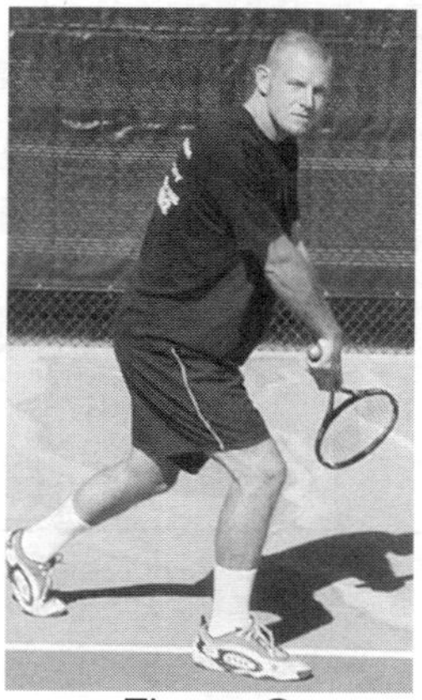
Figure C

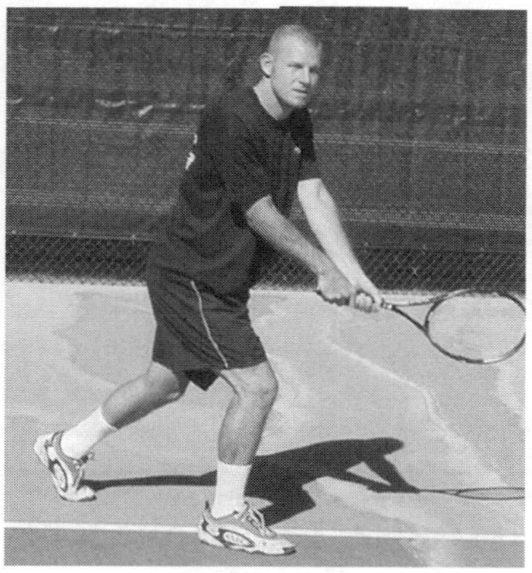
Figure D

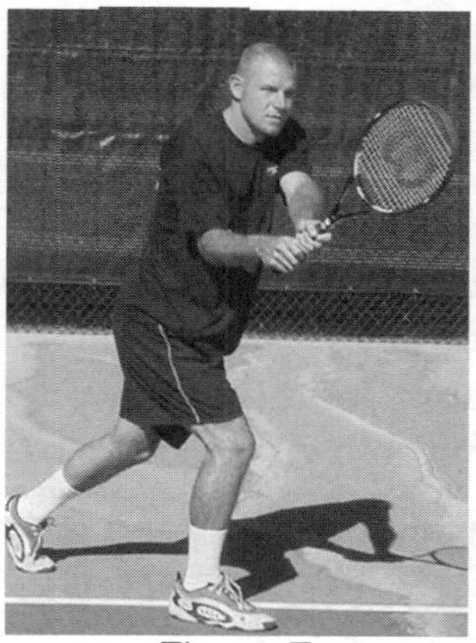
Figure E

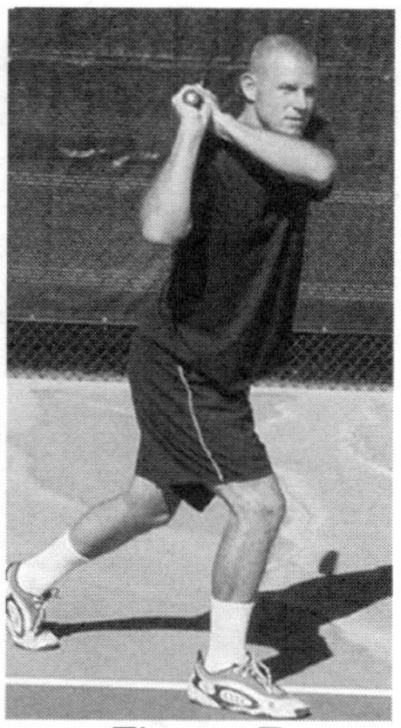
Figure F

In this sequence of pictures, notice the right shoulder's complete movement during the execution of the two-handed topspin backhand. The upper body makes one-quarter turn sideways followed by the same one-quarter turn back after follow-through. Notice, too, that the racket makes almost a 360-degree swing around the body in the process.

One-handed Backhand

Hitting the backhand with one hand offers some advantages in terms of reach and freedom of movement. However, as I have mentioned, these same advantages are the reasons that players who often learn the one-handed backhand never develop their backhand as a weapon. Because we can reach out and hit one-handed utilizing minimal footwork and generally poor form, players tend to not get in the right position for hitting the stroke…resulting in questionable technique. Likewise, because the one-handed backhand does not have the second hand on the racket for stability, one-handers, (who have not developed proper form and technique), often

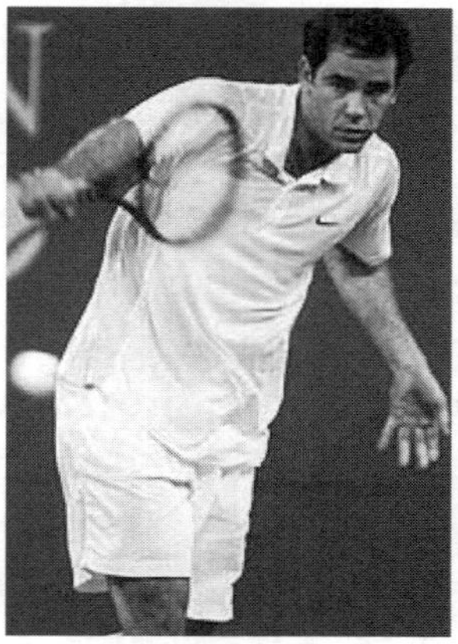
Figure 32
A skilled one-handed backhand is in many ways quite different than the two-handed backhand. Yet there are similarities between the two shots as well.

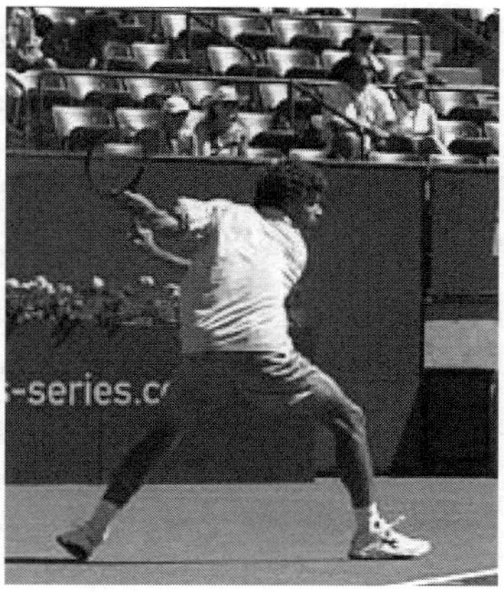

Figure 33
Gustavo Kuerten prepares his strong one-handed backhand by tuning his upper body, stepping into the shot with his right leg and an early loop backswing.

are seen slashing and hacking their backhand with little or none of the refinement we associate with a reliable backhand.

Because most beginners are now taught the two-handed backhand, we are seeing fewer and fewer one-handed backhands on tour. And those players hitting the backhand one-handed on tour often learned by hitting the two-handed shot first. Because there are still many beginner and intermediate players that began learning their backhand with one hand, those who wish to learn the two-hander have difficulty trying to make a change to the two-handed backhand. Thus, I am providing the proper techniques used to master the one-handed backhand here in this section for those who wish to hit one-handed.

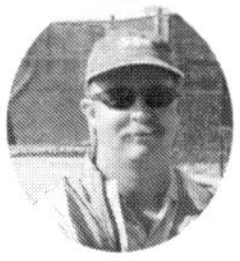

Author's Note

Many 3.0 and 3.5 players who use a one-handed backhand use such unorthodox form that they have to resort to unorthodox strategies when hitting it. If these strategies prevent the player from improving, I usually recommend "overhauling" their backhand. That is, start from scratch and develop the two-handed form described in this chapter. Even though this will take time and effort, it will eventually result in the player hitting a backhand that will provide sustained improvement in both the stroke and in the strategy they will be able to employ when they begin hitting a more formidable backhand.

BASIC ONE-HANDED BACKHAND TECHNIQUE

Much like the one-handed forehand, there is a great deal of variety exhibited among players who hit the one-handed backhand. Historically, the one-handed backhand has seen a shift from the continental grip (used predominantly in the 60's) to a full Eastern backhand grip used among many of the top players today. There are a few players on tour who do opt to use a continental grip for their one-handed backhand. However, most of the one-handed backhand players we see on tour now use the more powerful full Eastern backhand grip. (See Figures 32 & 33)

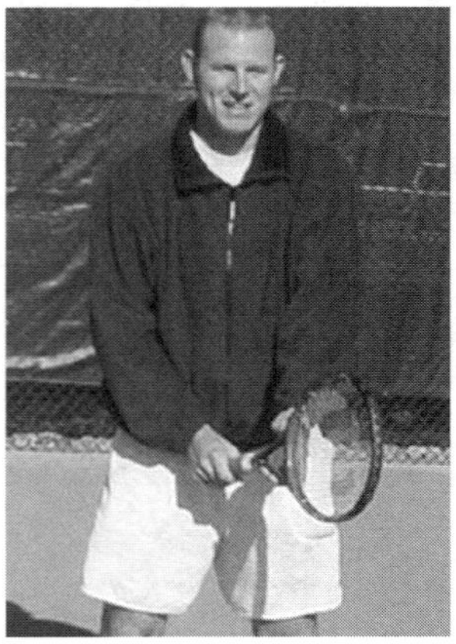

Figure 34
This is a neutral grip position featuring a Continental grip and the off hand cradling the racket at the throat.

Ready Position

There is no change in the ready position as described earlier in the two-handed backhand section. The player will want to make sure the off-hand is positioned at the throat of the racket to help facilitate the proper grip and backswing as will be described below. Because most advanced players today

In hitting the slice backhand, almost without exception, pros and skilled players alike use a continental grip. I will address the slice backhand later in this section.

change to the Eastern Backhand grip for their backhand, some players like to hold this position at the ready position. These players feel more comfortable making the grip change from the backhand to the forehand grip when the ball does comes to their forehand. However, some players prefer to hold either a neutral Continental grip or an Eastern Forehand grip and make the adjustment for the backhand during the backswing. (See Figure 34) Each of these grip positions is entirely acceptable for building your backhand foundation. The key is that any change should be done immediately during the backswing.

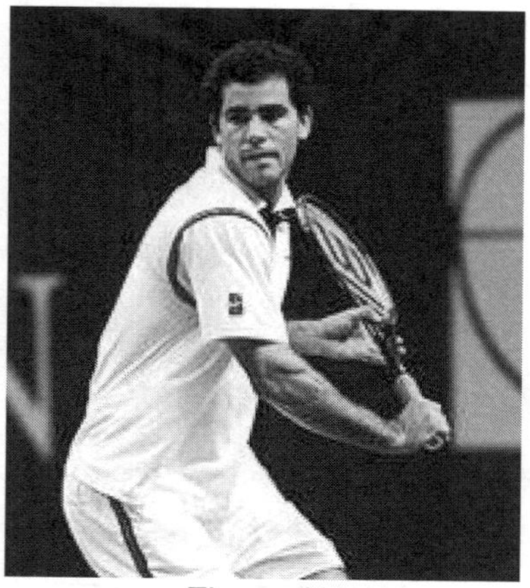

Figure 35
With the exception of the grip change to the Eastern backhand grip and the off-hand's position, the one-handed backswing has similar characteristics to that of the two-handed backhand.

BACKSWING

The one-handed backswing is similar to the two-handed backhand. I recommend that the player use the off-hand to help take the racket back. (Figure 35) This hand also acts as a stabilizer so the dominant hand can make the grip change if needed. Also, players who don't use the off-hand in making the backswing often lose control of the racket's head when making the turn. These players traditionally take the racket back too high or let the wrist flex or allow too much play in the racket head during the swing.

SHOULDER ROTATION

Because the two-handed backhand creates the proper shoulder turn during the back swing, little conscious control is needed to rotate the proper shoulder turn with that stroke.

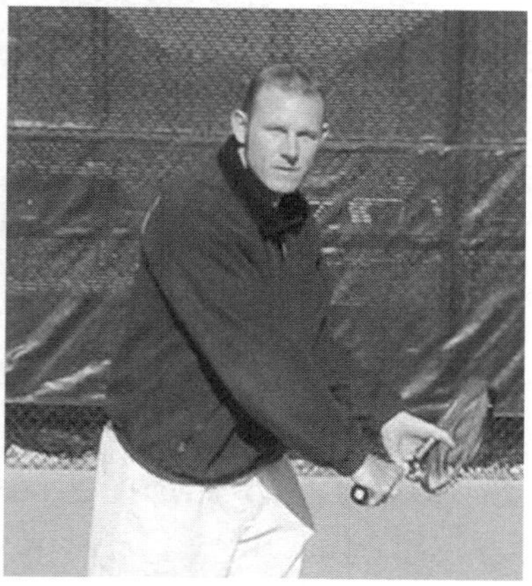

Figure 36
Here Scott starts his backswing by taking his racket straight back and turning the shoulders. Note the position of the racket face, slightly pointed down..

KEY POSITION POINT #6

While learning, it is a good tip to try and keep the racket face pointed slightly down during the backswing. (Figure 36) If the racket face is open (with the strings pointed up), the player will have to roll the racket face to a flat or slightly closed position just prior to contact. As I have mentioned before, the rolling of the racket through contact for any stroke will reduce the consistency and reliability of any shot.

However, with the one-handed backhand, players often only take the racket back with the arm and remain somewhat fixed in facing the net. Most top one-handed players will take the racket back with almost the same mechanics as a two-handed stroke. (See Figures 38 – 43 below.) Generally, the non-dominant hand cradles the racket at the throat throughout the backswing component. This position helps bring the right shoulder (for right-handers) sideways, pointing towards the target. This point of the backswing is critical in order to produce the proper setup for the remaining parts of the backhand. (Figure 37 & 38)

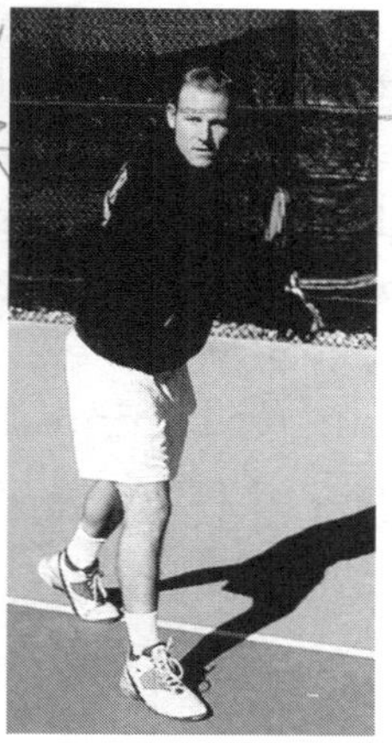

Figure 37
Proper shoulder turn on the backswing and the closed-step footwork pattern

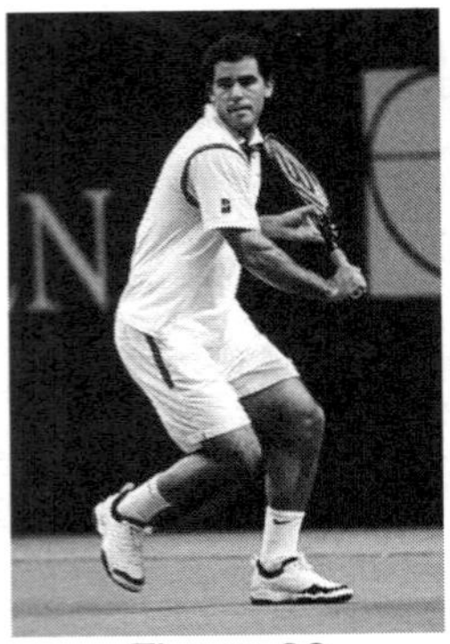

Figure 38

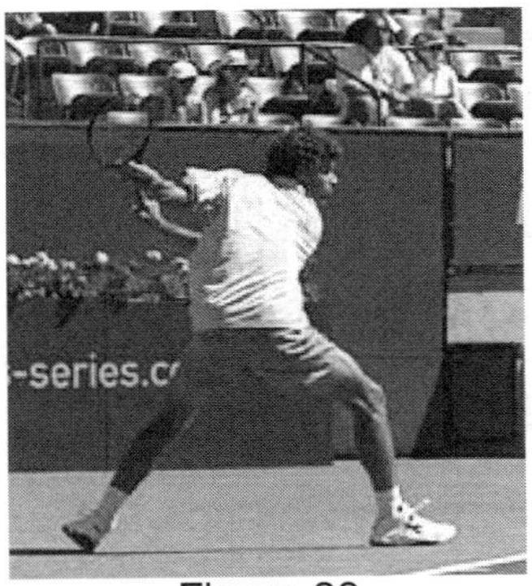

Figure 39

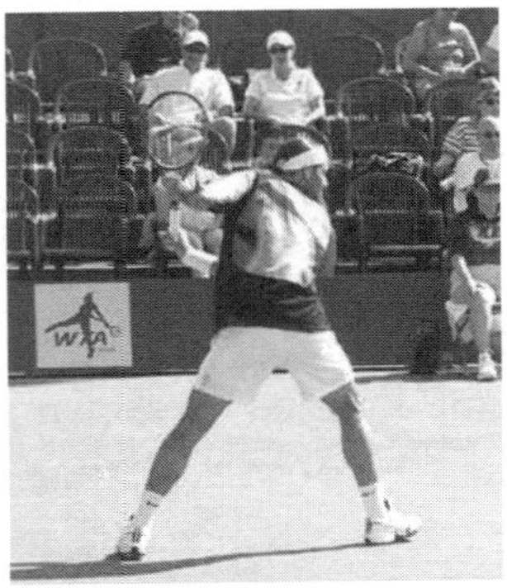

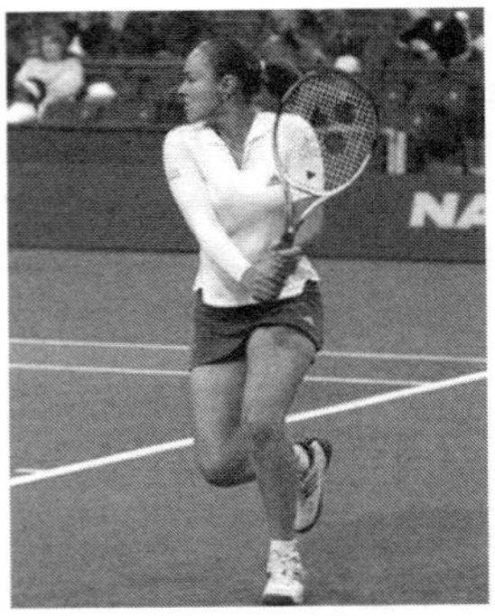

Figure 41

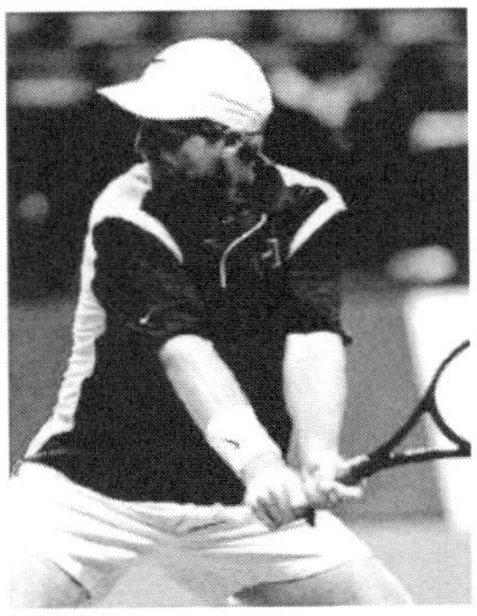

Figure 42

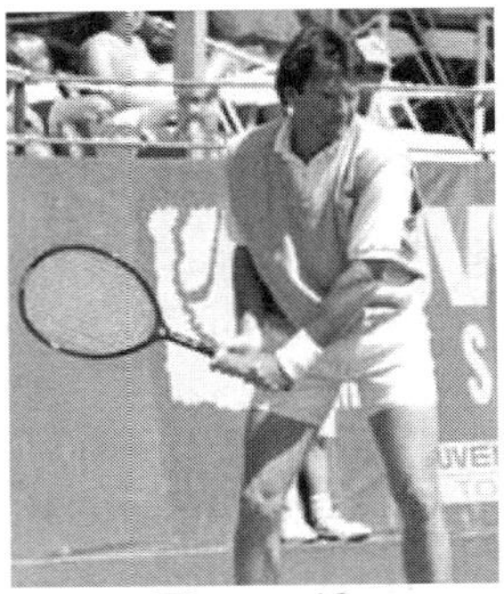

Figure 43

Note the similarities between the one-handed backhand backswing in the pictures above, (Figures 38 – 40) to the two-handed backswing in the lower pictures. (Figures 41 – 43.) Except for the off-hand's position, both backswing techniques are quite similar. The shoulder turn and the hips, the arm positions and footwork are all closely comparable to both swing patterns.

Contact and Footwork

Just like in any topspin stroke, the racket head must start below the ball prior to contact. As mentioned in the two-handed stroke, the racket head should drop down during the backswing with the wrist tilting down. It is at this point the wrist should lock and the racket motion should be generated by a combination of a firm arm and slight body rotation.

The contact point should be further out in front of the body than the two-handed backhand, anywhere from 6 to 10 inches in front of the front knee. (See Figures 45 & 46) Within these parameters, the more out in front contact can be made, the more the player can hit strong, sharp angle, crosscourt shots. At contact, the racket will be held almost at a 90 degree angle to the forearm with the racket strings moving up and through the center point on the back side of the ball. It is sometimes helpful to imagine hitting slightly around the outside of the ball. This helps create the proper stroke pattern. Many players will lead too much with the hitting hand causing the racket to make contact behind the hand resulting in late contact. (This error is one of the leading causes of tennis elbow!)

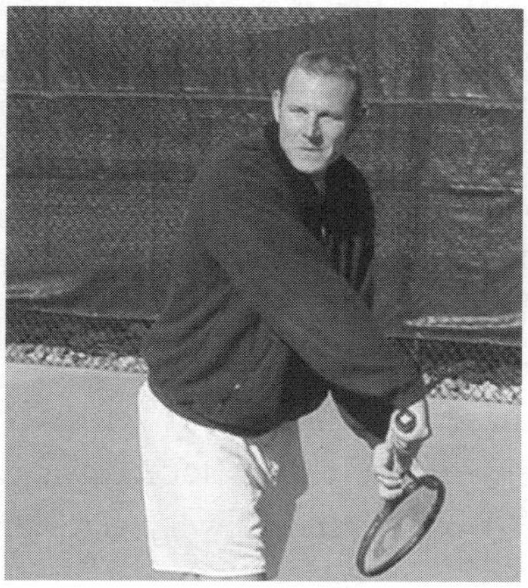

Figure44
With the full shoulder turn complete and the step into the ball, the racket will start down below the ball.

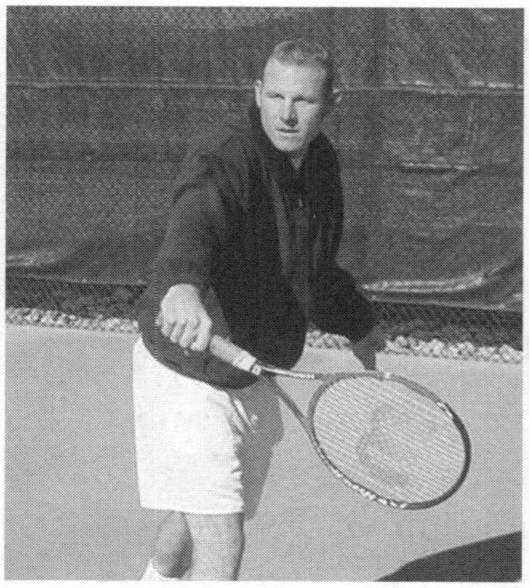

Figure 45
Contact with the one-handed backhand is much further in front of the player than the two-handed backhand.

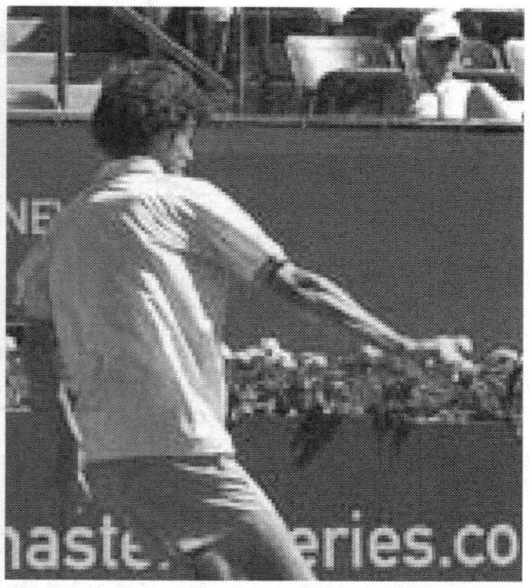

Figure 46
Gustavo Kuerten maintains a partially open stance in this backhand. Note the strong hitting arm position.

The footwork of the one-hand backhand can incorporate a closed crossover step or stance, (Figure 44 & 45) or an open stance. (Figure 46) I highly recommend the student learn and develop their foundation with the closed stance. This position teaches the player not to over-rotate during contact and helps create greater control on both crosscourt and down-the-line shots. Players who step out with the non-dominant foot for the backhand (open stance) tend not to get their upper torso turned enough sideways. However, it is fairly easy for players who have mastered the close stance stroke to begin hitting with a proper open stance backhand. In fact, it is another natural progression for most players who learn the closed stance backhand to evolve to the open stance backhand as competitive experience dictates.

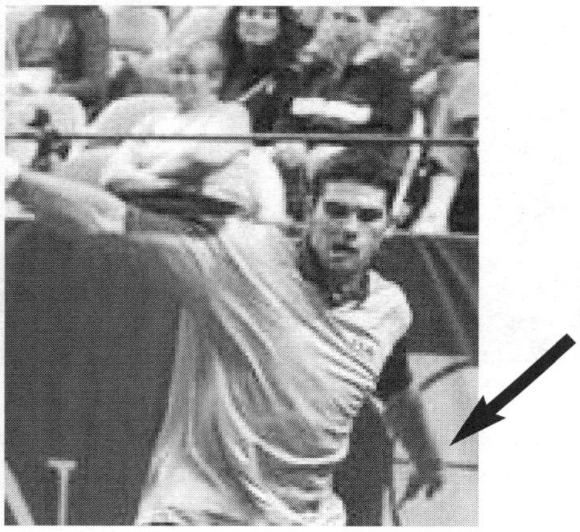

Figure 47
Observe the back arm extending back dramatically as the hitting arm drives up and out around the body.

KEY POSITION POINT #7

As a skilled player begins their swing up through their backhand, typically the non-dominant arm will move back. This move is similar to an umpire making an exaggerated "SAFE" signal in baseball. (See Figures 47 & 51) This move of the non-dominant arm helps keep the player from over-rotating through the shot. This movement of the arms is even more apparent during the slice backhand which will be discussed a little later.

"Keep the plane the same"

If I had to pick my favorite and most valuable condensed phrase, this is it. It literally describes the racket face as it should be during the contact point of virtually every shot in tennis. When hitting the one-handed backhand, one of the biggest faults made by players is the tendency to flick the wrist or roll the racket face over the ball at contact. It has been proven that the ball is not on the strings long enough that any of these movements will make a measurable difference in spin. What these extraneous movements actually do is create inconsistency at contact. Any movement of the racket face during contact will change the relationship of the strings to the ball on virtually every stroke. Thus, aiming will be of minimal help. (Figures 48 – 50)

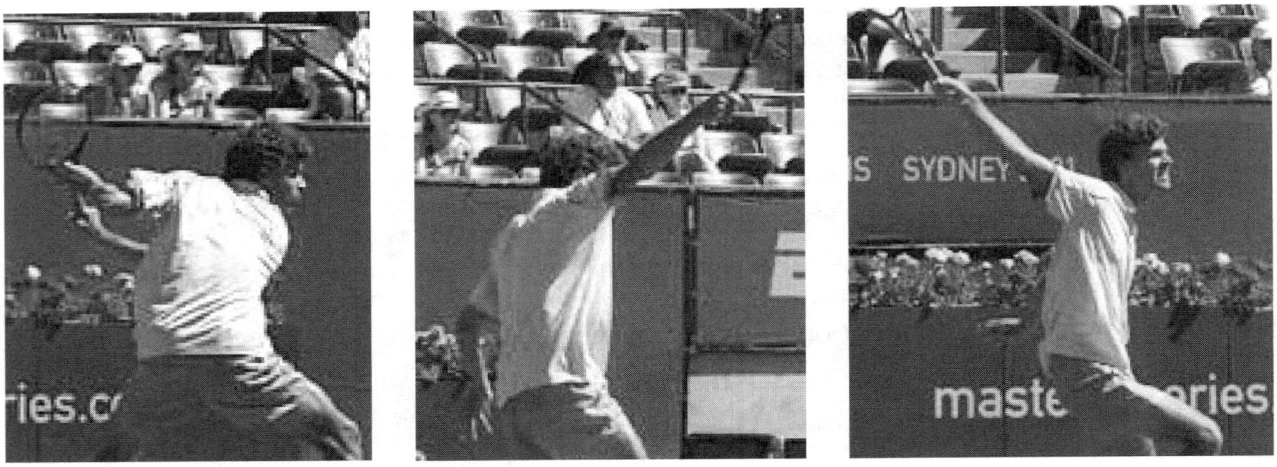

Figures 48 - 50

In this sequence of backhands by Gustavo Kuerten, note the racket face continues in the same plane from start to finish. Also look for these Key Position Points: Closed stance; shoulder rotation on backswing; sideways position through contact; toe drag after contact; body balance through contact; long finish well after contact.

Here is an example of why aiming is difficult when players roll the racket face through contact: If a player, hitting their backhand with the racket face rolling over the ball, hits the ball late, the ball will tend to go too high. (The racket face was too open at contact.) Seeing the ball go long or too high, our player now aims lower on the next shot. However, if on a subsequent backhand, the player hits the ball too early and the racket face has rolled too far and over the ball, the player's shot will end up going into the net. Thus, in this scenario, the player's attempt to aim was a lost cause.

This illustration certainly magnifies how a common fault can lead to a player's lack of confidence! The solution to this problem is to develop a swing pattern that keeps the plane of the racket (the string face) the consistent on each and every swing. Now, if a player hits the ball too high or too low (or too far left or right), the player can aim accordingly on subsequent shots and have a certain amount of confidence that the ball will do what they want it to do.

Follow-through

Because the contact point is further in front of the body and doesn't utilize the off hand to help drive the racket through and up the back of the ball, the follow-through is generally longer and not as much wrap around the body as the two-handed backhand.

For a solid topspin backhand, it is important that the follow-through is strong and full, allowing the racket head to generate momentum and acceleration through contact. Players who tend to cut their follow-through short generally have to decelerate the racket quickly. These players tend to push the backhand instead of driving the ball with topspin.

Similar to the two-handed backhand, it is important to keep your rear leg back through contact. Equally important is to not step out of the backhand early with the front foot. Both these moves open the body too early during the stroke. Most skilled players work to pause their feet at contact, in most cases, to maintain the integrity of the body during contact. (See Figures 49 & 51)

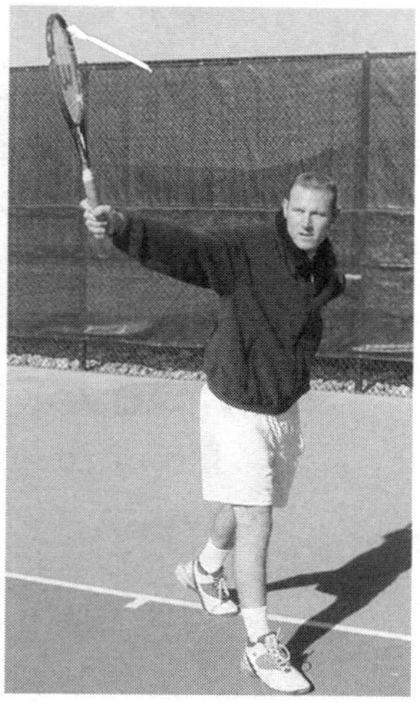

Figure 51
As the arm finishes the stroke, the body has remained sideways with the back toe still down on the ground.

During contact and follow-through, the off arm moves in the opposite direction from the hitting arm. This spreading apart of the arms helps maintain a solid sideways body position through the contact point. When players fail to use this hitting tip, they notoriously try to swing the racket through with their upper body, pulling the racket across themselves instead of up and through the target line.

Slice Backhand

Prior to this point, all the instructional backhand information has described hitting with topspin. Because topspin allows a player to hit balls that clear the net with greater error room and yet with high velocities, we see a far greater number of top players hitting predominately topspin backhands. However, the slice backhand also offers several advantages and strategies, making it a stroke that every good player should master. (Figure 52)

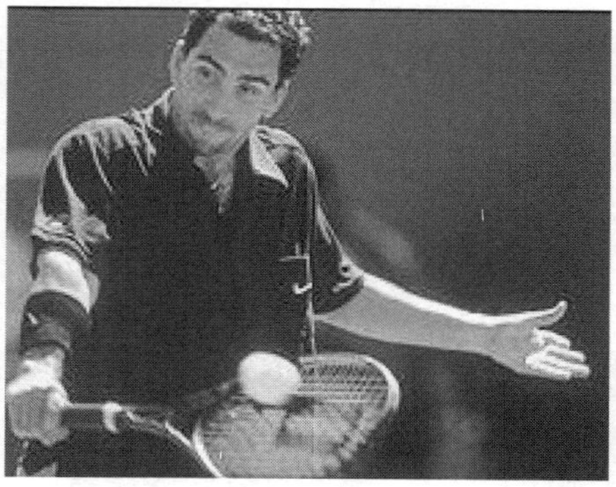

Figure 52
The slice backhand is very similar to a backhand volley. In most instances, the play will keep the dominant arm locked, the racket face open, and hit the ball with a downward, driving stroke.

INTRODUCTION

The slice backhand produces basically the opposite resulting spin on a tennis ball as the topspin. The aerodynamics, the biomechanics, and the ensuing results produced by slice shots offer many effective advantages that all players should understand, as well as be able to produce.

Mechanically, the slice uses gravity to assist the stroke. Because of the downward slicing action of the racket on the ball, gravity helps assist the racket speed through the shot. Also, because of this principle, players tend to maintain the racket head through the shot steadier and longer, helping produce more consistent results and improved aiming abilities.

The backspin produced by the slice backhand (and forehand for that matter) is very useful in approach shots as the ball stays lower after it bounces on your opponent's side of the court. If you are coming to the net, it is usually more advantageous to force your opponent to hit up to you at the net than to be able to drive down and past you with a topspin passing shot.

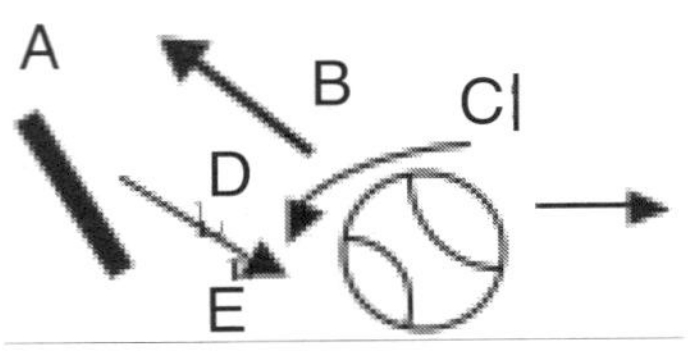

DIAGRAM A

When the racket (A) moves in a down and forward path, (D), the contact with a ball that is bouncing up from the ground, (B) will impart the same spin (C) that the ball already possesses. The only thing that really is changed on a slice is the direction of the ball (E).

Spin Advantage

One of the most unknown and unreported advantages of the slice is what I call the "Spin Advantage". This is the application of the same kind of spin to the ball that the ball already has as it comes towards you. With any slice groundstroke, the type of spin you apply to the ball will be essentially the same kind of spin that the ball already has. (Diagram A) This is because virtually every single shot hit to you from your opponent that bounces on your side of the net would have a significant degree of topspin after

the bounce. (A ball moving towards you will, by virtue of friction with the court, have topspin after the forward bounce.) By hitting a slice yourself, you are causing the strings of your racket to move in harmony with the spin that the ball already possesses. In comparison, hitting a topspin shot reverses the spin that the ball has prior to your contact with it.

This action of applying comparable spin to a spinning ball allows for an increase in controlling the shot. This spin advantage also increases the feel of the stroke for the player. While this advantage does not have a "Quantitative" figure in terms of the actual parameters of an advantage, the "Qualitative" feel and results of the shot are very real.

MECHANICS OF THE SLICE BACKHAND

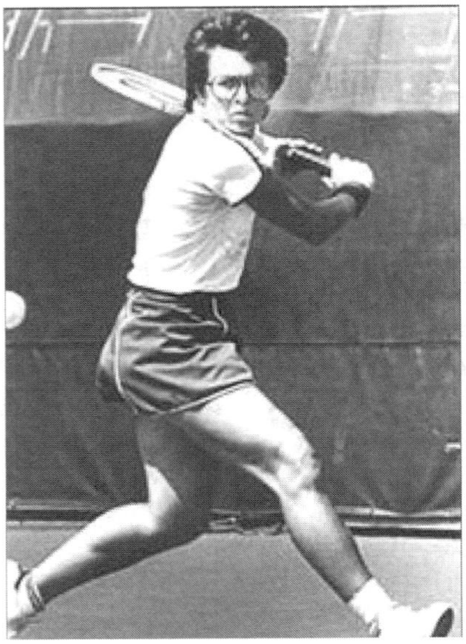

Figure 53
Billie Jean King used an effective slice to help her rule women's tennis in the 1960's. Here, you can see the classic preparation with the off-hand cradling the racket that is held high.

Essentially, if I were to summarize the slice backhand in one sentence, I would say that the shot basically emulates the backhand slice volley only with a full back swing and follow-through. (See Figure 52) With that said, I would recommend the study of the backhand volley discussed in Chapter 7.

Ready Position

As with all tennis shots, a player should attempt to be in a ready position with the racket held in front ready to hit any shot. When behind the baseline, because most shots anticipated will be groundstrokes, the ready position described at the beginning of this chapter (on the two-handed backhand) is a good place to start.

Backswing

Unlike the topspin backhand, the racket does not need to drop below the ball prior to contact. On the contrary, the racket needs to start much higher than the contact point on the slice backhand. (Figure 53 & 54) How much slice desired will dictate the height of the backswing once a player has mastered the foundation for the shot. Some players like to hit a big slice while others like to hit a flatter slice. Both shots are hit the same way with changes only in the racket height on backswing and in the amount the racket face is beveled open at contact.

The most important part of the backswing is the shoulder turn. Much like the volley, the best slice backhands are hit with the player standing sideways to the net at contact and beyond. Players who open up on the slice backhand will have a difficult time controlling the direction of the shot.

Take the racket back high with the off hand cradling the throat as you turn sideways to the ball. Because it is mechanically difficult to hit a slice with a two-handed backhand grip, a one-handed backhand with a Continental grip is recommended. Keep the hitting arm straight on the backswing, just as in the backhand volley. The difference between the volley and the slice backhand groundstroke at this point is that the racket is taken back further so it is basically pointing towards the back fence.

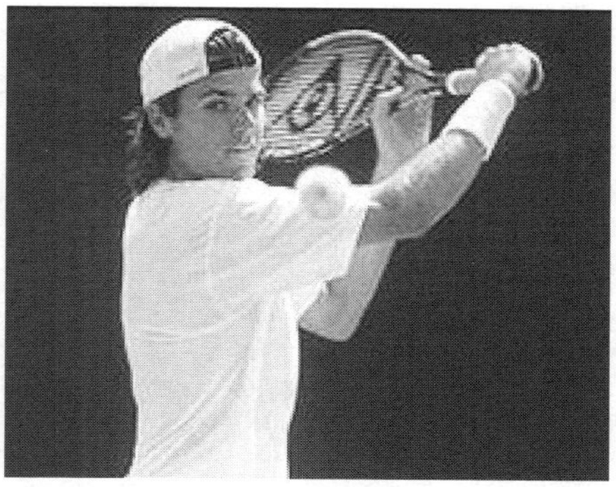

Figure 54
Here, Tommy Haas executes the backswing in preparation to hit a slice backhand. Note the high racket position and off-hand cradling the throat of the racket

The Slice Stroke

I always recommend that the slice backhand be hit with a closed stance. That is, the right foot (for right-handed players) will step across and towards the projected contact point.

As the ball approaches, the player will drive the straight right arm down and forward. The racket head does NOT catch up or pass the hand! It is very important that the racket position in relation to the hand and forearm does not change from backswing through contact and beyond. The contact point is generally even with the knee of the front leg. Do not try to swing early. This will cause the racket face to be open too much at contact. Keep your weight forward slightly, but don't lean so far forward that your back leg has to step around to keep from falling. The slice must be hit with good balance.

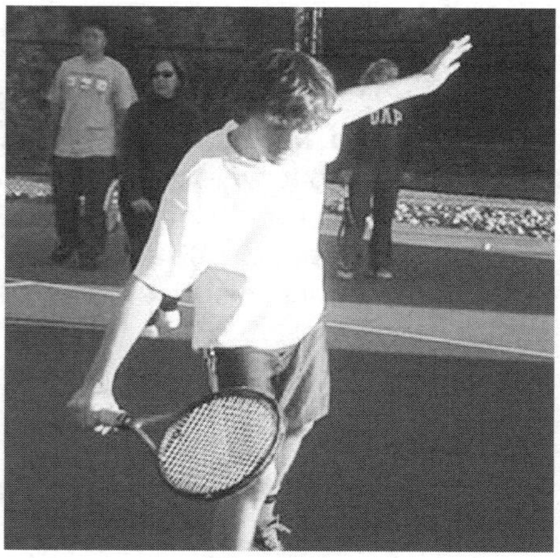

Figure 55
Notice the sideways body position held here long after contact. This position helps players keep from rotating around the slice as in the conventional topspin.

To help maintain the required balance, the off hand shoots back, simulating an umpire signaling "Safe" in baseball (as mentioned earlier). (Figure 55) This counter movement of the off hand helps maintain not only balance, but also it acts to keep the shoulders from over-rotating at contact. The player should remain sideways until long after the ball has left the racket. The path of the racket should be down and through the intended trajectory line. If the player opens up too soon, the slice comes too much across the body away from the intended target.

When hitting the slice as an approach shot, one of the biggest mistakes players make is that they try to start stepping towards the net too soon, causing them to step through the shot with their back foot. This will cause the body to open up too soon and the player usually will hit the ball into the net or too far to the right. Make sure you complete the backhand slice through contact before moving forward towards the net. Top players actually "glide" sideways through the slice, keeping their bodies sideways through contact, yet still able to move forward during the shot. This requires timing and discipline that will be learned better if the player pauses slightly during the shot, allowing the player's body to stay sideways.

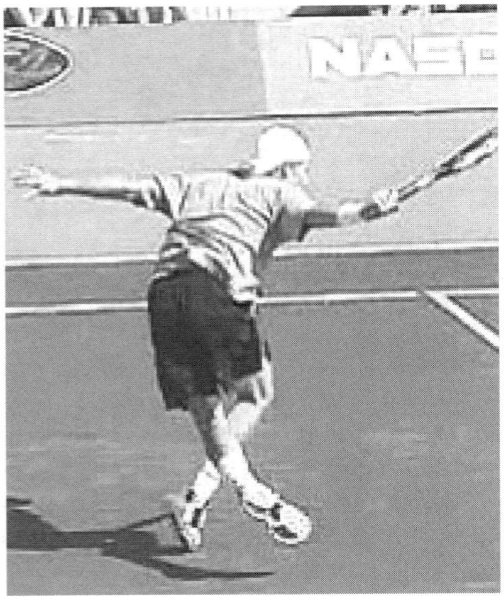

Figure 56
Here Lleyton Hewitt attacks the net while moving forward to hit a low, slice approach shot. Note his left foot moving in behind the right foot. This will allow him to put weight on this back foot and continue gliding forward with little or no hesitation. It also prevents him from rotating his hips toward the net too early.

Footwork in using the Slice as an Approach shot

As I just mentioned, in executing a slice approach shot, the player will want to remain sideways and "glide" through the shot. In order to accomplish this somewhat complex movement pattern, players need to learn the "Carioca Step." Described in the last chapter on volleys, the Carioca Step is where the back foot steps forward—but behind—the front foot usually during contact. For right-handed players, the left foot will step behind the right foot as the player continues to glide forward towards the net during the stroke. It is this move that allows for the player to remain sideways both at the hips and the shoulders even while moving forward. (Figure 56)

The Slice as a Defensive Shot

Because the slice is easier to manufacture, it is an excellent shot to use in a defensive situation. When an opponent has hit a very aggressive groundstroke, the speed of the ball will make a topspin stroke difficult and relatively inaccurate. A defensive slice is hit no differently than an approach slice in terms of the stroke. However, because the ball is coming faster, usually a shorter backswing is mandated. The firmness of the racket arm and wrist can utilize your opponent's power in a controlled slice return that won't necessarily get you in trouble. With practice, a player can control this hard hit ball with graceful, yet effective, pace as well as placement.

The Slice as an Offensive Stroke (Approach Shot)

The slice offers several advantages when used as an approach shot. Usually, the time for an approach shot is on short balls hit by your opponent. This usually means one of two things: 1) the ball is hit softly, and 2) the ball is hit very low. In both cases, coming in towards the net to get such a shot can present problems. First, the closer to the net you are when you hit the ball, the less airtime your shot has to drop into your opponent's court. (As you come towards the net, you are also coming closer to their baseline as well!) Thus, topspin shots don't do as well as they don't have enough air space to utilize the topspin nature of the shot to drop down in the court. Also, because these approach shots tend to be low in the first place, it is hard to generate the same amount of topspin as a ball that has bounce higher near your baseline. Finally, because you are perhaps rushing up to get the short ball, your forward momentum can increase the velocity of the ball beyond that which you can consistently control.

In each of these scenarios the slice allows for greater control and potentially greater effect against a potential passing shot. Because the slice stays much lower than a topspin shot, a slice approach shot makes an opponent have to hit the ball further up to clear the net. Also, against players who have severe western and semi-western grips, a hard slice that stays low will be even more difficult for these players to hit effectively. This is because such severe grips are designed for high bouncing balls, not for low, skidding balls.

The Slice as an Offensive Stroke (From the Baseline)

As you just read, the slice used against full and semi western grips is very effective as an approach shot. In recent years, the hard slice backhand to such western-grip forehand opponents can produce weak shots. This is because the semi and full western grips tend to close the racket face on low balls. (Most western grip players prefer higher bouncing balls.) Thus, a low ball to these grips invite miss hits or necessary changes in an opponent's forehand.

Ideally, the slice backhand should be hit more from the middle of the player's court. This will make the ball fade out wide to the opponent's forehand. Also, the anatomical position of the arm makes the slice backhand a little easier to hit fairly hard. This is because the arm is moving away from the player's body and not into the body as a forehand slice would. Players will want to work on hitting the slice with a tremendous amount of back and inside-out sidespin. The player starting the backswing further away from the body and sweeping down across the front of the body accomplishes this. The combination of underspin and sidespin will have an additional effect of keeping the ball even lower after the bounce on your opponent's side of the court. The result is a ball that is very difficult to hit deep, hard or accurately by an opponent.

After an effective slice backhand, you can often anticipate a short forehand return. This should open the door to hit any number of offensive shots. From approach shots, to dropshots, to inside out forehand winners, such a slice backhand can be an excellent shot used to set up a point.

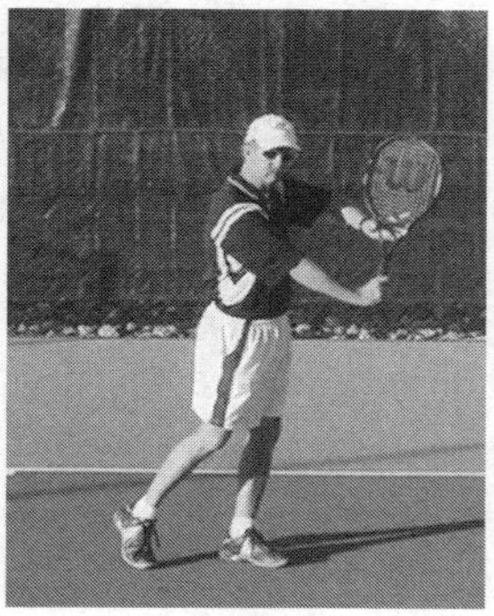
Figure 57

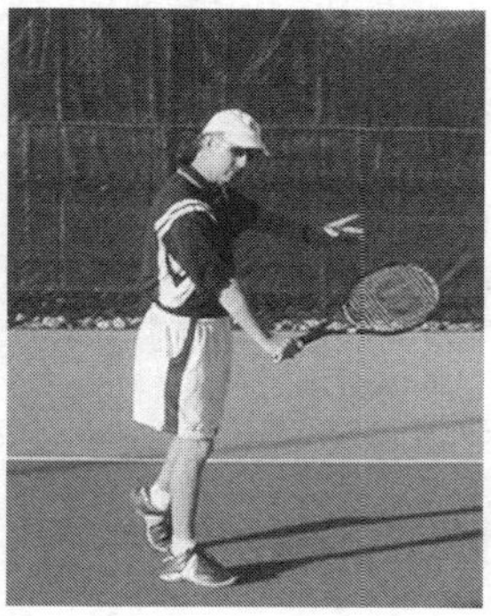
Figure 58

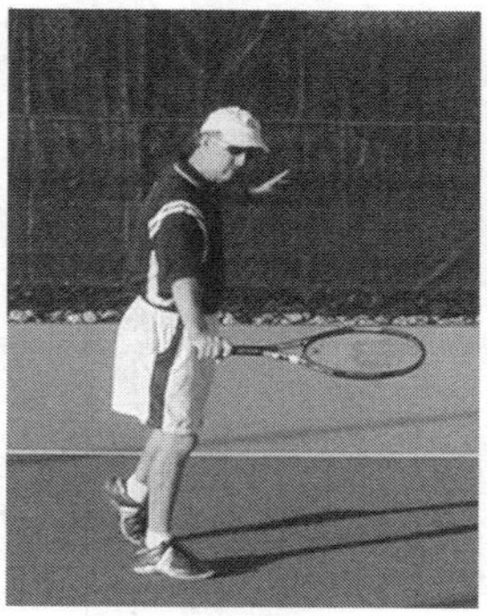
Figure 59

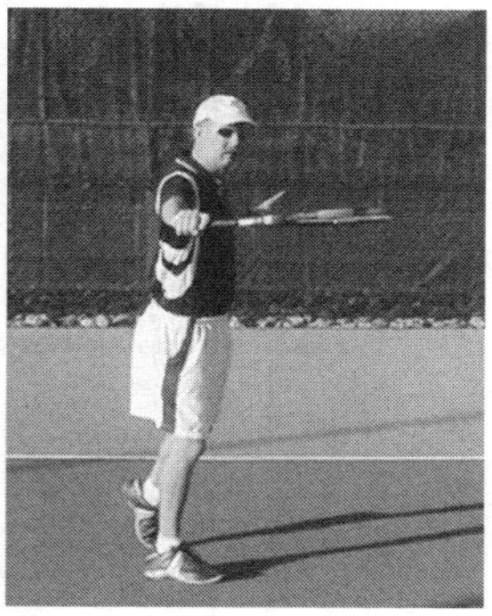
Figure 60

As with the volley, the slice drop shot starts with a straight dominant arm, racket held high and an initial shoulder turn (Fig, 57). As the racket comes down to meet the ball, the player will step in with a closed stance (Fig. 58). The stroke continues down and under the ball with the player remaining sideways (Fig. 59) The finish of the stroke will be in line with the target. Thus the player will separate the arms and keep the back foot down to prevent early rotation (Fig. 60)

The Backhand Drop Shot

The drop shot hit from the backhand side mirrors much of the same technique and pattern that is used in hitting the backhand volley. The main difference is that contact is made more on the underside of the ball as well as struck with a longer, softer swing than the volley. Ideally, the drop shot should be hit from inside the baseline as if hitting an approach shot. From here, you are closer to the net to hit a softer underspin stroke. Also, because this is also where you might hit an offensive approach shot deep, many opponents will be anticipating a hard hit ball instead of a drop shot. (There will be more on the strategy of hitting drop shots when the shot is discussed in the next chapter on forehands.)

Advanced Backhand Patterns

As a player develops the advanced foundation for their backhand, other effective derivatives of the shot can be learned. Strategically, players who begin to hit effective backhands look for ways they can move their opponent more. This "opening up" of the opponent's court provides opportunities to hit more winners.

Consider the hierarchy of strategy for any tennis player:

- Get the ball in over the net
- Get the ball in opponent's court
- Get the ball deeper in opponent's court
- Get the ball to opponent's weakness
- Hit the ball to opponent's corners
- Move opponent around
- Hit the ball harder

DIAGRAM B

Angular Advantages

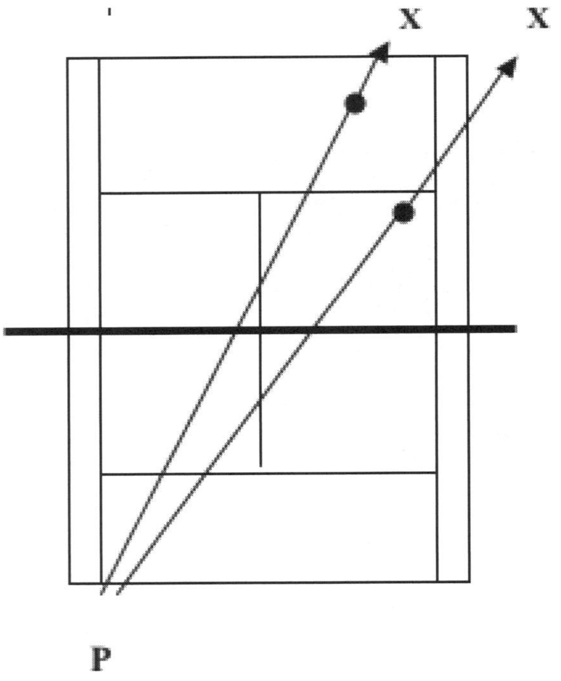

The geometric placements of a backhand (or forehand) crosscourt (in this example of a right-handed player's "P" backhand) can open up the court and force your opponent (X) to increase the amount of distance needed to retrieve your shot.

The ability to hit greater topspin will allow a player to hit more angles on a typical cross-court. By making the ball dip faster through the use of topspin, a player can hit a greater angled shot and still get the ball in.

The first four strategies deal only with minimal lateral directional differentiation. They mostly deal only with hitting the ball fairly straight in a direction over the net. As players develop their skill, placing the ball more into the corners is the next developmental strategy. However, if you study the geometry of angles as they relate to a tennis court, you can make your opponent run considerably longer by using shorter angles to the sides of your opponent's court. If you study Diagram B, you will see how a shot hit from the same spot but hit at a different angle will make your opponent move further to retrieve the ball.

Thus, one of the highest levels of tennis skill can be measured by a player's ability to hit greater angles. This ability requires an increase in ball rotation or spin. (See Diagram B)

As players advance, the ability to manufacture shots that have greater angle is a huge advantage. These advantages include:

- Opening up your opponent's court by moving them further from the middle
- Increasing the effectiveness and variety of passing shots
- Making your opponent work harder to retrieve your shots

However, by increasing the angle of your shots, you must also understand that your opponent is then offered greater return angles back to your side of the court. Players must learn to read their opponents and test their ability to respond to various shots. Obviously, the more effective your use of angles (as combined with speed, accuracy, and opportunity), the less likely your opponent will be able to get an offensive shot off against such angles.

It becomes clear to most players that without an Advanced Foundation, such offensive and geometric shots would be very difficult to accomplish. Players who tend to only push balls over the net, or those who can only hit slice shots or flat shots, will seldom be able to make such tennis shots with any kind of consistency.

Spend quality time working on your Advanced Foundation and these higher levels of shot-making skills will become available to you in time.

Sequence of Learning

In this, our checklist for mastering the backhand groundstroke, keep in mind that the more repetitive you can make your stroke, the more stability and reliability you will have in hitting your backhand. (Your ability to aim with greater accuracy will be greatly increased as well!)

TWO-HANDED TOPSPIN BACKHAND CHECKLIST

1. *Grips: Continental grip on the dominant, lower hand; Eastern forehand grip on the top, non-dominant hand*
2. *Backswing: Straight back and low. Loop swings will develop naturally once the general stroke has been mastered. Racket head is pointed down and back towards the back fence, the hitting surface of the strings, (racket face) is pointed down as well.*

ADVANCED TWO-HANDED BACKHAND CHECKLIST

1. *More or less topspin: Start with the racket higher on the backswing to flatten the backhand out. To develop a sharp-angled, dipping backhand, drop the racket head down lower and brush up the outside of the ball.*
2. *Open or closed stance patterns: Once the backhand stroke is established, players will want to experiment with open stance backhands in some situations.*
3. *Subtle grip changes: For players looking for greater topspin, adjust the grip to a semi-western forehand grip for the non-dominant hand. Experiment with various hand positions for personal needs.*

SEQUENCE OF LEARNING: ONE-HANDED TOPSPIN BACKHAND

1. *Quick turn and grip change: On a one-handed backhand, make sure you turn quickly and adjust your grip to the Eastern backhand grip*

2. *Movement: players must move quickly to get in the best position for the backhand stroke.*

3. *Deep shoulder turn: for both down the line and crosscourt, you will want to turn significantly so you don't end up pushing the ball away from you. Keep the racket head low on the backswing.*

4. *Contact: Make sure the racket is locked in the Eastern backhand grip.*

5. *Follow-through: While staying sideways, allow your racket to drive out to the ball and then brush up the outside portion of the ball. Keep your back foot back and remain balanced well past your follow-through.*

Conclusion

The backhand can be hit one-handed or two-handed, with topspin or slice or flat. While the forehand often can be quite varied, even among pros, both the one and two-handed backhands tend to be much more similar among top players. The bottom line is that the developing player must work towards creating a backhand that is stable, repeatable, and balanced. If these three things are accomplished, the student will have a reliable backhand that can be further developed. Such attributes will make it possible to improve the backhand through greater effectiveness and dependability. Such effectiveness will include greater placement (including depth and angles), greater pace and applied spin, and greater ability to aim. A flawed backhand stroke will prohibit, or at least diminish, the ability for the student to make these advancements.

CHAPTER 10

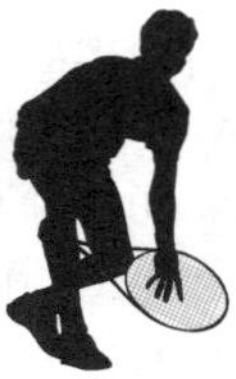

The Advanced Foundation – The Forehand Groundstroke

One and Two-handed Forehand Strokes

Historically for both the recreational player and the pro, the forehand groundstroke has been looked upon as the more confident—if not the more dominant—stroke for most. However, since the advent of the two-handed backhand now being employed by an ever-increasing number of players, we are seeing a trend in which many players are becoming more consistent as well as more confident with the backhand than the forehand. In some cases, players are even hitting more aggressively with their two-handed backhands than their forehands. Compared to the flawed one-handed backhands that so many individuals attempted, the one-handed forehand has been mechanically easier to hit correctly with more control and consistency. Traditionally, the power and perceived reliability of the forehand was relative only to the weakness of the player's backhand. Now that the two-handed backhand has been proven to be generally a more reliable, and for some, a more dominant stroke than its predecessor (the one-handed backhand), the forehand for many players is now the suspect stroke.

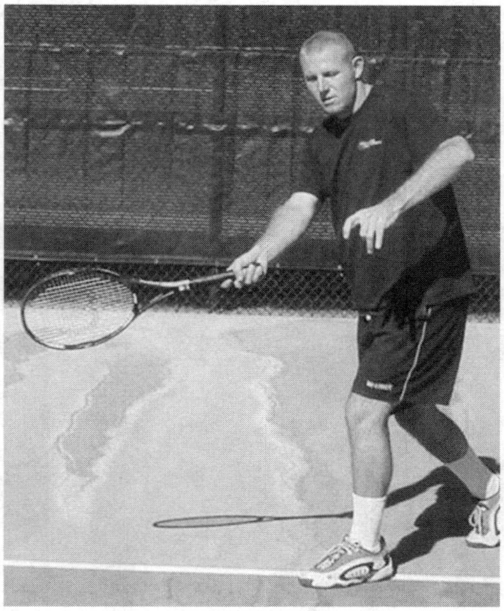

Figure 1
The "conventional" forehand groundstroke.

One-handed strokes (forehand and backhand groundstrokes) tend to provide a sense of freedom, one that can be detrimental to developing effective and reliable strokes. Like the one-handed backhand, conventional single-handed forehands (Figure 1) can be executed with less footwork and more reach. It has been argued for decades that it is this perceived lack of reach available to two-handed players that makes any two-handed stroke a liability. Yet, because players can hit the conventional forehand with relative success while utilizing poor or improper footwork, balance, and mechanics, players often are seen sacrificing position or form in favor of what they perceive as less effort. Sadly,

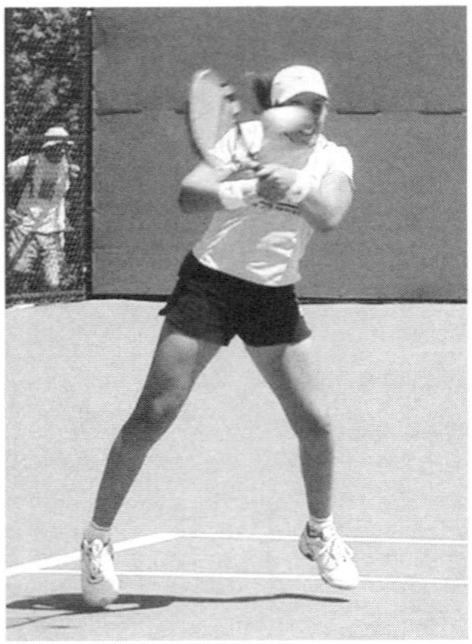

Figure 2
France's Marion Bartoli hits a two-handed forehand.
(Photo by David Smith)

through this process a great number of players, (even those with athleticism and talent), develop mediocre forehand strokes! More importantly, most of these players never fully develop the required footwork necessary to hit higher level forehands with consistency and reliability.

The rise of heavier topspin strokes and emphasis on topspin at earlier periods of player-development has created the need for players to learn how to specifically "brush up" on their forehand side. Today, there is a stroke emerging in greater numbers among skilled players: the two-handed forehand. Similar to the features of a two-handed backhand, the two-handed forehand offers an almost "self-working" topspin.

Having taught the two-handed forehand (Figure 2) for over 15 years, I have seen a value that the stroke offers to players similar to what the two-handed backhand did for those with weak or poorly developed one-handed backhands. As you will read, the two-handed forehand offers substantial value for both developing players and for those who are searching for a better forehand. Why has it taken so long for two-handed forehands to evolve? Considering that even now, while many two-handed players are emerging (and winning!) in skilled competitive arenas, this book is the first-ever clinical description on how precisely a player should hit the shot! With few knowledgeable pros understanding the process of hitting the shot, few students of the game are being offered the chance to explore the stroke.

Why Learn With Two Hands?

Before I discuss the advantages of learning a two-handed forehand, I want to address those of you who are set in learning or improving only a one-handed backhand. Without question, there are far more one-handed players all across the board. It would be both foolish and erroneous for me to insist or assume that everyone is going attempt to learn an "unconventional" stroke such as the two-handed forehand. However, it will be both interesting and informative to all that are reading this book to—at the very least—understand the components of the two-handed forehand presented here. Many conventional forehand players have experimented hitting the two-handed forehand. Most of these players have discovered, through the two-handed practice, specific improvements that have helped

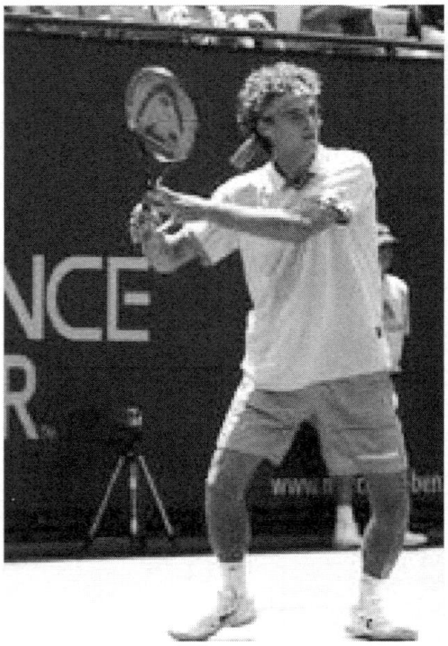

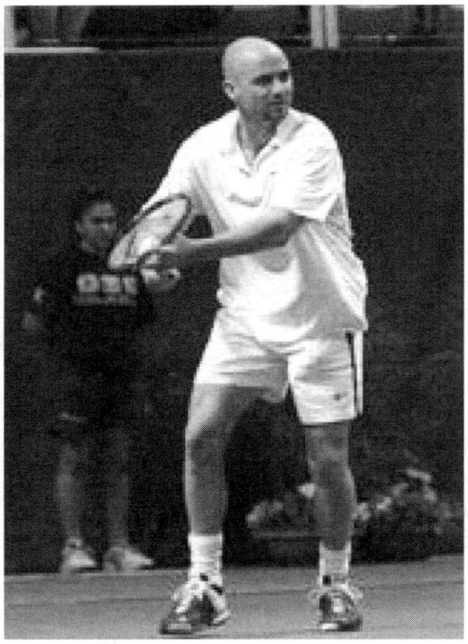

Figures 3 & 4
Gustavo Kuerten (above) and Andre Agassi (below) both set up their forehands with an identifiable two-handed position.

their conventional one-handed stroke! Many of these improvements might not have been discovered through conventional learning methods. However, you are more than welcome to move on to the conventional one-handed forehand that follows this two-handed forehand section.

Ironically, some of the best players in the world use two hands in parts of their conventional one-handed forehands. Note in Figures 3 and 4 pro players like Gustavo Kuerten and Andre Agassi both set up their turn and backswing using essentially a two-handed position on their rackets.

Unfortunately, the use of two hands in executing a forehand stroke has been criticized by a) those who are unfamiliar with the advantages of the stroke, and/or b) those who are ignorant of the learning and progressive nature of the stroke. It is interesting to note many of those who are indeed critical of the stroke identify three areas in which they the claim the stroke is limiting: power, reach, and response to pace. I believe they are wrong; the two-hander is NOT limited in these three areas, and it can be more productive in each area by almost all individuals.

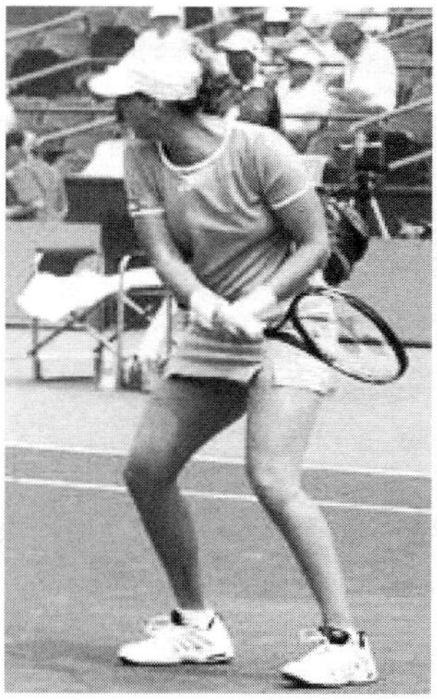

Figure 5
How different is the initial take back swing of such greats as Gustavo Kuerten and Andre Agassi (Figures 3 & 4) from that of Monica Seles true two-handed forehand? Notice how these players use their off-hand to help rotate their bodies sideways.

Power Under Control

Typically, those who berate the two-handed forehand claim the stroke has less power potential than the conventional forehand. This claim must be examined within the context of "controllable power." Using one hand, power or racket head speed can certainly be increased through the use of the wrist and even within a wild use of whole body movements. These procedures to increase racket head speed come at a substantial cost of control.

Using two hands to generate power, the two-handed forehand creates a stable-hitting pattern far more naturally derived within the biomechanics of advanced tennis strokes. The same thing can be seen with the two-handed backhand. While the outright power through the use of questionable or undesirable swing patterns can be achieved within an arguable margin using one handed conventional forehands the true test of the stroke will be exposed by a lack of controllable power.

Ironically, this argument of power using one hand over two hands can be dismissed in the analogies of other power-intended sports. Baseball batters, golfers, hockey players, and even cricket players, for the most part, use two hands for their swing patterns. Only badminton and racquetball use one handed swings in terms of swinging their implements. Interestingly, both badminton and racquetball employ a tremendous amount of wrist in generating their racket head speeds. Almost all tennis students, even beginners, know that tennis is NOT a wrist-intensive sport! The act of trying not to use wrist in tennis is difficult enough, especially when we are given the undesired opportunity to use the wrist through one-handed swing patterns.

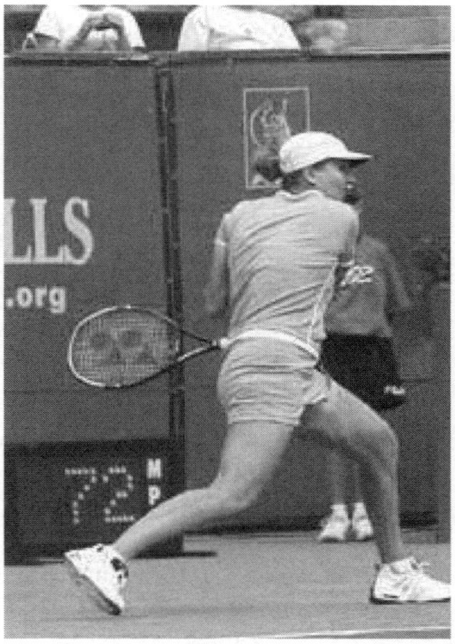

Figure 6
Monica Seles is able to hit her left-handed two-handed forehand with an open stance.

If power was both more controllable and more efficient using one handed swings, baseball players, hockey players and golfers would certainly be seen utilizing this method.

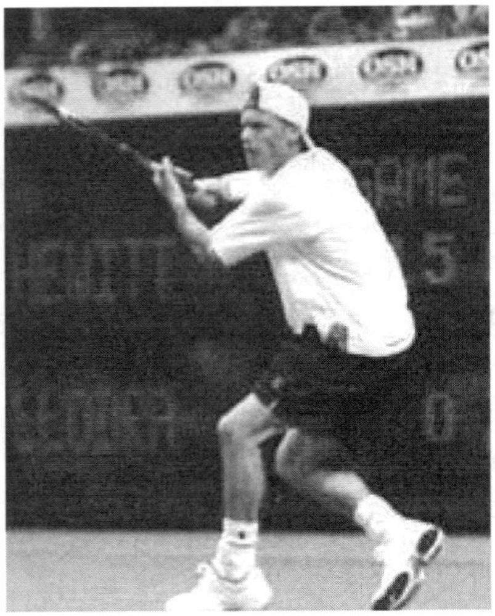
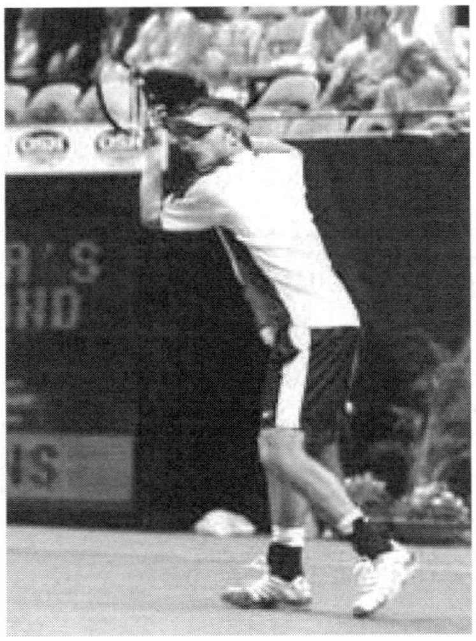

Figures 7 & 8
Lleyton Hewitt (left) and Andy Roddick both execute their one-handed forehands using a two-handed take back.

REACH: LESS IS MORE!

The issue of reach with any two-handed stroke has been argued for decades. Certainly, with questionable form most players can create far more reach with one hand holding the racket than with two. However, when we look at all the ways this reach is accomplished, we seldom see form associated with skilled play. Thus, the use of two hands on both the forehand and the backhand literally force players to use proper footwork associated with the stroke. I have seen how players using the two-handed forehand or backhand strokes improved their footwork patterns far faster than did those who elected to hit with one hand on either shot. Since 99 percent of shots in tennis are hit within the reach of any two-handed stroke—as long as the player has moved correctly—this argument against the two-handed stroke because of reach does not hold water.

Response to Pace

It is interesting to watch most of the top male players on tour hit their forehands. Almost without exception, all these pros use their off hand in some degree to take the racket back. It would seem that if the two-handed forehand had limitations due to the pace of shots hit to these top-level performers, these players would not be using this pattern to take the racket back! On the contrary, the short, compact stroke that the two-handed forehand usually produces is ideal in returning fast, hard-hit balls. Consider, too, that Monica Seles has maintained a top-5 world ranking longer than almost any women player has. Her ability to compete far better than hundreds of players below her with the likes of the William sisters, Jennifer Capriati, and a host of other hard hitting players, can be at least partially attributed to her two-handed forehand.

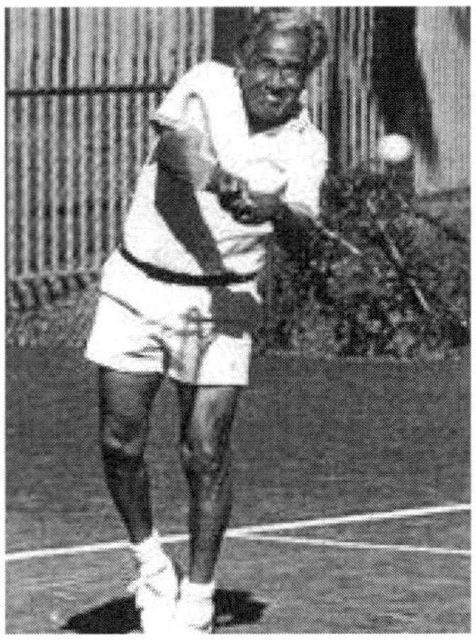

Figure 9
Pancho Segura was one of the first to introduce the two-handed forehand to the high-level game.

TWO-HANDED FOREHAND HISTORY

Before delving into the technical aspects of the two-handed forehand, it is important to understand that the stroke is far from new.

While its use has been far overshadowed by the sheer number of one-handed forehand players, the inarguable success of the two-handed forehand—among those who have mastered the stroke—has made a significant mark in tennis history.

Ironically, it was a male who first introduced the two-handed forehand to the modern game. Gene Mayer, a New Yorker, used a most unorthodox, two-handed stroke on both sides—placing his dominant hand above the other for both his forehand and backhand. Though Mayer reached number 4 in the world in 1980 as well as a number 2 world ranking in doubles, it would be another ten years before another world-class player would emerge using the stroke.

Yet, it was back in 1943 that Francisco "Pancho" Segura, an Ecuadorian, would introduce the significant potential of a two-handed forehand. (Figure 9) Segura reached a ranking of number 4 in the U.S. and won 14 North American tournament titles using the two-hander. Also in the 1940's there emerged a lesser-known doubles great, John Edward Bromwich, an Australian who was an ambidextrous player using a two-handed stroke on his right side. Even though not well-known, Bromwich managed to win two Australian singles titles and 13 other Grand Slam doubles titles including 3 U.S. Titles, two Wimbledon and 5 mixed doubles titles.

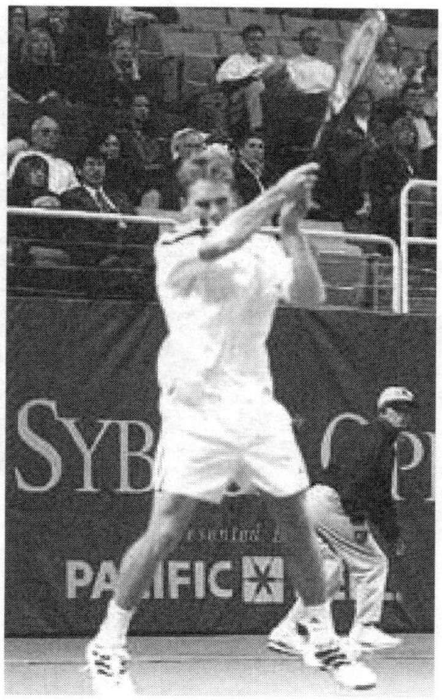

Figure 10
American Jan-Michael Gambill has shown that the two-handed forehand does just fine on today's men's tour.

A few might recall the South African Frew McMillan's two-handed play on both sides, earning him 9 Grand Slam doubles titles including three Wimbledon and two U.S. (mixed doubles). McMillian's triumphs came during the late 1960's and late 1970's.

Undoubtedly, the most notable competitor exemplifying the potential of the stroke is Monica Seles. Ranked in 1991 as the world's top female tennis player, Monica demonstrated what a weapon her two-handed forehand was at that time and continues to be today.

Today, on the men's tour, France's Fabrice Santoro and American Jan-Michael Gambill (Figure 10) have demonstrated that the stroke is not relegated to women's tennis only. Both players have been ranked in the top 50 in the world and have done well recently on the ATP Tour using their own brand of two-handed forehands. Other tour pros using two-handed forehands, emerging among the world's top players, include Marion Bartoli, a top ranked 18 year-old from France, (Figure 11) and Raemon Sluiter, one of the top men from the Netherlands.

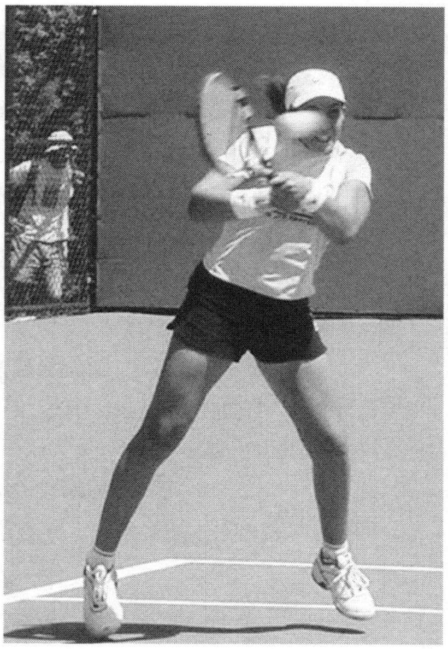

Figure 11
Marion Bartoli from France uses a two handed forehand and backhand. *Photo by David Smith*

Because very few teaching tennis professionals understand the working mechanics of the two-handed forehand, few are inclined to teach the shot. (We can recognize similar circumstances when the two-handed backhand was first emerging.) When Monica Seles proved the stroke could be taken to the highest level on tour (number one in the world), players began to see its potential. However, at the same time, many players and teaching pros branded Seles' stroke only as an isolated instance of success or a simple case of extremely rare achievement. (Incidentally, this was the initial critical response of Bjorn Borg and Jimmy Connor's two-handed backhands in the early 1970's as well!) Many pros simply refuse to study the stroke, assuming that few players would benefit from such technique. Yet, since relatively few players have been introduced to the stroke, it would be hard to draw such an empirical conclusion from such a small experimental field! Curiously, it would be interesting to compare this small—but growing—number of successful players

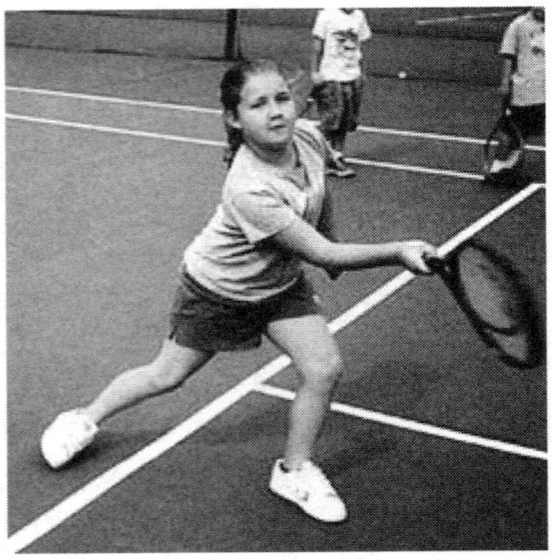

Figure 12
Children in general have difficulty controlling their forehand and repeating a reliable stroke pattern.

who currently are using the two-handed forehand to the vast number of players who use the one-handed forehand. As ratios go, it might prove to be quite revealing. Certainly over time, the question of the stroke's true validity will be revealed.

Advanced Forehand Foundation

While there is a wide discrepancy in the form and technical components of the top players in the world, the forehand (either the one-handed or two-handed methods taught in this book) consists of very dynamic and comparable advanced foundations and structure.

Interestingly, the two-handed forehand—as it is taught here—provides players with the same Advanced Foundation and general mechanics as the "conventional" one-handed forehand. That is, the two-handed forehand incorporates the majority of key position points utilized by an advanced single-handed forehand. As I have seen among the thousands of players I have taught, those who were introduced to the two-handed forehand at first generally made faster and earlier strides in hitting better topspin forehands as a whole than those who only learned hitting the one-handed forehand.

It is important to point out that I believe the two-handed forehand is not for everyone. While I do teach the stroke within four distinct student situations (listed below), I also teach the one-handed forehand to those individuals who exhibit appropriate abilities. There have been many examples of talented players, both adults and juniors alike, who quickly became comfortable hitting the two-handed forehand. However, as a guideline, there are four situations in which I specifically teach the two-hander:

a. Very young children who don't have the strength nor physical comprehension of what their racket is doing.

The two-hander provides significant strength and a natural swing pattern that makes it relatively easy to learn a proper topspin forehand and build a repeatable stroke pattern.

b. Adults and juniors who have learned the one-handed forehand yet are having difficulty creating consistency and/or ample topspin on the forehand groundstroke.

Even intermediate players who knowingly hit a suspect forehand will immediately experience a higher level of topspin and consistency. It is far easier for players to repeat a consistent swing pattern with the two-hander. This is especially true for players who don't generate topspin on their forehands.

c. Seniors or adults who have pain associated with their arm, wrist, or elbow.

Two hands obviously share the stress and impact vibration that would normally be absorbed by the joints, muscles and tendons of the single arm of the one-handed forehand.

d. In a beginning group setting.

In a group of beginners, the two-handed forehand provides everyone, regardless of ability or potential, a foundation on which to build a successful forehand. It automatically incorporates better footwork, swing patterns, and body rotation.

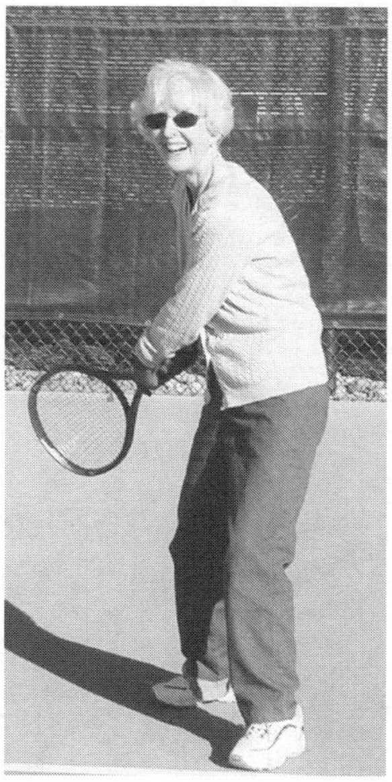

Figure 13
Senior players can enjoy the feeling of hitting solid forehands with much less stress to the body

Among top players we still see a dominance of one-handed forehands. We will probably see this for a long time. However, as we have seen the acceptance of the two-handed backhand as a potent weapon over the last thirty years, I believe we will see a significant shift of top players utilizing the two-handed forehand over the next decade or two. The reason I believe this is because it is already being utilized very effectively at the advanced junior levels. In tournaments and team play we see a growing group of top juniors utilizing the two-handed forehand. Certainly not yet as prevalent (because of the still-favorable mechanics for many players executing topspin properly with only one hand), the two-hander, however, is already being recognized as a viable weapon and as a terrific learning tool for a great number of players.

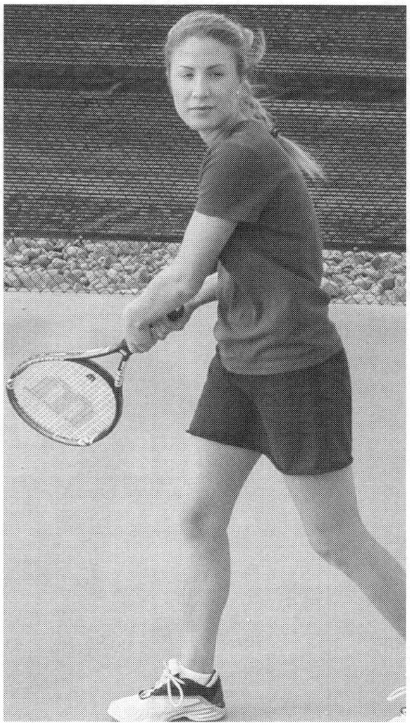

Figure 14
Players who have trouble creating a solid topspin forehand can accomplish excellent strokes with the two-handed forehand.

Two-hands as a Learning Tool

Over the years I have found the two-handed forehand a remarkable learning tool for players of all ages. Initially, I used the stroke to teach little kids and high school girls who were having difficulty creating topspin with their forehands. I found that players who had trouble knowing what their racket was doing on the forehand oftentimes swung down on the ball. Consequently, most of these players could not brush up the back of the ball to create the desired topspin.

Upon introduction to the two-handed forehand, these students quickly developed a progressively advanced forehand foundation. Most of these students (nearly 70%) stayed with the two-handed stroke for their career. Without question these players developed a dominant topspin forehand faster than if they had never been introduced to it at all. In addition, those players who elected to switch to the one-handed forehand found that they had a better foundation through learning the two-handed forehand first. Certainly, these players developed a true and progressive one-handed forehand faster and with a better overall foundation than those players with similar difficulty did who didn't learn the two-handed forehand first.

Adults and Senior Players Using Two Hands

It wasn't long ago that I found that older people have an equally positive response to the two-handed forehand.

While I was providing tennis clinics for the Huntsman World Senior Games here in my hometown of St. George, Utah, I discovered what an impact this stroke had on the "50 and better" tennis playing population! I had nearly 30 participants in my final clinic of the week, a clinic advertised as a "revolutionary approach to the forehand." Of course, none of these players had any idea what the revolutionary technique I would be teaching would be. I began the clinic feeding four lines of players each about a half-dozen shots to their forehand. I had the others watch the group that was hitting. Then I would rotate and repeat this scenario for each group. It was an amazing thing that each of these players witnessed: No two players seemed to hit the same forehand! My only instructions were to hit a topspin forehand to a target. Ironically, some players who hit slice forehands actually thought they were hitting topspin! Some hit flat, some hit open stance, some closed, some fell backwards as they swung, some stepped through with their back foot during their swing, and some slapped at the ball like racquetball players.

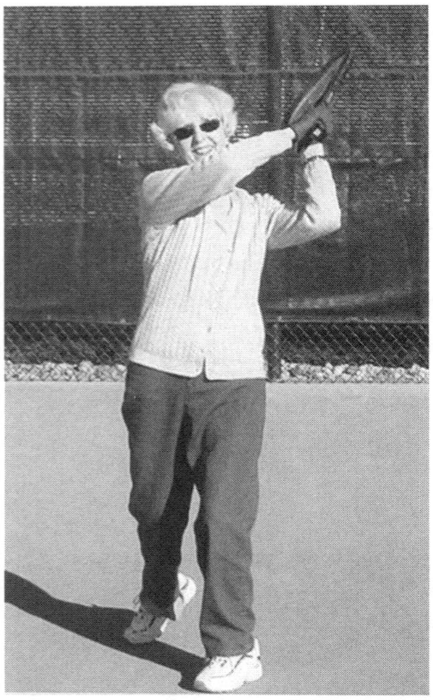

Figure 15
As a whole, senior players develop much better form with greater effectiveness using two hands on their forehands.

After a ten-minute introduction to the two-handed forehand, I had players mimic the swing pattern for a few minutes and repeated the drill with players watching each group as they hit. What transpired over the next fifteen minutes was indeed revolutionary. Every single player hit topspin. Every single player hit with better balance and proper footwork. Every single player saw how each player's stroke was certainly more congruent with what they knew as a more refined swing pattern. Many of these players hit topspin for the first time in their tennis-playing career! Many developed a far better topspin stroke than they had ever done previously. Seeing the smiles of joy from many of these players, each finding something new and effective, was gratifying to say the least!

SOLVING FOREHAND PROBLEMS

Look at the following forehand problems:

Can't hit topspin
Erratic control
Inconsistent forehand

If you possess any (or all!) of these forehand problems, the two-handed forehand is a must for you. Understand the following:

1. *If you learn the two-handed forehand, you will develop a swing pattern that will improve your one-handed forehand in every problem area listed above.*
2. *If you attempt to hit the two-handed forehand, you won't suddenly lose your existing forehand (as many seem to fear anytime change is explored!).*
3. *If you stay with the two-handed forehand for several weeks, you will not only improve your forehand, you will improve your footwork and balance throughout the course of developing the two-handed stroke.*

The following instructional portion will be dealing with the two-handed forehand. Because the one-handed forehand is still the dominant stroke as viewed by most players, I will follow the two-handed forehand instruction with a complete description of how to hit the conventional one-handed forehand correctly. Understanding both strokes is helpful for players developing either forehand. The footwork, racket swing-path, and the action of the strings are essentially the same for both strokes.

Two-Handed Methods

During my 15 years of teaching the two-handed forehand, I have had the pleasure of discussing the stroke with several authorities on the shot. Interestingly, those who have used the stroke effectively have actually utilized distinctly three different two-handed methods. Through study of the stroke, I have researched these three basic and distinct methods. Each method has advantages and disadvantages that should be discussed. Understand that while there are three distinct methods to the shot, only one method has multiple advantages over the other two. This will be discussed further after I introduce the three methods. It would be a good idea to have a tennis racket available to simulate each method. This will make you more familiar with each concept.

Here is a summation of the different two-handed models that are currently being hit by players:

METHOD #1: NO FOREHAND...TWO BACKHANDS

One method is simply to not hit a forehand! That is, the player switches his dominant hand so that he is hitting either a left-handed backhand or a right-handed backhand. (See Figure 16) In terms of mechanics, this is really the easiest to "hit"... however, the hardest to be ready for. That is, the player must switch both hands up or down depending on what side the ball is hit to them. I have seen a few players become proficient at this, learning how to prepare the hands to make the transition in a quick manner.

The obvious disadvantages include the switching of the hands and the fact the player will still need to learn and master a one-handed stroke on each side to hit slice ground strokes.

The mechanical advantage to this method is that it places the hand of the arm crossing over the front of the body at the bottom of the racket. This allows for greater reach and length on the backswing.

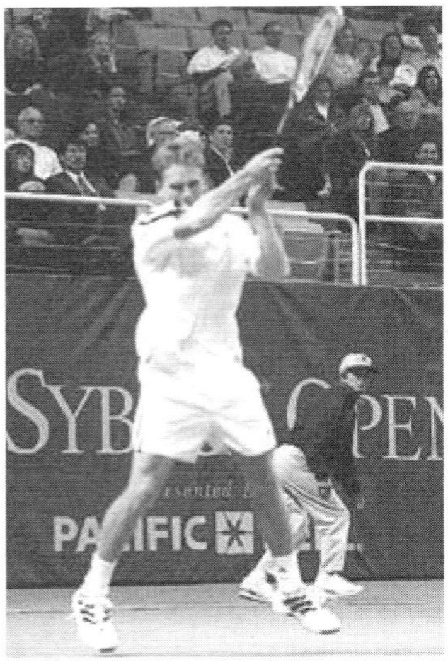

Figure 16
Jan-Michael Gambil, a right-handed player, moves his right hand up and places his left hand at the bottom of the grip. He essentially has two, two-handed backhands!

Method #2: Dominate Hand on Top

Gene Mayer, a two-hander on both sides who achieved a world ranking as high as #4 in singles and #2 in doubles, used the method of placing his dominant right hand on top of the left hand for his forehand. (See Figure 17) This model is basically hitting as a left hander. The forehand is actually a left-handed backhand (like the model described above), but the backhand side is technically a left-handed forehand with the right hand on top. In other words, there is no switching of the dominant hand. It stays on top. (This will make more sense after we discus the third and most reliable method below.) This method does not require the hands to shift on groundstrokes. However, for volleys, serves, and overheads, the right hand must move to the bottom of the grip (from its position above the non-dominant hand). This transition is somewhat difficult, especially for players who come to the net.

Method #3: Dominate Hand on Bottom

This is by far the most emulated swing pattern among top players today. Former world number one player Monica Seles (Figure 18) hits her forehand this way. The dominant hand remains on the bottom of the grip and the off-hand stays on top, essentially the same grip as the two-handed backhand with minor adjustments. This is the stroke that I will present to you. If, by chance, you seek to explore the other methods I just mentioned, you can experiment using the information offered throughout this section.

There are many advantages that this stroke offers: all will be described in detail within the following pages.

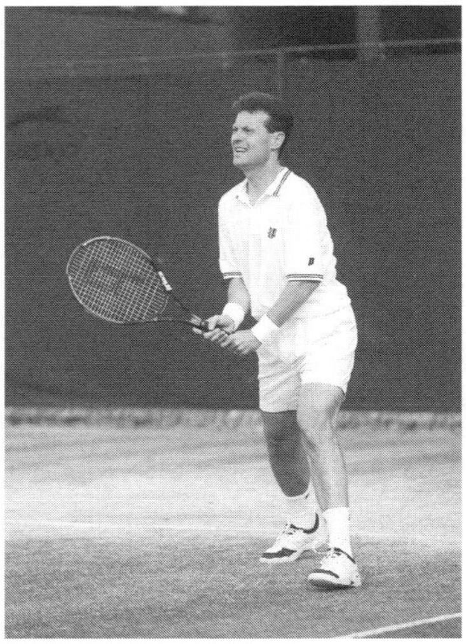

Figure 17
Gene Mayer, a right-handed player, hit both forehand and backhands with his right hand on top of his non-dominant left hand.

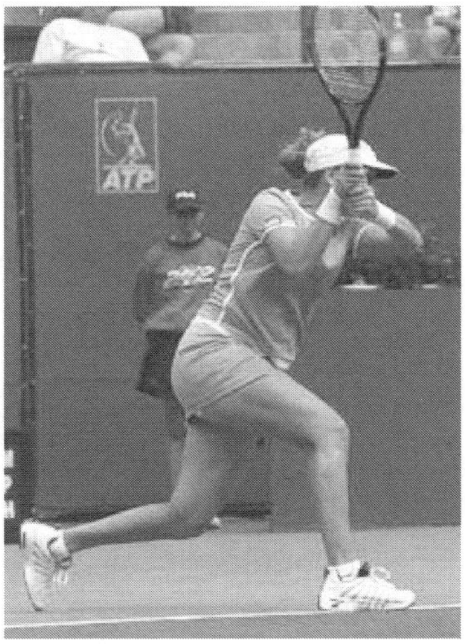

Figure 18
Monica Seles, a left-hander, hits her two-handed forehand with her dominant left hand at the bottom of the grip.

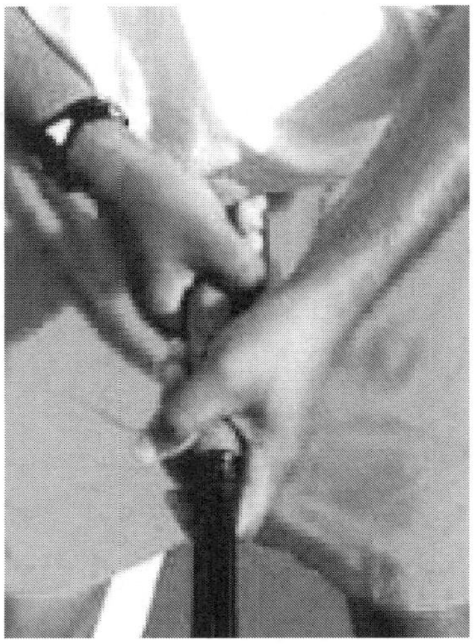

Figure 19
The right-handed, two-handed grip: The dominant hand is placed at the bottom in an Eastern forehand position. The off-hand is above also in an Eastern grip.

THE TWO-HANDED FOREHAND MECHANICS

Grip

The dominant hand on the two-handed forehand is no different than that used in executing the one-handed forehand. I prefer an Eastern forehand grip for the dominant hand and usually an Eastern forehand grip on the upper, non-dominant hand. (Figure 19 & 20) Because of the shortness of the reach due to the off hand on the top of the racket, it is not only more comfortable to keep an Eastern grip with the non-dominant hand, it also helps produce a smooth topspin motion for the two-handed forehand.

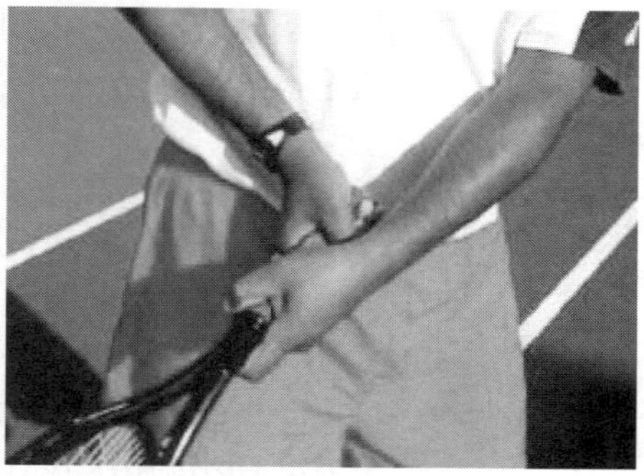

Figure 20
The two Eastern forehand grips allow for a natural take back on the back swing. Here, notice the hands don't cross over at the wrists.

There is no switching of the positions of the hands on the grip. For right-handed players, the right hand stays at the bottom, the left hand is on top. I have encountered a few players who actually switch their hands and hit basically a backhand on both sides of their body (as described previously in Method #1). While this is not as impossible as it sounds, the switching of the hands in competition is cumbersome. I don't recommend this method as it does not lend itself to a good forehand foundation.

Many top players who hit with both hands on both sides maintain these hand positions for both their two-handed forehands and backhands. Most players who learn to hit with these grips make subtle grip changes as they evolve into more prolific two-handed players. My recommended grips will give you the foundation to either stay with these grips or make your own slight variations to suit your idiosyncrasies as you become more skilled.

TWO-HANDED FOREHAND HITTING SEQUENCE

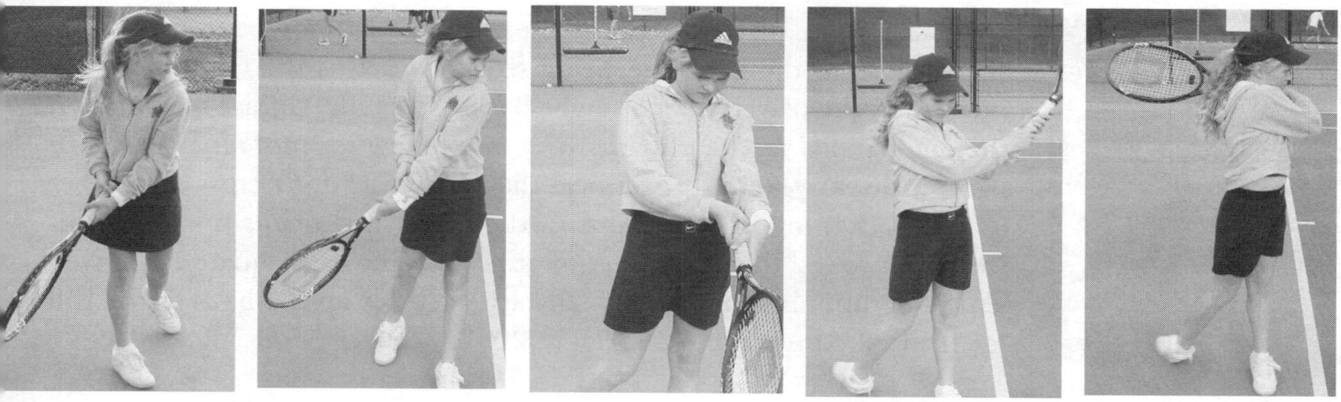

A B C D E

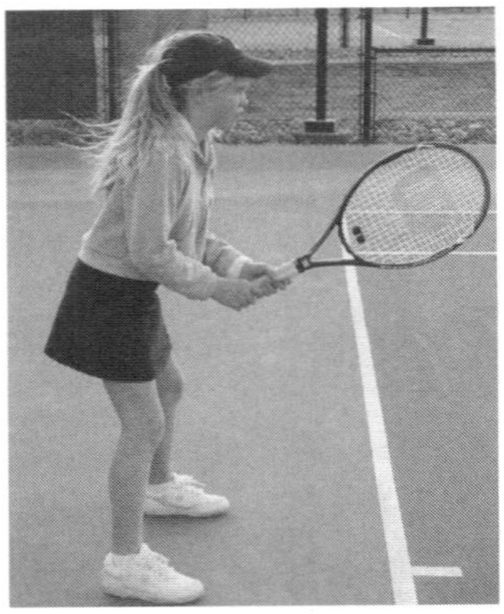

Figure 21
Ready Position

Ready Position

Like the two-handed backhand, the ready position of the two-handed forehand is identical. The racket head can be held high or low in anticipation of a groundstroke. (Figure 21)

A. Preparatory Backswing

Once the desired stroke is determined to be a forehand, two swing patterns are initiated: a) the shoulders turn so that the left shoulder (for right-handers) is pointed towards the net; b) the racket starts its backswing with the racket head pointing down and back. (Figure 22) The hands stay close to the right hip at this stage.

Advanced players tend to create a loop backswing, starting the racket high on the backswing as opposed to the "straight back" pattern described here. As I have mentioned, many top one-handed players use some aspect of a two-handed backswing on the forehand. (See Figures 3, 4, 7, & 8) The two-handed forehand can be hit with or without a loop backswing.

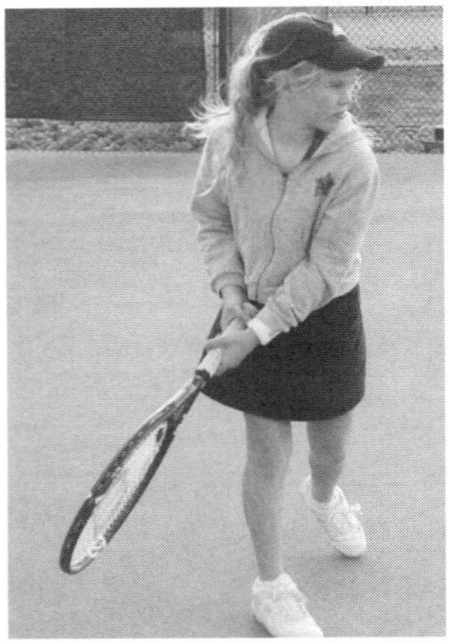

Figure 22
The preparatory backswing is a simple extension of the shoulder turn.

KEY POSITION POINT

Key Position Point: During the backswing, the right elbow bends and pulls back. This is very similar to the one-handed forehands of Steffie Graff, Pete Sampras and many other top tour professionals. (See Figure 23) For a bigger backswing, bend the right elbow and turn the shoulders more. This pulling back of the elbow is similar to the act of "elbowing" someone standing behind you.

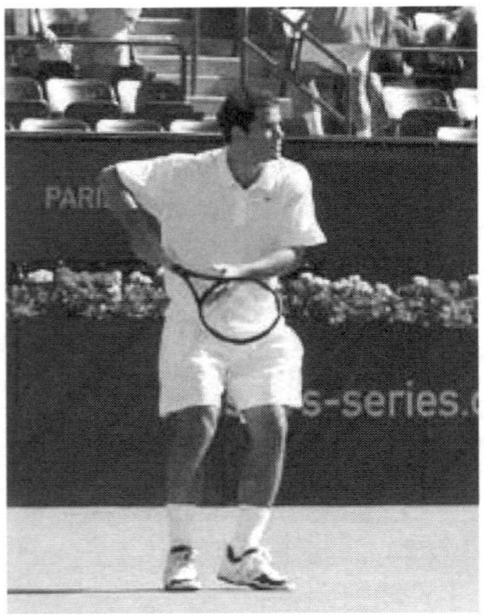

Figure 23
Note how Pete Sampras pulls his elbow back to start his backswing on the forehand. This is a very similar move to that of the two-handed forehand.

Backswing Notes: Because the two-handed forehand is usually shorter due to the left hand being stretched across the body, I recommend that the player use a Straight Backswing only. (Please see notes on the one-handed forehand backswing that follow for more information.)

Cautionary Note: It is critical that the wrists don't cross each other on the backswing. If this happens, the racket face opens up and forces the player to roll the racket over in order to come back square at contact. This will diminish the player's capacity to brush up the back of the ball for the desired topspin. (See Figure 20, 22, & 24)

B. Full Backswing and Step

As the ball approaches, the player steps into the shot with the left foot. (Figure 24) The racket has reached its full backswing position here. Notice the racket is almost pointed back at 180 degrees from the ready position. This is enough backswing needed to generate ample power. However, some players who want more racket head speed and distance will want to turn the arms and shoulders even more.

KEY POSITION POINT

Notice the chin rests almost upon the top of the left shoulder. Also, note that the left arm creates almost a straight line through the racket's center to the end of the racket head. These two points can help a player identify their position. (Figure 24)

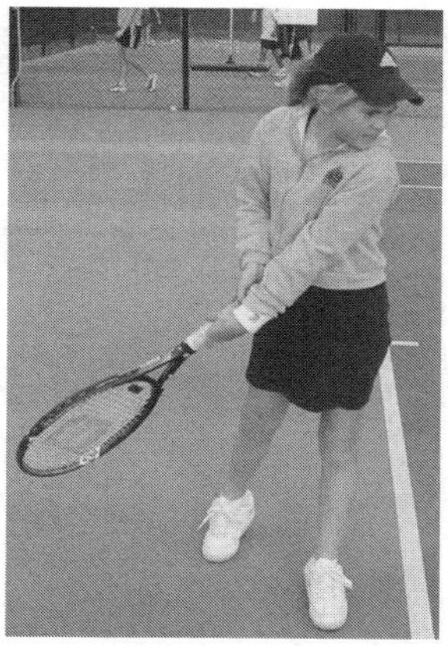

Figure 24
Prior to initiating the forward swing to contact, the right leg steps into the shot.

C. CONTACT POINT

Here, the racket head has come up to meet the ball in a low-to-high swing pattern. The racket is laid back in the right hand and the left hand is riding along at the top-front portion of the grip. The natural motion of the left and right hands driving up through the ball is what makes the two-handed forehand such a dynamic stroke for topspin. (Figure 25)

The use of the left hand through the stroke assists the right hand in brushing up the back of the ball.

During the backswing the hips and shoulders begin a one-quarter turn back towards the net. This turn is not big.

$E=MC^2$

THE KINETIC CHAIN AND ANGULAR MOMENTUM

As with every full-swing stroke in tennis, this transfer of the "kinetic chain" (the movements starting from the legs and hips ending up with movements of the shoulders, arms and racket) produces the initial swing pattern. However, similar to movements associated with the forehand groundstroke and serve, this initial rotation should diminish just prior to contact. If not, the racket will be swung with the turn of the body and not the rhythmic speed of the arms moving through the stroke. As in cracking a whip, the large muscle groups stop, allowing the hand holding the racket to speed up.

It is this transfer of movements that produces "Angular Momentum"...increasing the speed of an implement through rotating body components.

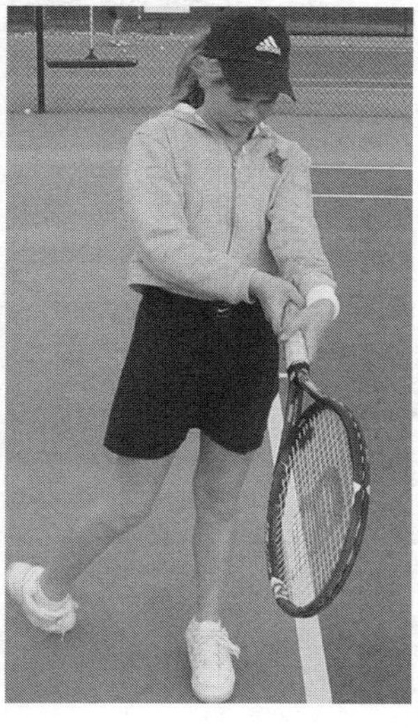

Figure 25
At contact, the racket is slightly closed as it brushes up the ball. The left hand contributes to the racket's upward motion through contact.

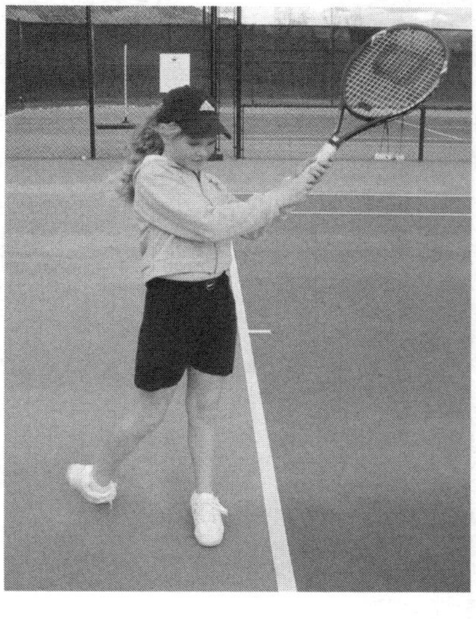

Figure 26
Note that while the racket has continued through the contact zone and is starting to finish its swing, the hips and mid section of the body are still sideways to the trajectory. Players who over rotate at this point will end up pushing the ball towards the target.

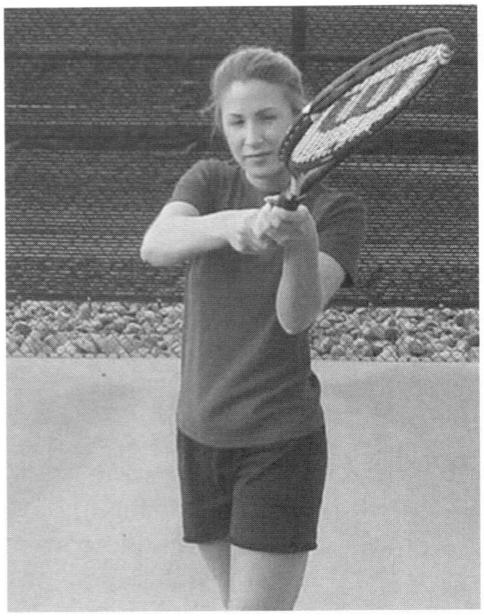

Figure 27
Observe the left arm's position after contact. By keeping this off-elbow close to the body, the player will generate excellent racket head speed while driving through the ball.

D. Primary follow-through sequence

As the racket continues up through the ball, the body remains partially sideways, allowing the racket to rotate both through the trajectory line longer and up the back of the ball. If a player over rotates here or rotates too early, the swing slows down. (Figure 26 & 27)

Note that the racket face has remained in the same plane from start to finish. As with all consistent strokes, the longer the plane is kept the same through a stroke, the more reliable the swing pattern.

KEY POSITION POINT

Like the backhand, the pivot point is the elbow of the inside arm. Here the left elbow remains close to the body as the right arm drives the racket up and through the ball.

The left forearm in coordination with the right arm pulls the racket up over this left elbow position. This sequence makes the two-handed topspin forehand almost self-working! (Figure 27))

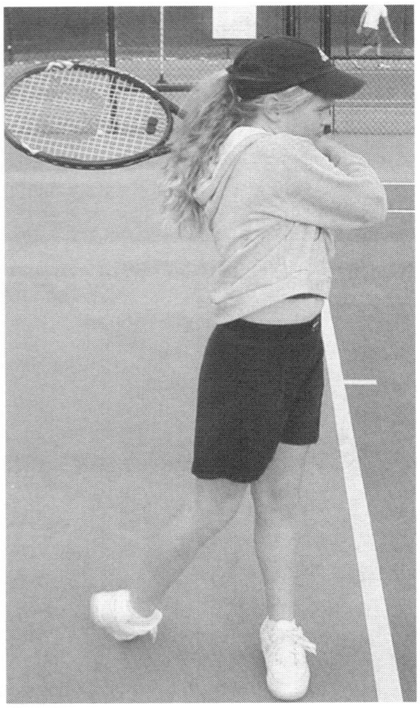

Figure 28
As the stroke finishes, leaving the toe on the back foot down helps prevent over rotation.

E. Full follow-through

The relaxation phase of the swing occurs during the follow-through of the stroke. The arms complete the swing by the inertia of the racket literally carrying the racket on around the neck (called a "wrap finish"). The body stays balanced at this point with the important "Toe-drag" of the back foot.

At this point, the arms lift due to the upward force of the racket brushing up the back of the ball.

KEY POSITION POINT: Toe-Drag

When a player swings, he has a natural tendency to allow the back leg to swing around (or the front leg to pull away). This movement usually makes the player rotate early. It also signifies an imbalance in the player after contact. Players should hold their follow-through for a fraction of a second before re-establishing the ready position in time for the next shot. Many pros can be seen holding this position after many strokes.

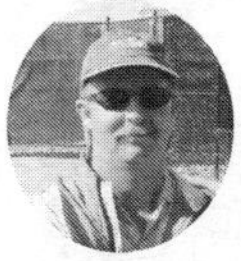

Author's Note
Recovery Step or Brake Step on the Forehand (Figure 29)

After contact has been made, advanced players will incorporate what is called a "recovery step". This movement is releasing the toe-drag foot and allowing it to swing around. The player can immediately push off this foot to recover back into the court. A problem occurs when players bring this leg around during contact. If this occurs, the swing speed is reduced and players tend to pull the ball to the left on right handed forehands.

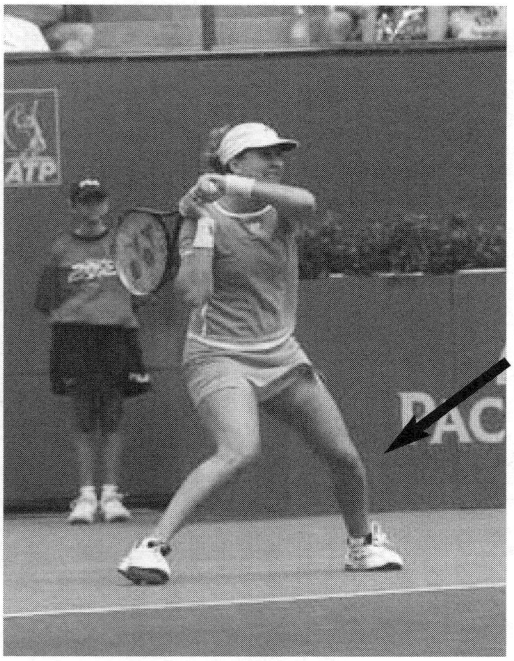

Figure 29
Often, skilled players, following the toe drag, will then swing the back leg through in order to push off in the other direction. Here, Monica Seles follows her left-handed forehand with her back, left leg swinging out after contact (Arrow). This allows her to "brake" her body's inertia and prepare to recover to a desirable ready position.

The One-Handed Forehand

Obviously, more players still use the one-handed forehand as their main stroke on the forehand side. Using the two-handed forehand as a learning tool will improve most players' ability to hit a solid one-handed forehand if they choose to do so. However, many players will still elect to hit only the one-handed forehand, both in the formative learning period as well as during the accomplished and competitive stage of play. You will notice that almost all the key elements found in the two-handed stroke mimic those of the one-handed forehand.

ONE-HANDED FOREHAND SEQUENCE

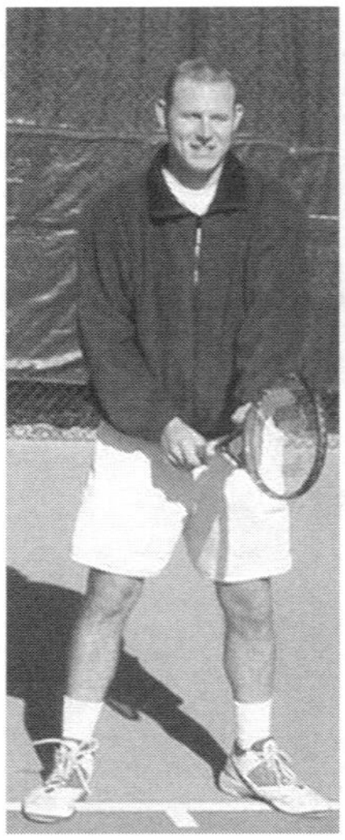
A

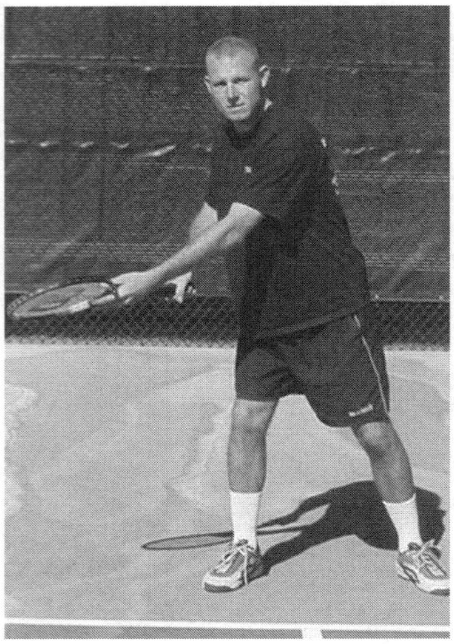
B

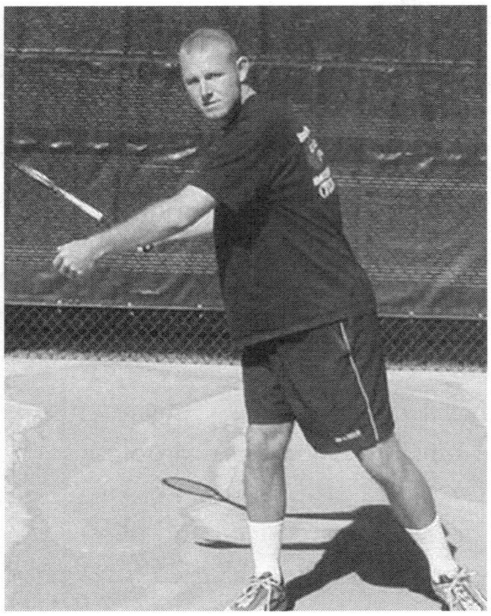
C

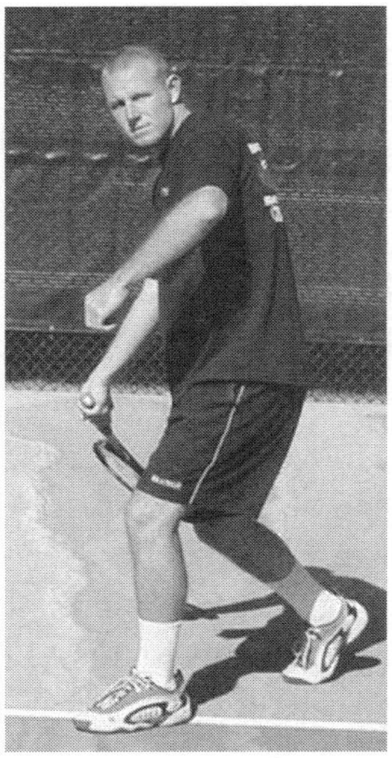
D

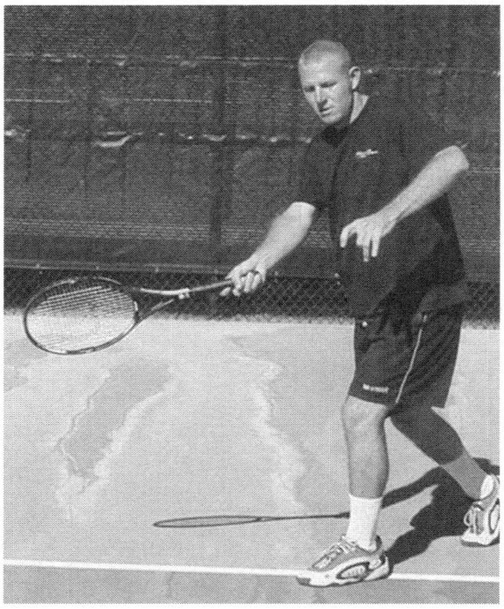
E

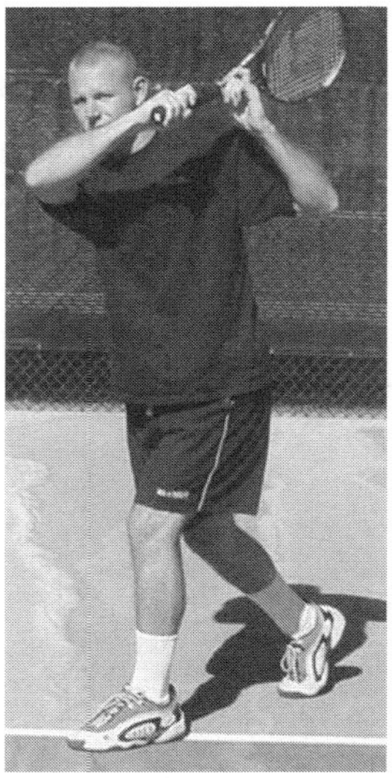
F

ONE-HANDED FOREHAND MECHANICS

Grip and Ready Position

More than any stroke in tennis, the one-handed forehand is the most diverse among top players. This diversity results from the wide range of grips top players utilize in accomplishing their stroke. There are basically four main grips that can be utilized when hitting a forehand:

- Eastern Forehand (Fig. 30)
- Semi-Western Forehand (Fig. 31)
- Full Western Forehand (Fig. 32)
- Continental (Fig. 33)

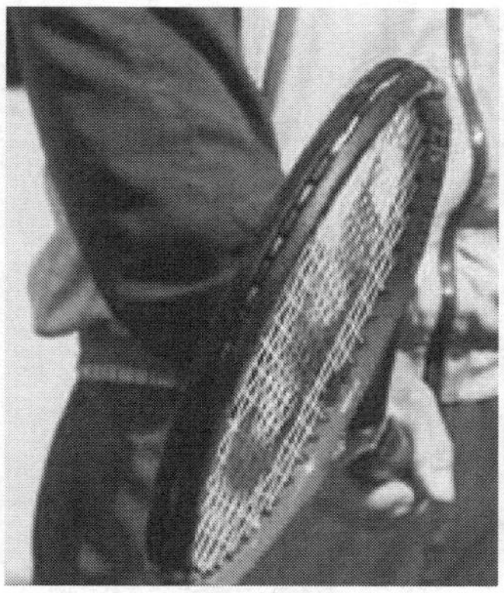

Figure 30
Eastern Forehand

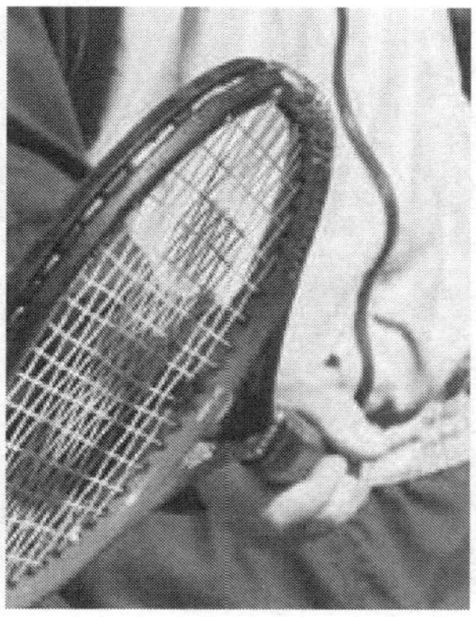

Figure 31
Semi-western Forehand

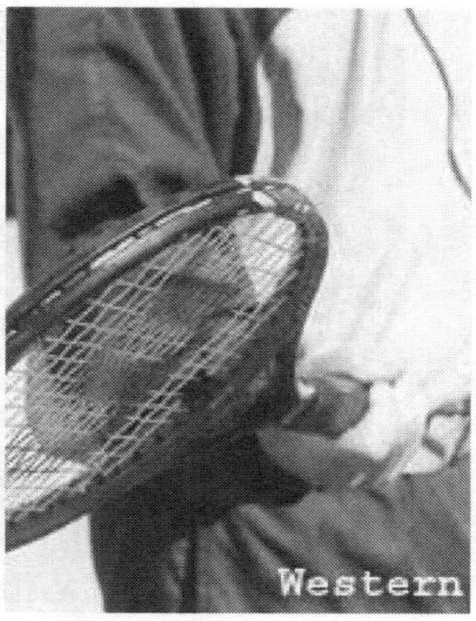

Figure 32
Full Western
Forehand Grip

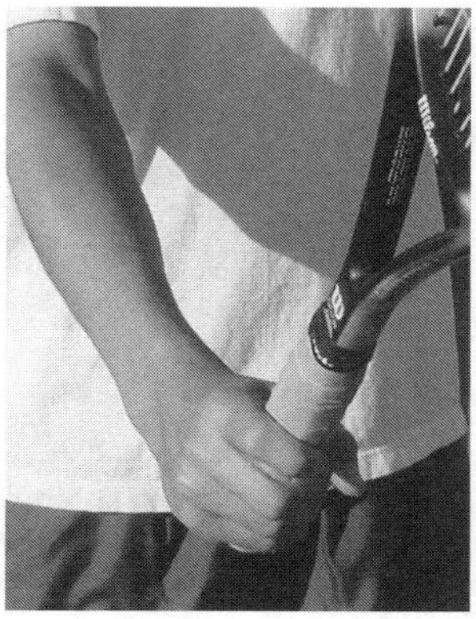

Figure 33
The Continental Grip centers the racket. Today, the Continental is used primarily for volleys, serves, overheads and slice groundstrokes.

Photos 30, 31 & 32 by John Yandell (TennisONE.com)

Each of these grips usually dictates a particular swing pattern that will be most accommodating for each grip. An entire book could be written about the use of each grip and its accompanying swing pattern. I have found that the Eastern forehand grip provides for an advanced foundation for the one-handed forehand while, at the same time, allowing each player to evolve into a more topspin/offensive grip as desired. The Eastern grip does not seem to prevent a player from evolving their forehand topspin stroke. In fact most of my players automatically begin utilizing the Western grips as they master the stroke associated with topspin. While the Continental Grip was used almost exclusively in the first 100 years of the game, it now is used only to volley and hit slice strokes by most of today's top players. (Figure 33)

Someone might ask then, "why not teach the Western grips at the onset of learning?" The answer is that the Western grips are very dependent on the proper stroke and timing sequence; realistically, most beginners would have great difficulty in being able to achieve such a stroke pattern. In addition, the angle of the racket face using the Western grip is so closed that beginners have a very difficult time just making contact on the strings! By using the Eastern forehand grip, players develop both the stroke pattern and the string action on the ball (of brushing up). Thus, they can, with relative ease, evolve their grip to these more extreme positions with minimal or no frustration as they develop.

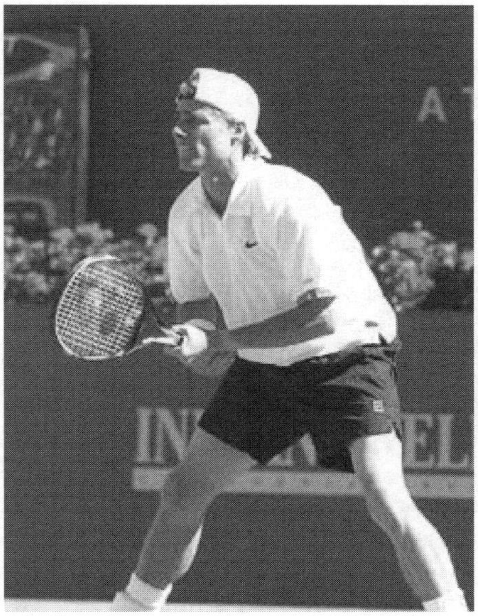

Figure 34
Layton Hewitt maintains a low center of gravity and a neutral racket position.

Ready Position (Figure 34)

As mentioned before, the ready position consists of a balanced position, allowing the player to move in either direction. Some players prefer to hold a backhand grip in the ready position, others prefer to hold their forehand grip (an Eastern, Semi-western, or full western). Either way is correct. The key position is to have the left hand on the racket at the throat or in the two-handed position. This will allow the player to use the non-dominant hand to steady the racket as the player shifts to the desired forehand grip.

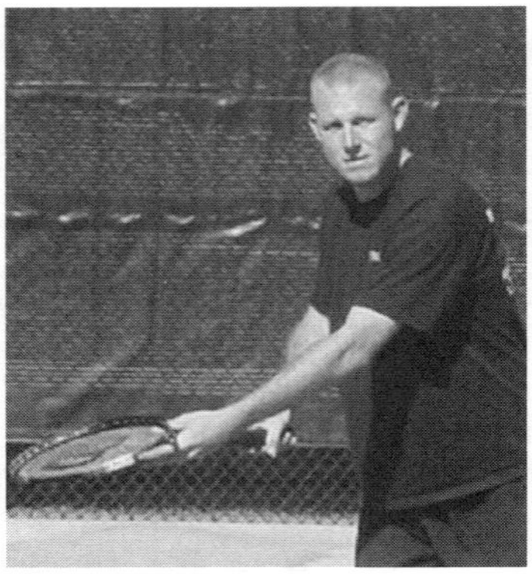

Figure 35

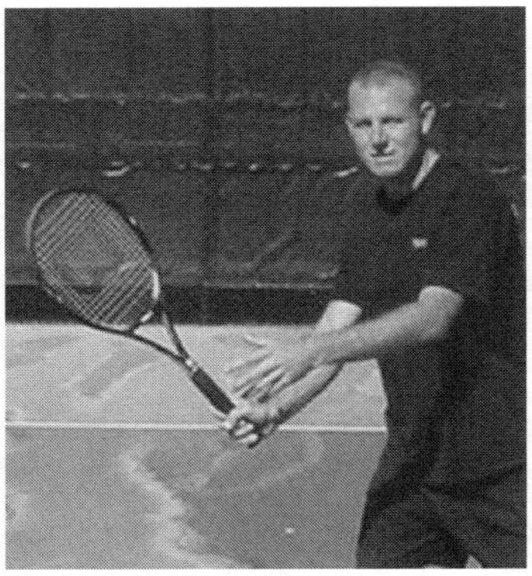

Figure 36

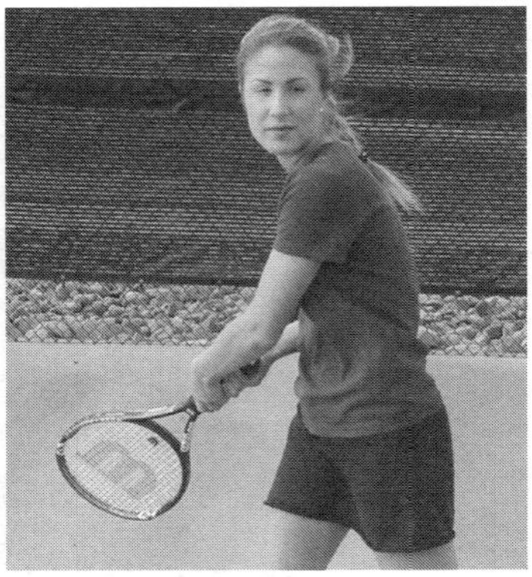

Figure 37

Note the similar movements of the one-handed forehand groundstroke (Figure 35) to that of the forehand volley (Figure 36) and to the two-handed forehand (Figure 37) A proper one-handed forehand groundstroke utilizes the off hand in creating the proper shoulder turn.

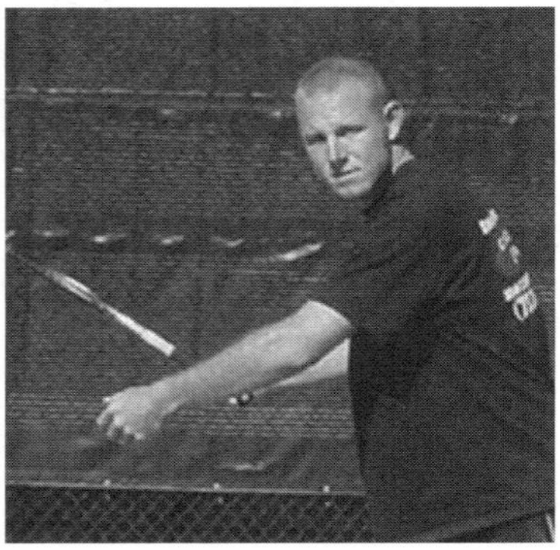

Figure 38
The "straight back" backswing is a common learning tool for the forehand.

Turn (Figure 35)

Notice how similar the turn of the one-handed forehand is to that of the two-handed forehand stroke. Like in a volley, a skilled player will use the shoulders to initiate the backswing. Thus, the hands are basically in the same position as that of our two-handed forehand player (Figure 37) as well as that of a player preparing to hit a forehand volley. (Figure 36)

Backswing (Figure 38)

There are three basic backswing techniques:

a) **Straight Back:** (Figure 38) This method is the most basic and simplistic; however, it sometimes is not as natural for most players. When taking the racket back, the player keeps the racket head low and points the racket down and directly behind them. This method simplifies the timing of the stroke in that it gives the player ample time to start the contact phase of the swing with minimal need to take the racket back or down prior to this phase. The straight back swing keeps the racket head pointed down below the contact point. From this point, the player only needs to decide when to hit the ball. Because the racket is below the ball, the player will generally always have a low-to-high swing pattern. This pattern is obviously needed to brush up the back of the ball and subsequently to produce the desired topspin. Two of the most prolific players to use the straight back backswing were Jimmy Connors and John McInroe.

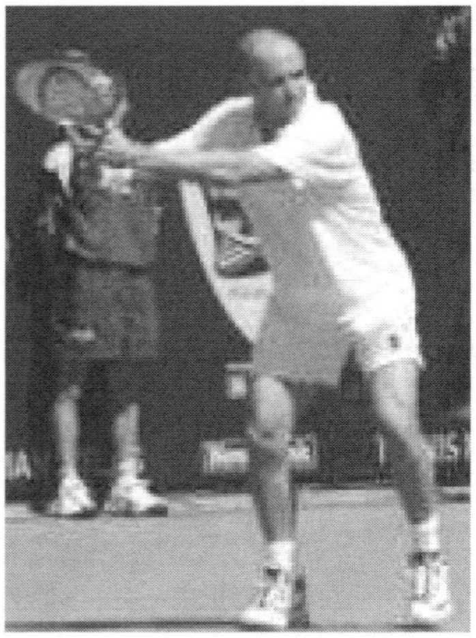

Figure 39
Andre Agassi uses a half-loop backswing.

b) **Half-loop Back Swing:** The racket taken back about shoulder height characterizes the half-loop swing. Here the player begins to utilize gravity in the rhythm of hitting the ball. By using any loop swing, the player keeps the racket head above the ball prior to the stroke. As the player begins the hitting phase, the racket is able to drop down and then sweep back up (hence the name "loop") in one continuous motion. The initial swing pattern integrates the force of gravity in starting the racket's movement. (Figure 39)

c) **Full Loop Back Swing:** As the name implies, the player creates a full loop pattern in the forehand swing. Starting well above the shoulders, skilled players will often pause here as they wait for the ball. (Figure 40) Because the swing pattern is more complex (due to the distance the racket must travel down prior to moving back up to brush the ball for topspin), this backswing is more difficult to time. It is recommended that players first adopt the Semi-Loop backswing prior to expanding to this more efficient, yet more skill-dependent, swing pattern.

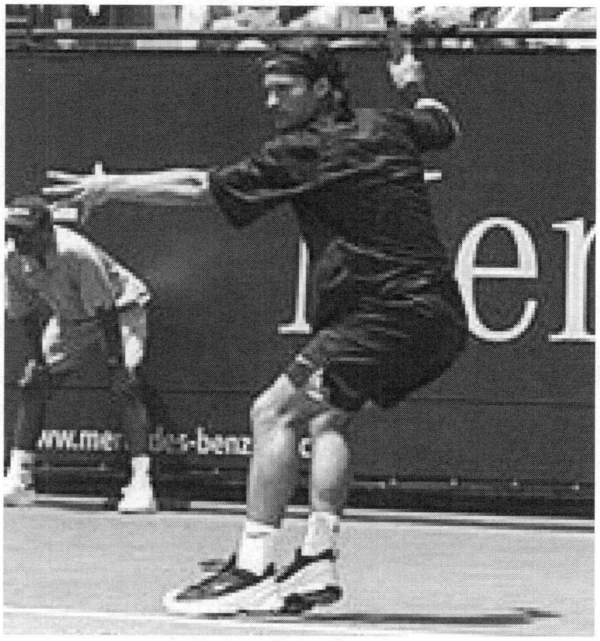

Figure 40
A full loop backswing starts with the racket high. This swing uses gravity to start a loop pattern to contact. The racket will drop from this position to a point well below the ball. With a continuous movement, the racket will then brush up the back of the ball for the desired topspin stroke.

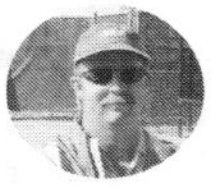

Author Comments on the "Loop" Backswing

There are three recognizable backswing patterns. However, when learning the forehand, most players will create a more congruent swing pattern if they learn the straight backswing style mentioned in this section first. I must mention however, that, almost without exception, each player will develop or "evolve" a backswing pattern that meets the player's personality and need. Every player I have ever taught has developed an individual swing pattern although each was taught the straight back pattern initially. Occasionally, I will cue a player to try the loop swings when they have demonstrated the proper racket position prior to contact. However, this is very rare as most players will develop some aspect of a loop pattern on their own as they progress.

Proponents of learning the loop swing at the first claim that since most skilled players incorporate the stroke pattern, players should learn it first. While in theory this might make sense, in practice it seldom works. Since learning the low-to-high pattern is developed faster among most beginners using the straight back stroke, I have found that in the real world of training students, this method is far better suited than learning the loop swing first.

Pros who identify students who can emulate stroke patterns faster can introduce the loop swings earlier to students who demonstrate a readiness to do so. Even so, I still would recommend all students first pursue the more conservative straight back swing as an initial learning technique.

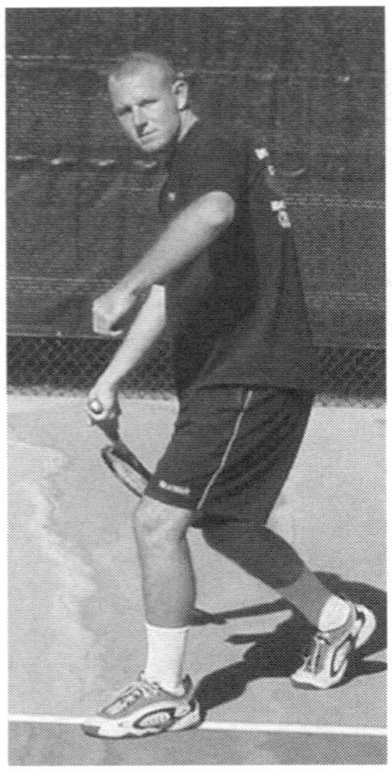

Figure 41
The closed racket face drops well below the contact point. Here also, a right-handed player will step into the ball with their left foot.

Racket Drop and Step; Closed Stance (Figure 41)

Regardless of what backswing technique you use, the racket head must drop below the ball prior to contact if you are attempting to hit a topspin forehand!

The traditional forehand that all players should learn to hit incorporates a "closed stance" footwork pattern. Like the forehand volley and the two-handed forehand, the right-handed forehand has the left foot stepping in and across the body prior to contact. This helps the player rotate the body sideways, a critical move in executing an effective forehand.

Note the racket head position here. The racket head is well below the ball and the racket face is closed. As the racket moves up to hit the ball, this racket orientation to the arm will be maintained from this point until well after contact.

Contact (Figure 42)

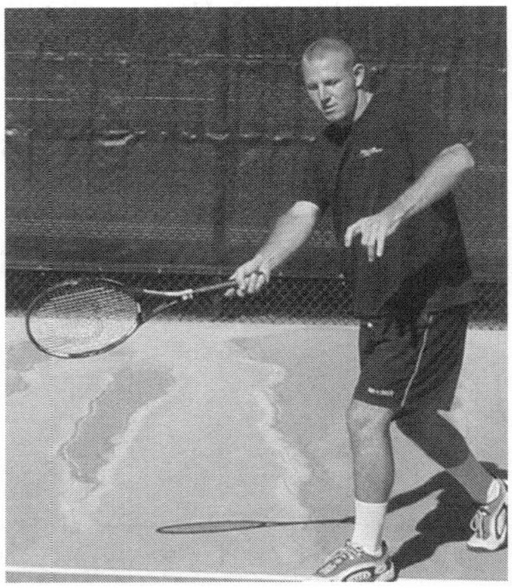

Figure 42
At contact, the racket is locked at the wrist and drives up the back of the ball.

At contact, the racket is reaching its acceleration peak with the racket head moving up the back of the ball. Notice how the shoulders have opened up slightly at this point to allow release of the racket arm through to contact. At this point the rotation of the shoulders stops, allowing the arm and racket to literally whip through the ball. If the shoulders were allowed to continue rotating, the swing speed would slow down. This is due to the fact that by over-rotating, the player would pull the shot too far to the left. The body subconsciously recognizes this and lays the racket back to counter this undesirable turn. Usually, the player who opens up too early must push the ball towards the target. In addition, swinging at a speed equal to the speed of the body turning is incredibly slow! It is the combined rotation to contact and the subsequent brake of this upper body rotation that provides for the kinetic chain to release the stored energy of the body from the coil at backswing.

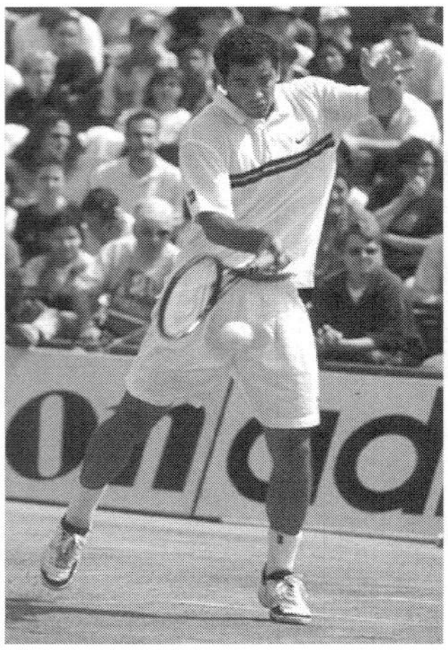

Figure 43

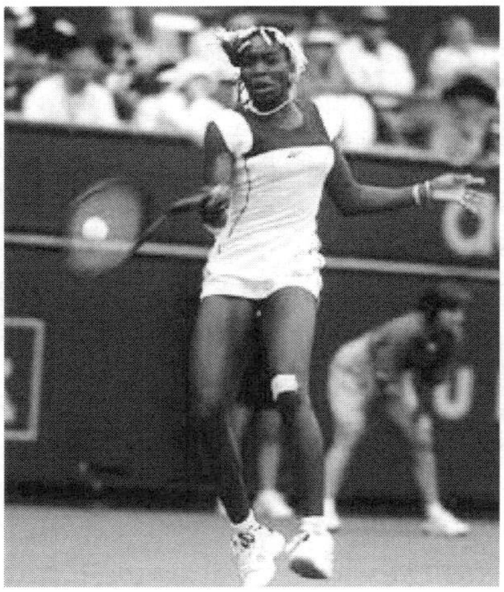

Figure 44

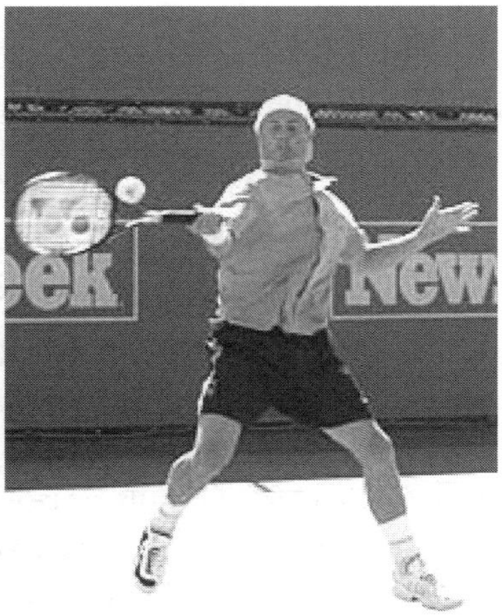

Figure 45

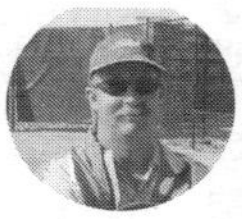

Author's Note – Contact Point
(See previous page figures 43-45.)

While each player has begun to rotate out of his or her sideways position, (established from the coil on the backswing), you will notice that each player here is still at an approximate 45-degree angle to the target. This can be ascertained by the fact that each player's hips are facing the camera (which is off to the side of the court in each shot) and not facing the net.

Follow-through (Figure 46)

The follow-through can often be an indubitable sign of proper or improper mechanics. A player who has utilized flawed technique prior to the follow-through will be hard-pressed to finish the swing in such a way as I am describing here.

Obviously, the topspin follow-through provides for a continued upward swing pattern. (If the racket was moving up at contact, this pattern will be retained through much of the follow-through.)

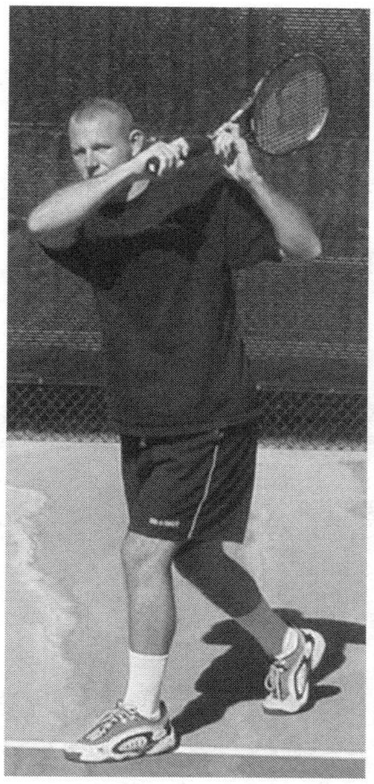

Figure 46
As the racket finishes high and over the shoulder, the off hand can be used to catch the throat of the racket

KEY POSITION POINT

The right elbow and the butt cap of the racket point to the target area. The back of the hitting hand is near the left cheek of the player.

In addition, the back foot remains down at the point for a moment before releasing and swinging around to provide a "Brake Step" for the player. The off hand can catch the racket at this point.

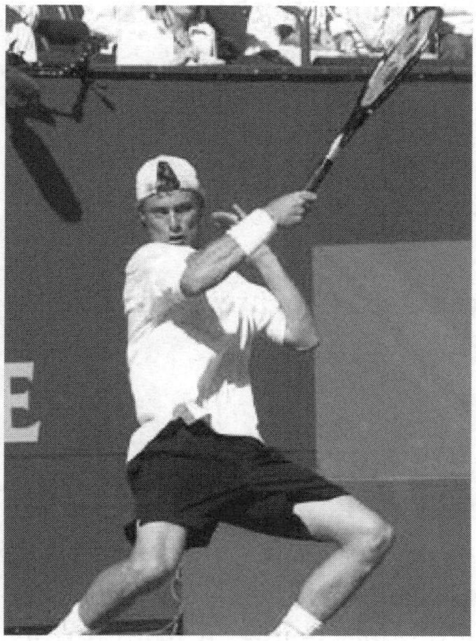

Figure 47

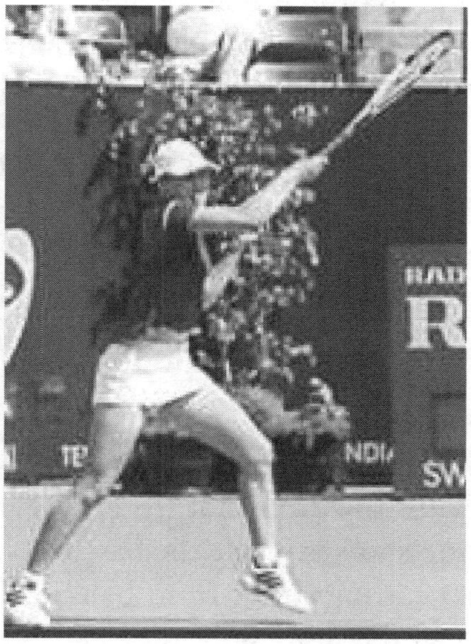

Figure 48

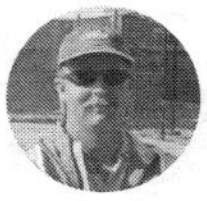

Author's Note –
Use of the off-hand

Many top-level players will use their off-hand in finishing the follow-through. Here, Lleyton Hewitt (Figure 47) and Martina Hingis (Figure 48) keep their off-arm up and fairly close to the body. By practicing the "catching the racket" in this off hand, (Figure 46), players can learn to use this hand effectively in producing a proper forehand. Many beginners and intermediate players end up dangling this off-arm down at their side.

"Finish" (Figure 49)

The end of a proper forehand is amazingly similar for most skilled players, regardless of grips and backswing. Most players end up with what is called a "Wrap" finish. This position, (Figure 49 & 50) has the hitting arm's elbow pointed towards the target. In addition, the butt cap of the racket also points towards the target. While the wrist remains locked through contact, this wrap finish is a relaxation tool for many players.

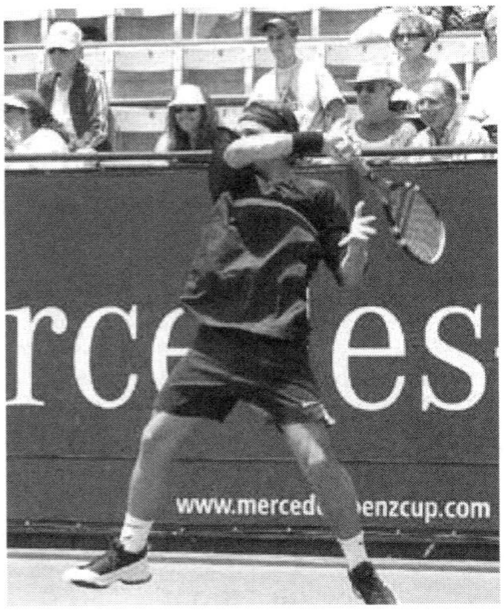

Figure 49
The classic "Wrap" finish by Carlos Moya with a reverse pivot step.

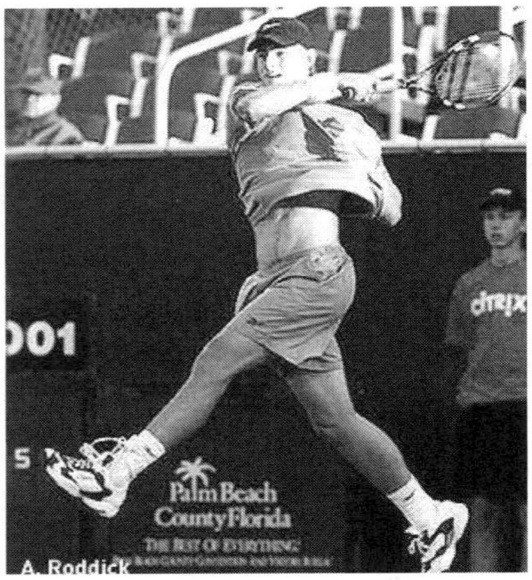

Figure 50
Andy Roddick finishes his forehand with the wrap finish and a crossover closed stance while on the run.

The Slice Forehand

The slice forehand at the pro level is almost non-existent. This scarcity can be traced to one major factor: most pros attack even low forehand groundstrokes with topspin.

Occasionally a pro or skilled player will hit the slice forehand as a blocking type shot when a hard hit ball is hit directly at them, or they will hit the slice forehand as a drop shot. Because of the scarce use of this shot, few books today cover the slice forehand. I believe that many players end up developing a decent slice through an extension of learning the forehand volley. Because the two shots are almost identical in intention (that is, a linear stroke with emphasis on a slicing motion), players often do very well in hitting a slice forehand after they have mastered the correct forehand volley.

At the club and recreational level, players often resort to the slice to help keep balls in the court. Because many have not mastered the topspin stroke, these players find that by slicing the ball they can control the pace of the shot. This is true. However, most players who execute the slice for this purpose seldom hit it with skilled form, and, thus, can't progress in hitting the slice with greater effect. Generally, players who use an Eastern forehand on their volley tend to have difficulty hitting any slice forehand as an approach or from the baseline. This is caused by the natural inclination by players who use this particular grip to drop the racket head when trying to slice the ball. This type of stroke resembles more of a chop or a hack. As with the proper volley, the racket head should remain above the wrist through contact.

FOREHAND DROP SHOT

The slice forehand comes into play at the higher levels in the execution of the drop shot.

The drop shot can best be described as a slightly longer volley stroke with emphasis on touch and backspin.

Drop Shot Position

Many intermediate players end up hitting drop shots from the wrong position on the court. Typically, they hit the drop shot from too far back. The most advantageous place from which to hit drop shots is inside the baseline about half way to the service line. The reason for this is that hitting drops from behind the baseline provides opponents with more time to run down the shot (since the ball is in the air longer being hit from further back). Also, from behind the baseline, a player hitting a drop shot will obviously have to hit the ball harder to get it to the net. This means the ball will either bounce higher or bounce more forward towards the on-coming opponent.

Closer in, three advantageous principles come into play:

1. *Since players typically hit aggressive approach shots when they get a short ball, opponents have a tendency to be anticipating a harder hit ball. They end up momentarily on their heels expecting to be hit a harder approach shot.*
2. *Because the player hitting the drop shot is closer, the distance to the net is shorter. Players can use a great deal of finesse from a closer position and not have to hit such a perfect drop shot from close in.*
3. *By hitting drops shots from a closer position, closing in behind the drop shot is easier and more natural. (The strategy of following a drop shot to the net will be discussed in Chapter 14 on Single's Strategies and Chapter 15 on Doubles Strategies).*

Drop Shot Technique

One of the most important points to remember when hitting a drop shot is to keep the racket, arm, and wrist fairly firm. While hitting a drop shot requires touch, the need for greater control of a player hitting drop shots with wrist and elbow movements is increased. The ability to develop a consistent drop shot is dependent on the player's ability to replicate the stroke over and over the same way. As in any shot in tennis, when the wrist is allowed to move in the context of any stroke, the control factor is greatly reduced.

The racket is taken back much like a player hitting a volley. The shoulders turn and the racket is held high. From this point, the player can hit a driving slice approach or the drop shot. The differences between the hits are that the drop shot is hit more under the ball and it is hit much softer. A sideways position must be maintained since, like the volley, the drop shot is a linear stroke as well.

The ideal height of a drop shot is difficult to describe. This is because of two things:

1. *If you hit the ball too low, the ball might not go over the net. If you do make it, the forward trajectory of such a low shot will bounce and move more forward towards your opponent as opposed to a ball hit higher.*
2. *If you hit the ball too high, it will obviously bounce higher giving your opponent time to run it down. However, a relatively higher drop shot will tend to bounce more straight up, as opposed to bouncing forward like a lower drop shot might.*

This issue of height combined with softness are what make drop shots either very effective winners or sitting ducks with which your opponent can punish you! Thus, every player must practice their drop shots with regularity if they hope to execute a decent one in match play.

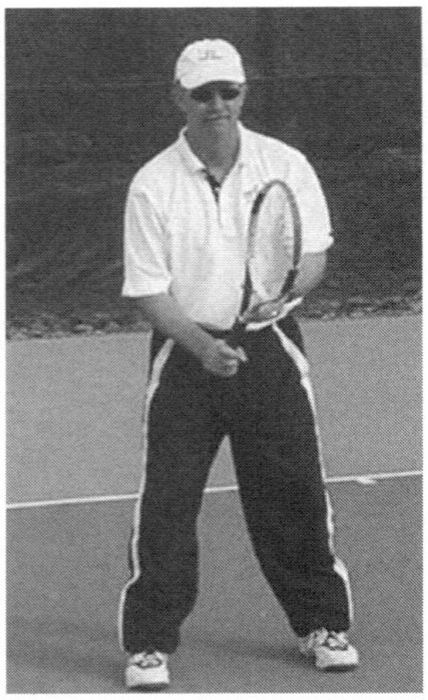

Figure 1

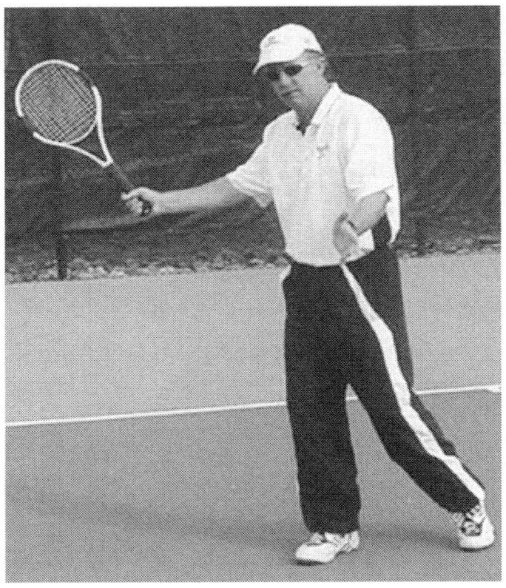

Figure 2

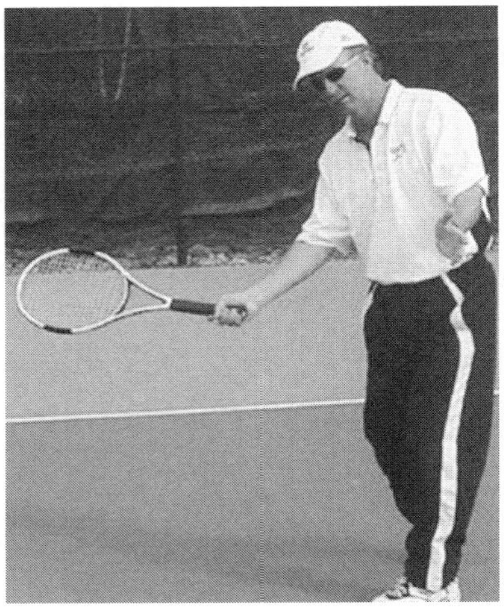

Figure 3

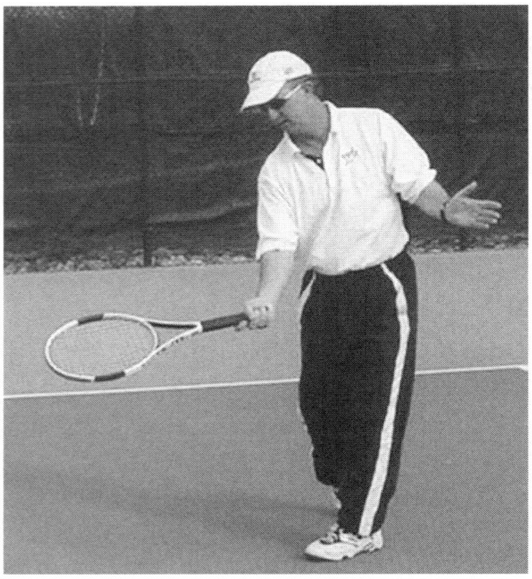

Figure 4

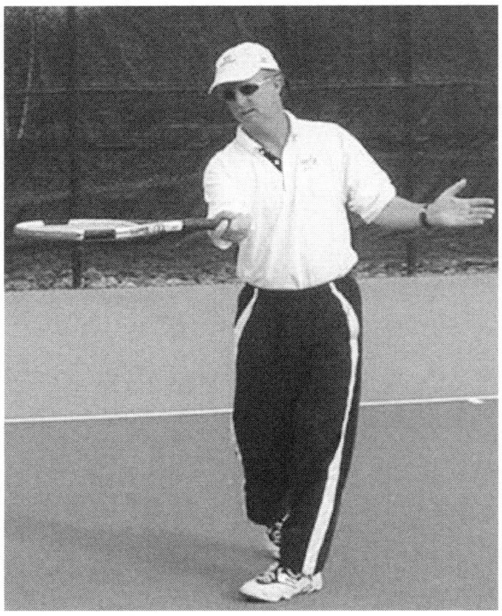

Figure 5

The Drop shot

After the ready position, (fig. 1) the shoulder turn is initiated with the racket held high on the back swing. (Fig. 2) As the racket moves down through the stroke, the racket face remains open. (Fig. 3) The body stays sideways as the racket continues down and brushes under the ball. Contact is made even with the front knee. (Fig. 4) Follow-through is in line with the target. Thus the racket will open up as in the final figure. (Fig. 5)

Photos by David Smith

Forehand Conclusion

As mentioned, there is more diversity in skilled players executing forehands than any other shot in tennis. This diversity is related mostly to the variety of grips afforded to skilled players. Players who learn to hit the forehand as described in this chapter will easily and naturally evolve their personal forehand style with minimal necessary attention to making any specific changes. I have found that when players learn this Advanced Foundation, they are free to explore subtle idiosyncrasies that they themselves find helpful in executing more effective strokes that fit their individual style.

Most importantly, players who seek skilled play will need that initial blueprint from which to build a quality forehand. A solid foundation will insure greater consistency and reliability.

CHAPTER 11

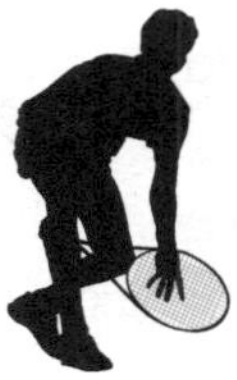

The Advanced Foundation
The Serve

Introduction

The serve has always been viewed as either a weapon or a liability for most players. Players who possess highly effective serves have a substantial edge in competition: they already have half the games well in hand! Consequently, a level of confidence seems to follow good servers into competitive arenas. However, weak servers possess a sense of dread when it comes time for them to serve. These players often elect to receive first, even though they may have won the choice of serve or side, just to delay the mortification of displaying their contemptible serve!

In theory, the serve, perhaps more than any other stroke, should be every player's best shot. Why? Because the serve is the one shot in which:

- *The player dictates when they will hit the ball*
- *The player dictates where the ball will be when hit*
- *The player dictates where he or she will stand while hitting the ball*
- *It can be practiced with or without a partner*

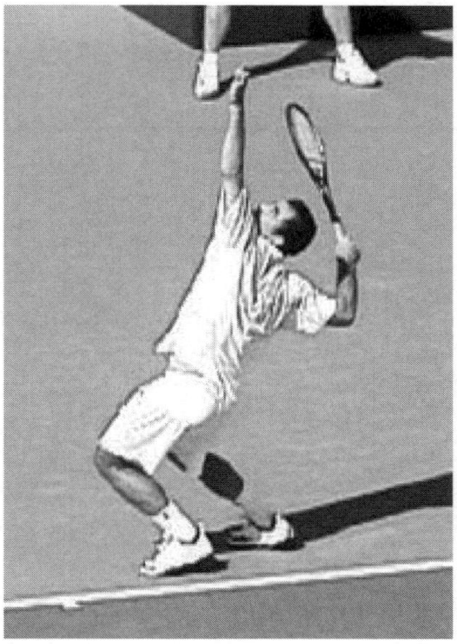

Figure 1
Men and women alike must learn to use their body, legs, and arms in a synchronized, explosive movement to create an effective serve. Here, Pete Sampras stores up his angular momentum in preparation of an explosive release of this power.

It is critical, however, that even dedicated players—who intend to practice their serve—learn how the serve should be hit correctly. Any player who is uncertain or has been given faulty service advice will surely meet with difficulty and doubt, creating, most likely, a questionable service motion in the process. It is interesting to observe that most recreational players possess a wide range of serving motions, most of which don't bear any resemblance to serves that are associated with championship play! From "paddy cake" serves to "leaping-leaners", from windshield wiper swings to tosses nearly reaching sub-orbital status, most recreational players who have minimal or no understanding of the proper service process

It is interesting to observe that most recreational players possess a wide range of serving motions, most of which don't bear any resemblance to serves that are associated with championship play

!

unequivocally put the ball in play using some pretty bizarre methods!

Like teaching the volley, many tennis instructors, authors and professionals, tend to teach the serve in a transitional pattern. The belief that a more basic model for serving should be taught and mastered before the more generally accepted advanced service motion is attempted, seems to be common among most books and instructors. While this teaching philosophy may or may not speed up the ability for students to successfully hit the serve into play, it most definitely will hinder these players in developing a more advanced serve with power, pace, spin and control.

It has been my experience that players, given the right tools for learning the serve, can easily establish an advanced foundation for this stroke. With few exceptions, almost every student I have taught was able to develop the proper service motion, grip and technique needed for this advanced foundation in essentially the same amount of time it took others to learn the more rudimentary serve taught by others.

The following instruction will provide you with the tools and knowledge to practice correctly. Such practice will result in your eventual possession of a highly effective serve.

The Serve: Advanced Foundation

The advanced service foundation is based on the mechanics that will provide the player with four critical components:

- *Racket head speed*
- *Spin*
- *Control*
- *Continued, progressive improvement*

Serves that are established on "elementary" foundations tend to lack the first two of these elements in varying amounts. (Elementary service motions include the Eastern forehand grip, players facing the net, and the player's hitting hand in front of the racket head at contact.) Without these two components—racket head speed and spin—an advanced serve, one that has pace and effectiveness, is virtually impossible. It is easy to spot players who don't possess the foundation for producing racket head speed and, even more important, spin. They attempt a supersonic first serve (usually out by several yards!) followed by the proverbial paddy cake serve in which even the spectators can read the label on the ball as it crosses the net! One of several defining characteristics that separate the 3.0 and 3.5 players from much higher developed competitors is the effectiveness of the second serve. Generally, more advanced players have not only acquired the proper advanced foundation described in this chapter, they also understand the relationship of the four components mentioned above that make up the advanced foundation.

It is critical that students learn the relationship of spin and speed of the ball in how it relates to successful serves. Understanding the various kinds of spin and their effect on the flight of the ball and its subsequent bounce from the court is also critical.

If the player is not able to produce desired racket head speed, the amount of ball rotation (spin) will be severely handicapped. Likewise, if the player is unable to create the appropriate spin, the ability of the player to hit faster serves accurately into their opponent's service court will be greatly diminished. When a player lacks the ability to produce the right kind and amount of spin, the player will usually become a serving "dinker". As mentioned, these players tend to hit astronomically fast first serves (with equally extraordinarily poor results) and second serves that are as slow as the name "dink" implies. With proper spin, not only are faster, more accurate first serves possible, but consistent and more effective second serves are possible as well.

When a player lacks the ability to produce the right kind and amount of spin, the player usually become a serving "dinker"

!

One of the problems with serves based on "elementary" methods is that they don't allow for "continued, progressive" improvement. This means that basic service motions will reach a point where no more improvement can occur. However, a serve based on an advanced foundation will allow the player to improve EVERY aspect of the serve. Greater spin, more speed, better placement, more effectiveness, and increased consistency are all available to each and every student of the Advanced Foundation.

THE "SECOND-SERVE ADVANTAGE"

Players who have a mastered an effective second serve gain two distinct advantages. The first one is obvious; your opponent won't be able to tee-off on your second serve if it isn't weak! The second advantage is less obvious but equally important. If you have a confident second serve, your freedom to go after your first serve more aggressively WITHOUT the fear of either double faulting or having your opponent drill a return off a weak serve, is substantial!

The aspect of developing a good serve quickly is greatly enhanced by learning spin first. The prospect of providing players with the opportunity to go after first serves with an aggressive swing—without the fear of a weak second serve—creates many potential easy points for the server.

Reasons for Spin

Like the age-old question "what came first, the chicken or the egg?" it is sometimes confusing for players to determine if they should learn to develop spin first, or should they learn to develop racket speed first. In my experience, it is absolutely imperative for players to learn how to hit spin first. There are several reasons for this:

- *Players who develop racket head speed first tend to have difficulty controlling or knowing what their racket is doing during the course of the serve.*
- *It is much easier for players to add velocity to their serve after learning how to generate proper spin first.*

- *Players who hit inconsistently with high racket head speeds tend to hit exponentially slower second serves in response to the fear of double faulting.*

There is an obvious relationship between spin and racket head speed. Certainly, if the goal is to generate greater spin (and hence take advantage of the characteristics provided by this spin), players must increase racket head speed to do this. However, it is advisable for players to first learn the "swing pattern" of the spin prior to attempting to increase the speed of the swing itself. The reason for this is simple. Players who try to swing hard don't have the capacity to maintain racket head control. Thus, a hard swing will usually follow a path that is most familiar to the player. This familiar path, in most cases, is far from the more complex path that players need to develop for an effective spin serve. As in learning any skilled movement, practicing slow, deliberate moves will increase the likelihood of the student gaining control of desired moves. Watch anyone trying to hit a tennis ball, golf ball, baseball, or other implement-related object. If they swing hard, the results are usually exponentially disastrous.

Types of Spin

There are basically three distinguishable spin serves. However, it should be noted that all three are based on a similar "advanced foundation", one that will allow the player to explore all three with minimal changes. (Flat serves also have spin. I will discuss the "flat" serve later in this chapter.)

SLICE SERVES

This is the starting point for all three spin serves. The slice serve is excellent in helping the student learn how spin effects the trajectory of the ball. In simple terms, a slice serve mimics the rotation of the earth on its axis. The ball is "brushed" with the strings moving across the equator of the ball creating sidespin. (Please see Diagram 1.)

Diagram 1

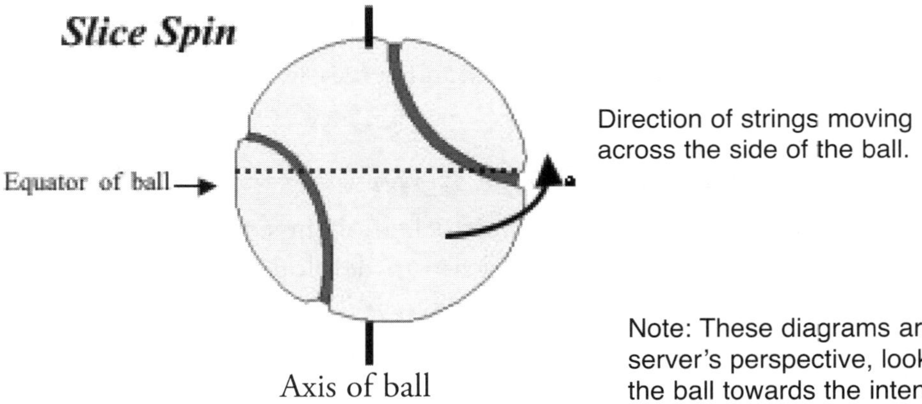

Note: These diagrams are drawn from the server's perspective, looking at the back of the ball towards the intended target. These are viewed as a right-handed server would see and hit the ball.

For right-handed players, the slice serve will cause the ball to curve from right to left as it travels through the air. The action of the spinning ball against the air will create friction on the right side of the ball and lower air pressure on the left. (Review Chapter 7 on the "Physics of Spin".) A true slice serve will have a slight dropping action on the ball, causing the ball to also dip slightly down as it curves to the left. However, this apparent downward movement is due to the fact that the forward velocity of the ball is slower compared to a ball hit with an equal amount of force but with little spin. The majority of the downward movement of a slice serve is still influenced more by gravity than by the spinning action of the ball.

Diagram 2

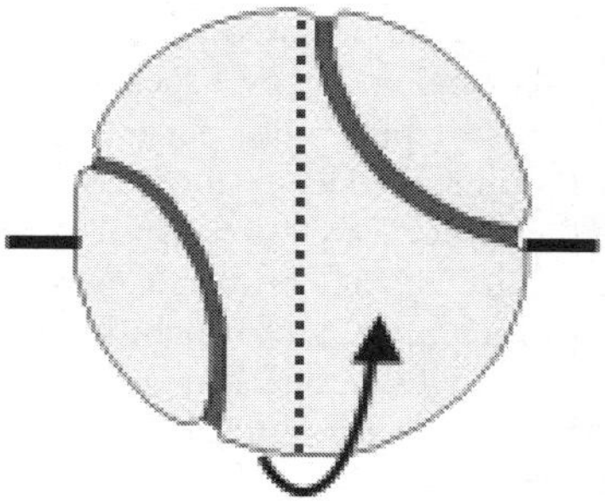

TOPSPIN SERVES

The topspin serve is actually a misnomer. The action on most topspin serves is actually a combination of slice and topspin. Most players will have a most difficult time creating true topspin on a serve. In order to hit true topspin on a serve, the strings of the racket must move directly up the back of the ball at contact. Because of our anatomy, this action is almost impossible for most people. (See Diagram 2)

In reality, most skilled players brush up the ball at an angle from lower left to upper right (for right-handed players.) Or, using a clock analogy, the strings brush up from 7 or 8 o'clock to 1 or 2 o'clock. (See Diagram 3)

Diagram 3

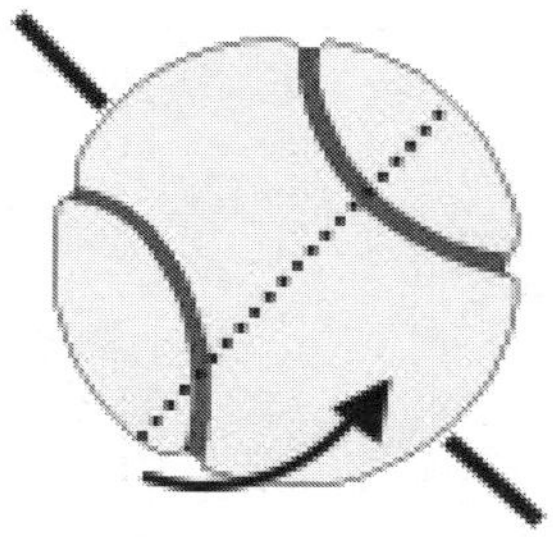

Combination slice and topspin action.

The action of a "topspin" serve (or combination slice and topspin) helps bring the ball down into the court using the physical properties of the spin. In addition to gravity, a ball moving with topspin will have additional help in arching down into the court (just like topspin groundstrokes do). This action allows a player to hit the serve with more velocity and have a relatively greater margin for error over the net. In addition, the topspin action will cause the ball to bounce higher off the ground than the slice or a flat serve with minimal spin. This makes the return generally a more difficult shot for the returning player.

The combination of slice and topspin will produce a bounce that resembles both: a dipping serve with a higher bounce that also curves right or left (depending on left or right-handed spin). As players develop their tennis abilities, advantages of making the ball curve and bounce differently on their serve provide greater diversity and, consequently, greater difficulty for opponents!

KICK SERVE

The third kind of spin serve is called a "kick" serve. It is by far a more difficult serve to execute for most players, but is quite effective when developed. The spin of a kick serve is produced by a player hitting up on the inside or left edge of the ball as opposed to up the back as in the topspin or around the outside edge as in the slice. (Decades ago, this serve was often referred to as an "American Twist." However, the follow-through action of the modern kick serve is different than the old Twist serve. This will be mentioned later as we get into the instruction of the serve.)

Unlike the slice in which the ball is spinning from right to left in relation to its direction from the server, the kick serve spins up slightly from left to right. The racket strings

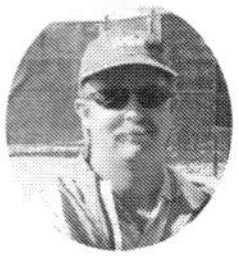

Author's Note – Left-handed Servers

For those of you who are left handed, you have a nice advantage built into your game: Left-handed serves obviously curve and bounce to the opposite direction as right-handed serves. The advice of developing spin over speed is even more of an advantage to you lefties! It is simply foolish not to take advantage of this benefit. If you are a left-handed player, focus on developing a spin serve as described here and your serve will be far more difficult to return than if you simply hit it flat. A "flat" left-handed serve is, for the most part, no more difficult to return than a flat right-handed serve.

Another advantage of left-handed serves is that on the ad court, the left-handed server can use an effective slice serve to the typical right-handed player's backhand. This is a very difficult shot for many right-handed players to hit back effectively.

The bottom line is that as a left-hander you will utilize these advantages far better by developing a spin serve. A flat serve will not be much more difficult for opponents to negotiate compared to a comparable right-hander's flat serve.

brush up from below the left side of the ball and finish higher and to the right of contact. This action causes the ball to spin with its rotation from left to right. The result is a serve that curves slightly to the server's right and bounces up and to the left of the returning player. Since topspin and slice serves bounce up and/or to the right of the returning player, the kick serve, with its leftward bounce, can be quite difficult to return.

For right-handed servers, learning to serve a kick serve is easier to develop on the left-hand court, serving to the ad service box. Since the kick serve is a more "advanced" serve, it is important to establish an advanced foundation before moving to this serve. It will be much easier to learn and master the kick serve if this foundation is first developed.

The "Advanced Foundation" Serve

GRIP

As with all playing foundations, the serve begins with the proper grip, one that will be used in developing an advanced serve. Beginners, intermediates, and advanced players—all who seek to serve well—should utilize the same grip when developing their serve.

As most books and teachers recognize, the Continental grip is the preferred choice among all skilled or advanced players. Those who learn the serve with the more basic Eastern forehand grip will have several components in their service technique that differ from those who serve utilizing the Continental grip. This is one of the reasons why players who learn the more basic serve pattern using the Eastern grip have extreme difficulty making the transition to a service motion that uses the Continental grip. Not only is the grip different, but many other service components need to change as well.

READY POSITION (FOR RIGHT-HANDED PLAYERS)

The stance for the advanced foundation is similar to a closed-stance forehand groundstroke at contact. The position starts sideways with the left foot in front, the right foot back and slightly behind the player. Notice how this position (Figure 3) mimics a closed-stance forehand groundstroke.

The racket is held with the Continental grip and the hitting side of the strings is facing slightly up. (Figure 4) This is accomplished by turning the wrist

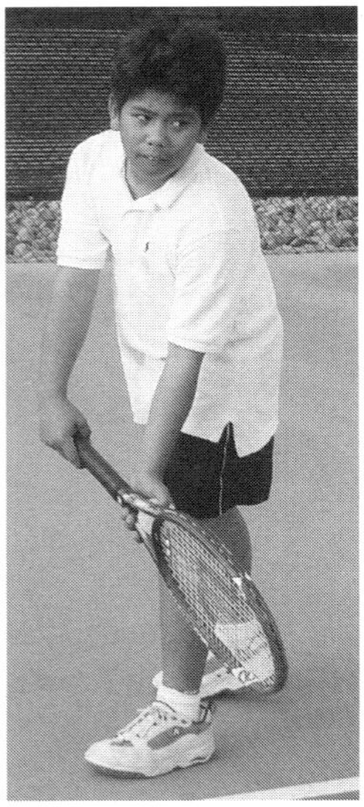

Figure 2
The Advanced Service Foundation can be achieved at any age.

of the hitting hand in towards the server. The left hand cradles the throat of the racket.The ready position also includes several initiating moves for most players, such as bouncing the ball, letting the arm swing freely and loosely, and a pause prior to starting the swing sequence. I will address these important additions to add to your advanced foundation at the end of this segment.

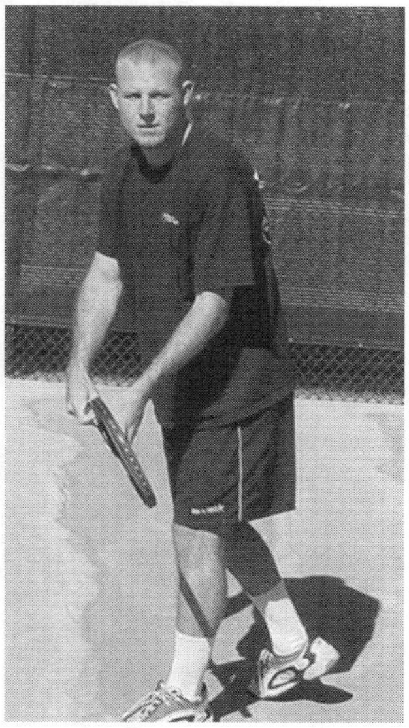

Figure 3
A proper ready position includes a strong, distinctive preliminary stance.

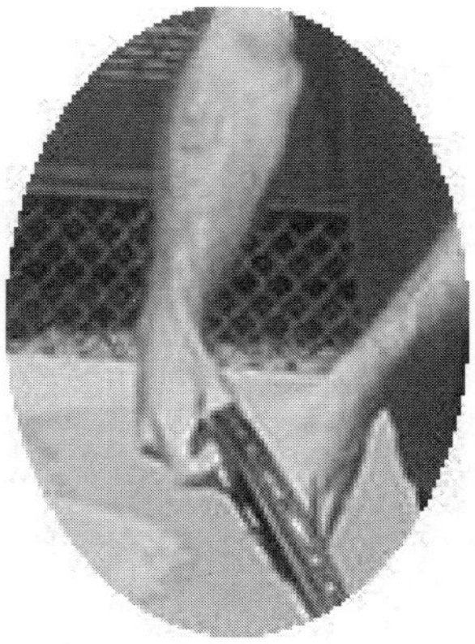

Figure 4
Note the open racket face at ready position.

SWING SEQUENCE

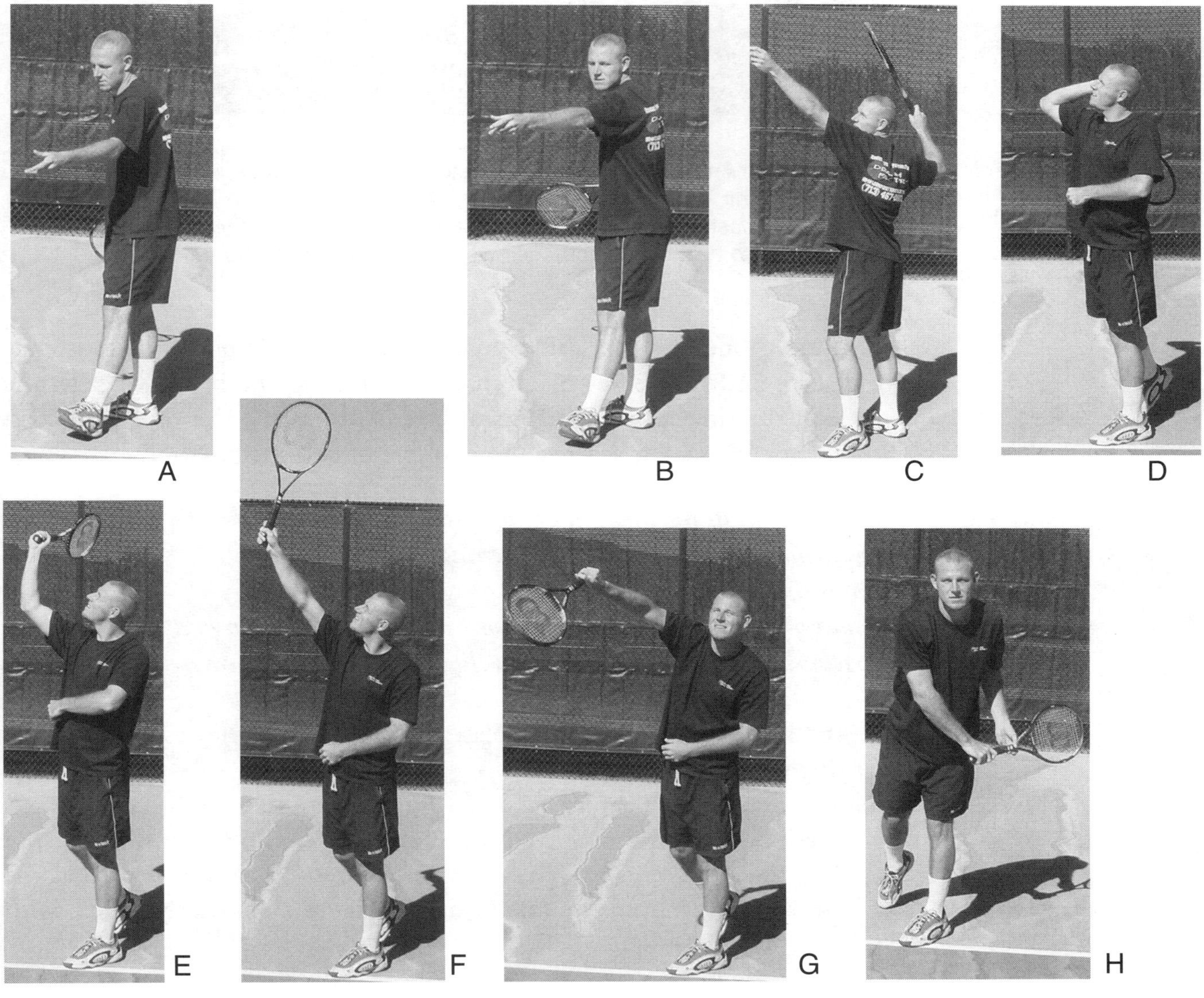

KEY POSITION POINTS

A & B The Toss (Figure 5 - 8)

Here, the weight of the player has shifted to the back foot. The tossing arm is held straight and slightly to the right. The hitting arm begins to drop back, but the racket face stays facing the player's hip. (Figure 6)

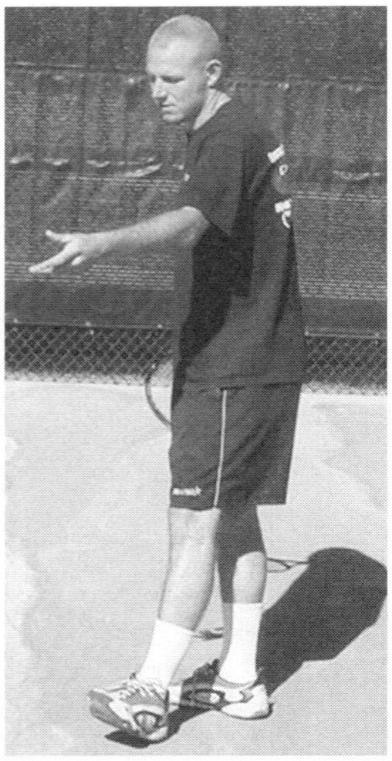

Figure 5
Note the rocking back of the player's weight to the back foot as the toss is initiated. The racket arm drops down and back. The face of the racket does not lay open.

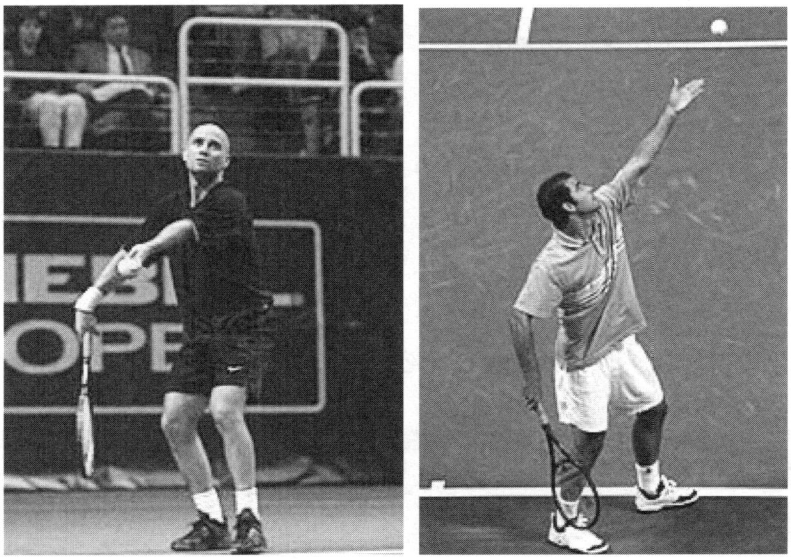

Figures 6 & 7
Observe both Andre Agassi (left) and Pete Sampras (right) as they begin their service toss. The racket arm is held loose, the tossing arm pushes up the ball to the player's right, and their body begins to coil. In addition, their weight moves back to the back foot.

The toss is one area that causes many players trouble both in consistency of the serve and in the actual mechanics of hitting the ball. Typically, the major contributing factor to an inconsistent toss is the use of the wrist in "flicking" the ball upward. I recommend one of two toss methods:

a. Hold the ball in the fingertips and "push" the ball upward with the arm. Release the fingers by opening the hand palm up as the arm lifts the ball.
b. Hold the ball as if holding a glass of water. Use the thumb and first two fingers to hold the ball as the arm lifts. (See Figure 8)

Both of these methods will decrease the player's tendency to use the wrist in making the toss.

Notice the toss arm is forward and to the server's right. This position sets up the desired toss required for both a slice and a combination slice/topspin serve. Notice in the sequence of the serve pictures (Figures A – H) that the extension of the arm from the toss position (Figure B) is nearly in line with the racket at contact (Figure F).

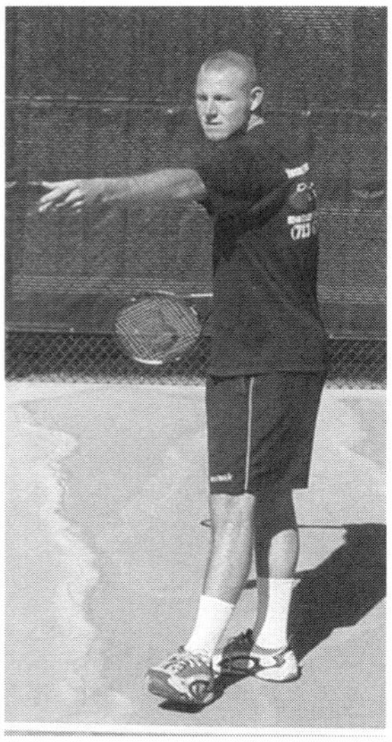

Figure 8
The toss release

C. Backswing Continuation (Figure 9)

As the tossing arm continues up, the racket begins to rise. Notice the face of the racket is still leaning forward. This is important. Do not lay the racket back. (Figure 14) This typically causes the palm of the racket hand to rotate and face upwards. As a general rule, keep the same wrist position as in the ready position through the backswing (with the wrist turned in slightly). This will prevent the notorious "Palm-up" position later in the swing!

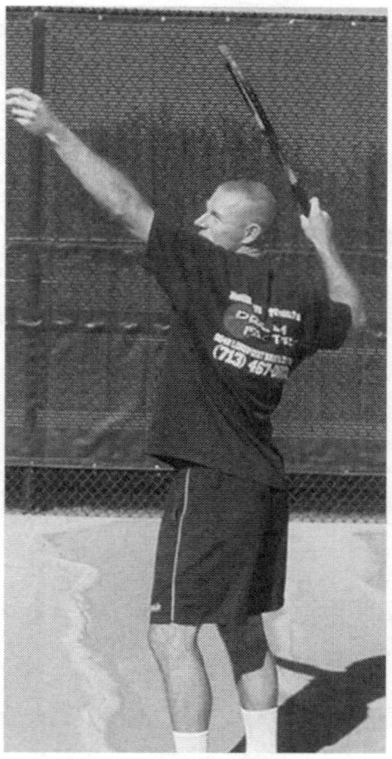

Figure 9
As the backswing continues, the right elbow moves back as the racket moves higher.

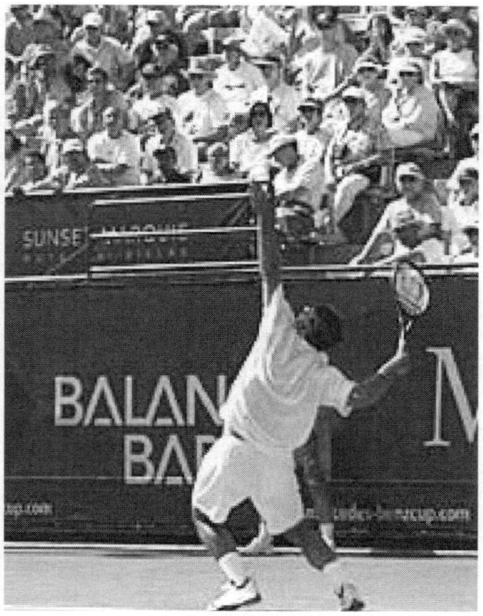

Figure 10
Note the racket head pointing up, the weight still back, and the deep knee bend.

Notice that as the toss is completed, the body is turned further sideways to the net, almost to the point of the back facing the net. (Figure 10) This foundation is required for players to maximize power and body rotation without the prospect of rotating too early or too much. At this point, the toss arm is fully extended and the hitting arm is cocked at the elbow. The elbow, at this point, is held up away from the body. Many players tend to drop the elbow here creating a hitch in their service motion.

Also note the position of the hitting palm. Typically, players who use the rudimentary Eastern forehand grip will be in the "Waiter's" position, holding the palm flat, facing the sky (as if holding a tray! Figure 14). Holding a Continental grip will keep the palm of the hitting hand more sideways nearly facing the player's head.

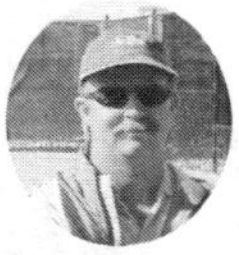

Author's Note

Notes on Swing Pattern Prior to Contact

A number of instructors stress the importance of a particular backswing pattern. Some say to bring the racket down near the ground and then up in a wide arc before collapsing behind the player's back. Others will tell you to bring the racket straight up from in front of the server and over the head. The main issue in developing the best serve within a player's ability is hardly ever the result of how a player learned the backswing. What I have found to be of primary concern is the player's ability to make the strings of the racket make contact in a specific and desirable manner. Thus, my emphasis in serve development is not on the backswing but on the action of the racket at contact. If we look at all the historically great servers in tennis, we find that few players had the same backswing pattern. However, they all made contact with the ball within almost identical parameters with their racket. Make sure you too are making contact with the ball as described in this chapter.

D. Preliminary Contact Sequence "Collapse" (Figure 11)

At this point three distinct actions take place: 1. The toss arm drops and is held near the stomach area; 2. The hitting arm has come forward with the elbow leading; 3. The racket has completed its "collapse" behind the player's back.

This sequence is completed as a continuous motion. The combined movements of the elbow moving forward and the racket head dropping to the collapsed position creates the necessary movements for maximum racket speed. The sequence creates a similar

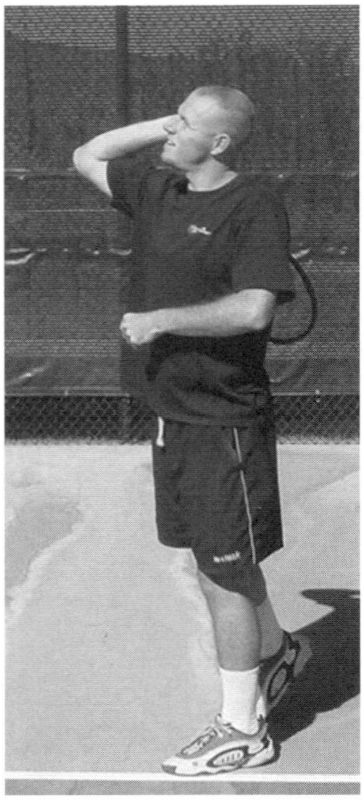

Figure 11
The "collapse". The racket drops down as the elbow moves forward.

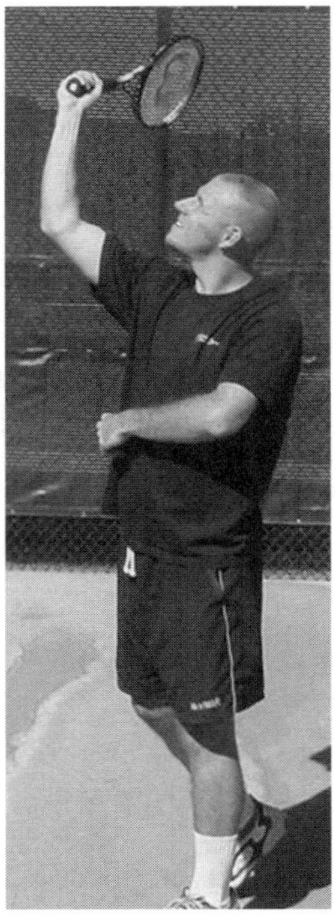

Figure 12
"Edge-on" The player leads the racket forward with the butt-cap just prior to the brushing contact on the right edge of the ball.

motion to throwing a ball or cracking a whip.

It is at this point that many players who use the Eastern forehand grips for their serves commit an error: they tend to hold the racket in a "palm-up" position. (Figure 14)

E. Pre-Contact "Edge-on" position (Figure 12)

As the elbow continues forward, the racket begins to "whip" up from its collapsed position. When the elbow reaches this position, the racket moves up with the edge of the racket leading. This position makes it look like the player is going to hit the ball with the edge of his racket instead of the strings, (which is why we call it the "Edge-on" position!). Key points include that the butt-cap of the racket is nearly facing the target. The palm of the serving hand is still turned in as opposed to facing the sky (as most players will do if they are using the Eastern forehand grip. See Figure 14).

At this point, notice the slight rotation of the shoulders from their closed position. Many players over rotate at this point. Players who use an Eastern grip on the serve tend to face the net prior to contact. (Figure 14) This diminishes the rotational power (from angular momentum) and limits the racket distance during the key acceleration phase. Our advanced foundation of using the Continental grip will utilize a body rotation DURING contact as opposed to BEFORE contact.

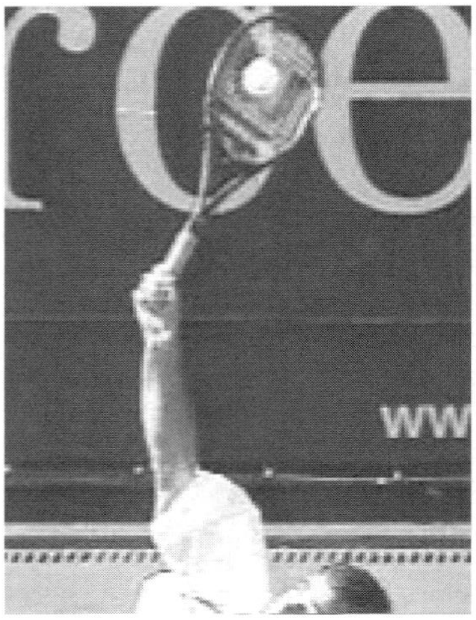

Figure 13
Note the racket attacking the right side of the ball.

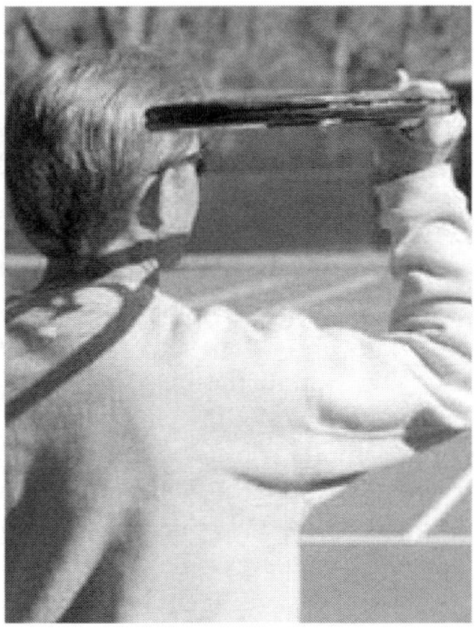

Figure 14
The notorious "Waiter's Grip" and serve position.

F. Contact (Figure 15)

At contact (and just prior to) the racket face is beginning to pronate towards the ball. (Figure 12 &15) During the sequence that leads up to contact, the swing pattern will dictate the type of spin the player wants to apply to the ball. For more slice, the racket will be hitting more across the outside edge of the ball. For topspin, the racket will be moving up the back of the ball. For a kick serve, the racket will move up the ball from the back and slightly on the left inside edge of the ball.

Note that the contact point is almost at a full extension of the arm. With most spin serves, the contact point will be slightly below the full extension point as the racket will still be moving up or across the ball. Contact made at the very apex or top of the player's reach will reduce the capacity of spin potential. (However, it should be noted that a great majority of beginning players tends to let the ball drop too low prior to contact. It is not uncommon to hear pros tell their students to "reach higher" when hitting the serve.)

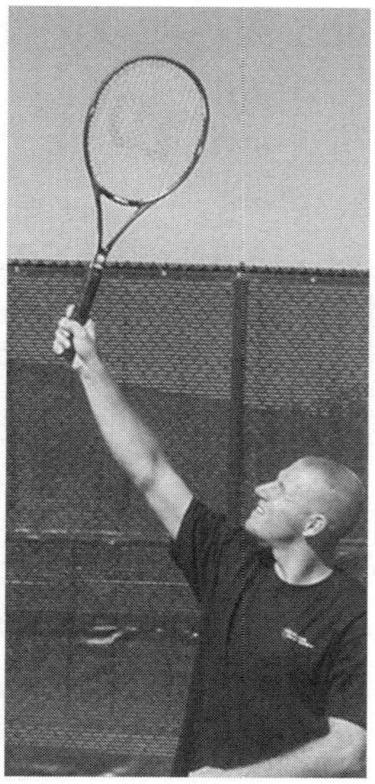

Figure 15
Contact of the ball is almost at full extension of the arm. Pronation of the forearm brings the racket face to the ball. On spin serves, the stings will be moving across the ball at contact.

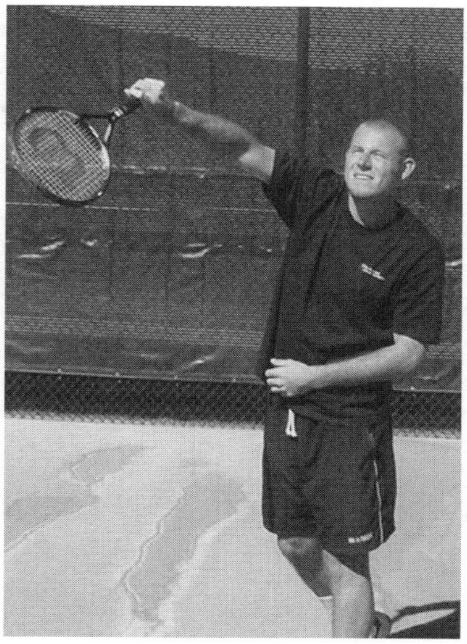

Figure 16
Maximum racket speed is generated when the racket continues to pronate. If the player attempts to swing from the arm, the racket head speed is reduced. (Note the position of the upper arm compared to Figure 12. There is very little movement of the arm as the racket is pronating.)

G. Pronation of the forearm. (Figure 16)

This is a critical point for developing racket head speed. As the contact point of the racket addresses the right side of the ball, the racket head is pronated to the right. (This makes it look like the racket is hitting the ball to the right instead of to the left! However, the ball has left the strings at this point. Here, relaxation of the racket occurs after contact begins.) This movement generates tremendous racket head speed. An important point to remember here is the fact that the player will want to address the right side of the ball prior to the pronation. If the player pronates too early, the ball will be contacted too flat or on its left side. Remember the foundation serve is based on a slice serve.

Notice the toss hand and arm is still held across the stomach area during contact. (Figure 16 & 17) As in many shots in tennis, this action helps prevent the player from over rotating. Also, the hips still face to the right slightly, demonstrating that the rotation of the body and hips is only one-quarter of a turn. Compare this position of the hips with that of their full coil in Figures 9 & 10.

Another point should be mentioned here. Notice the upper arm position in Figures 12, 13, 15, 16, and 17. In Figure 12, just prior to contact, the upper arm position is exactly in the same position as in Figure 16 (and Figure 17 of Pete Sampras), just after contact. This is an example of how the serve is not an "arm" swing as much as it is a forearm rotation (pronation). There is a kinetic chain of muscle movements in this sequence that include the shoulders and the upper

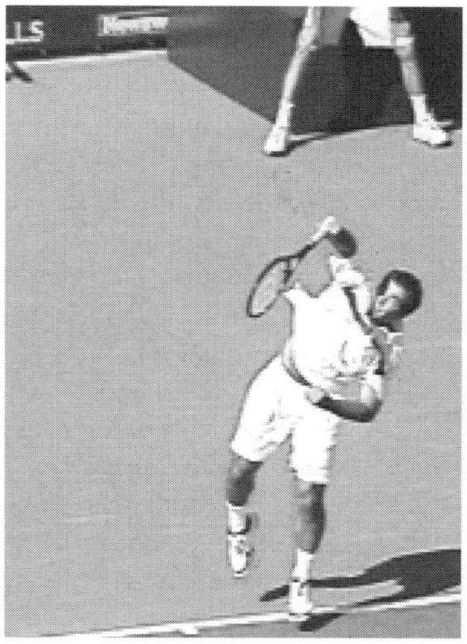

Figure 17
Pronation of the forearm has occurred, bringing the racket face to the player's right

arm slightly. However, the vast majority of beginning and intermediate servers tend to over-swing with their arm at this stage (pulling their elbow down and forward prior to contact) and not gain the explosive power available when the upper arm stays relatively still. This minimal movement of the upper arm allows the forearm and wrist to pronate correctly producing the whip-like action of the racket through the ball.

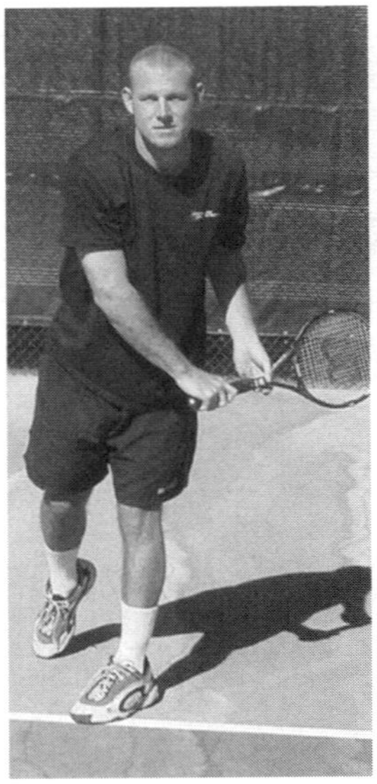

Figure 18
Follow-through is a relaxation phase of the serve

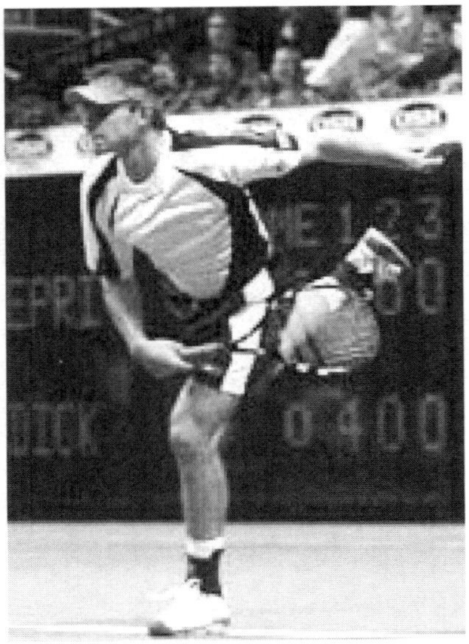

Figure 19
Here, Andy Roddick lands on his left front foot. His back leg kicks back before coming forward and stepping into the court.

H. Follow-through (Figure 18)

The follow-through of the serve is a relaxation of the hitting arm. Notice the arm moves down and across the front of the server. Players who use too much arm-swing in trying to generate power tend to finish on the right side (the wrong side!) of their body. This is because the arm is pulling down through contact with such force that the player can't maneuver the racket across the body.

At this point, the weight is forward, but still on the left foot. Like many shots in tennis, do not let the back leg swing around until long after contact! This is a common fault among beginning and intermediate players. By swinging or stepping into the court with the back leg, the hip and shoulders tend to rotate too early and too much. The player who does this will tend to push the serve instead of creating a full stroke. (See Author's Footwork Notes, left.)

Stance Variations

There are basically two distinct stances used by skilled players. They are the "Platform Stance" and the "Pinpoint Stance". Both are used effectively by top pros but there is a debate as to which one is most preferred and advantageous to the student. I will provide a description of both stances and explain the key points of each.

PLATFORM STANCE (FIGURE 20)

This stance is demonstrated within the sequence of pictures that have been used in the description of the service motion. Basically, the platform stance places both legs on the ground about shoulder width

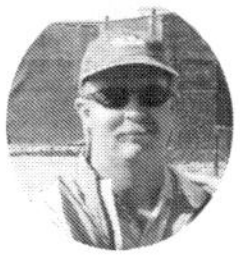

Author's Footwork Notes

On the serve, top level players push off on their front foot (left foot for right-handers) and land on this same foot after contact. (Figure 19) As players use greater upward thrust in generating additional power, the push off the ground is with this front leg. For years, there has been an argument among teaching pros of whether this is the best way for players to get to the net following the serve. Some pros believe stepping through with the back foot during contact and thus landing on this foot speeds up the movement of the player to the net. However, this is false. In addition to the problems this technique creates (as I have mentioned regarding rotating the hips too early), it does not offer any advantage to a player who wishes to advance to the net. This is because the relationship of the body at contact dictates movement towards the net. Thus, a player who is stepping in with the back foot at contact lands one step in just after contact. In order to take a second step, the player must change the direction of rotational inertia of the body in order to get the next step in to the net. A player who pushes off and lands in the court with the front foot also has one step in just after contact. However, the natural rotation of the body's inertia continues to bring the back leg around in the same movement allowing the second step to be in sync with the body's natural rotation after the serve. One final note, at last inspection, not one top player on tour steps through with the back leg until landing on the front foot!

apart without any major movement of the back leg until contact. Andre Agassi and Pete Sampras favor this position.

The platform stance seems to allow greater body coil on the backswing providing more angular momentum through contact.

PINPOINT STANCE (FIGURE 21)

The pinpoint stance is characterized by the server sliding his back foot up to or next to the front foot prior to contact. Many top players including Mark Philippoussis, Greg Rusedski, Gustavo Kuerton and Layton Hewitt favor this motion. Even as the pinpoint stance provides for less body coil of the hips, many players are more comfortable with this position. Also, it is theorized that the pinpoint stance allows the player to push with both feet during the swing as opposed to just the front foot. However, in analyzing high-speed video of these positions, the extra power or speed produced through this position is negligible.

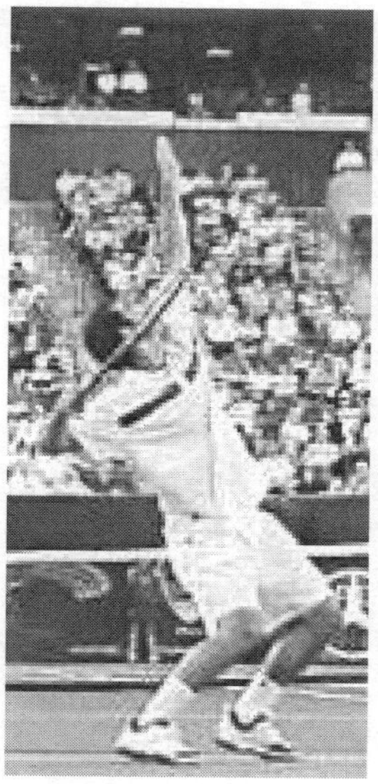

Figure 20
Serving, Pete Sampras maintains a "Platform Stance" during his serve

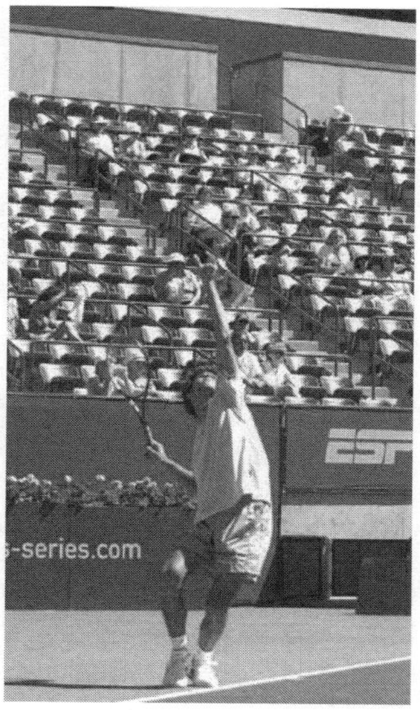

Figure 21
Gustavo Kuerton uses the "Pinpoint Stance" where he brings his back foot up to his front foot.

Advanced Service Progressions

Once the Advanced Foundation on the serve is developed, more progressive and effective serves can be developed without any major changes in technique. Here are some advanced progressions that you will want to work on once your foundation is mastered.

1. ADVANCED PROGRESSION: GREATER USE OF LEGS

As you can see from the sequence of pictures of the serve exhibited throughout this chapter, there is minimal movement of the legs. However, as a player develops, the legs play an important role in adding pace to the serve. But, if the legs are used improperly, every aspect of the serve can be negatively affected. This is one of the reasons I have not addressed the legs up to this point.

The legs emphasize three directional components during the serve: upward, forward, and rotational movements. (Upward and forward movements are both termed "linear movements.") If a player capitalizes by adding these three movements in proper correlation with other service components, they can improve their serve's effectiveness dramatically.

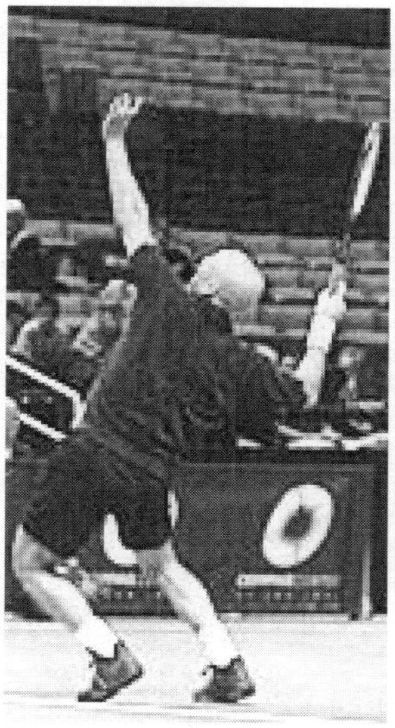

Figure 22
Legs flex during the toss and prior to contact of the serve. Here, Andre Agassi prepares to attack his serve.

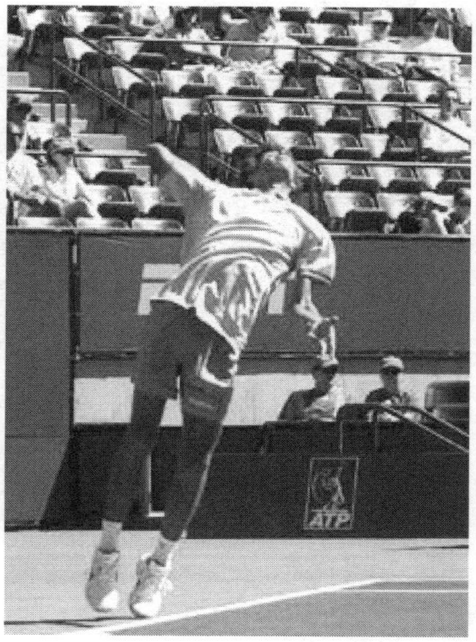

Figure 23
Upward Trust will propel players upward through contact.

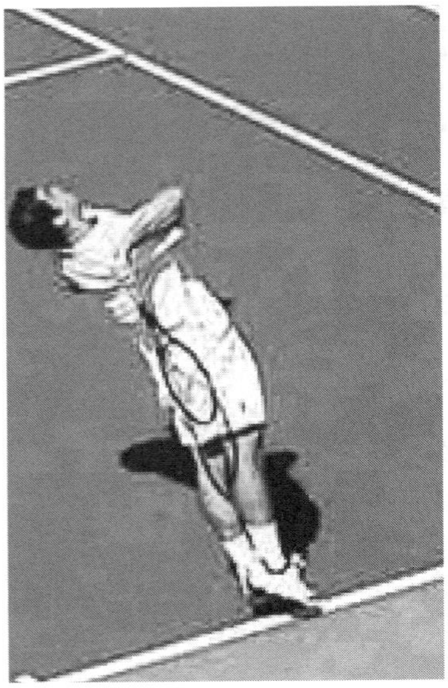

Figure 24
When players lean in to generate power, they lean in SIDEWAYS, so they don't end up rotating forward too early.

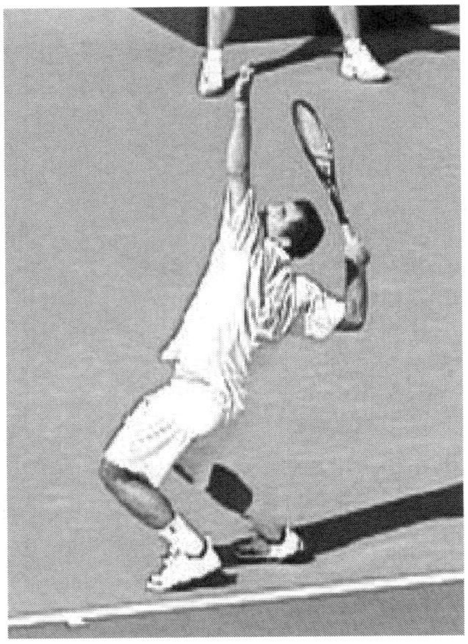

Figure 25
Here, Sampras rotates nearly 180 degrees in relation to the net.

A. Upward Thrust

By flexing the knees (see Figure 22) and thrusting upward at contact, the body can add inertia and force to the serve. Notice the body position and leg flexion prior to contact.

The result of this contraction and subsequent extension of the legs propels the server upward. The player is not intentionally jumping to hit the serve. The result of a powerful extension of the legs during the serve results in the player being lifted off the ground. (See Figure 23)

B. Forward Thrust

By tossing the ball towards the net on the serve, the body can lean forward to hit the serve. However, this movement must be done correctly. The body must stay sideways as it leans forward. (See Figure 24). Most players who have not mastered a proper service motion will rotate their shoulders to face the net when attempting to hit a ball-toss further forward. This will flatten the serve out or result in the player pulling the serve out wide to the left. Players should lean forward over their toss arm's shoulder.

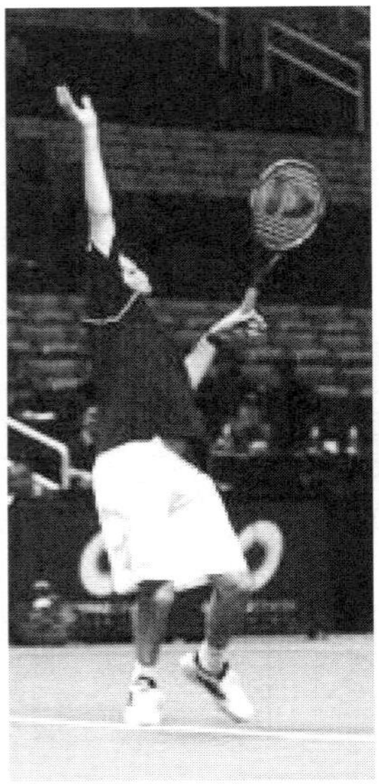

Figure 26
Note the loose, open fingers of Greg Rusedski on the backswing of his serve.

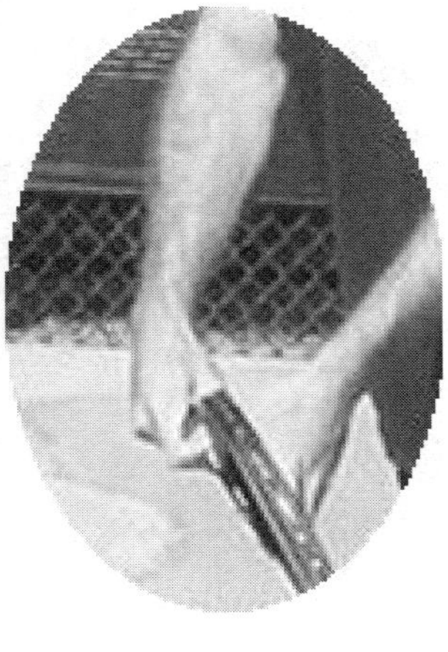

Figure 27
A relaxed hand turned slightly inward creates the proper position and feel for developing high-speed serves.

C. Rotational Thrust

By coiling up more on the backswing, the player will be able to generate more thrust by the uncoiling of this available rotation. Some players rotate almost 180 degrees in creating this coil. (See Figure 25) This movement can cause the player to actually turn their back towards the net on the backswing.

2. ADVANCED PROGRESSION: INCREASED RACKET SPEED

Obviously, a faster moving racket will impart greater speed to a ball. Here are a few tips that can give a player greater racket speed.

A. Loose wrist and fingers (Figure 26)

By relaxing the hand and fingers, the wrist and forearm can have greater flexibility and range of motion. Many top players actually open their hand slightly on the backswing, allowing the hand to relax prior to the acceleration of the racket towards contact.

Beginners and even some advanced players must be careful not to let their grip change during this relaxation stage. This is especially common among players who are trying to change from the rudimentary Eastern forehand grip to the more advanced Continental. Players notoriously (and usually unconsciously!) switch grips in mid swing!

B. Greater rotation of the wrist on the backswing.

Turn your wrist in towards your hips at the ready position. (See Figure 27) The more you can turn the wrist in, the more range of motion the racket will be able to create in the serve. This usually creates more slice for most players initially, generally sending the ball too far to the left. However, as a player begins to set up by aiming more to the right, they eventually will gain greater racket speed on the serve.

"Flat Serves"

The term "Flat Serve" is a misnomer. There is virtually no such thing as a perfectly flat serve. Whether intentional or not, every serve hit will have some amount of spin.

The idea of a flat serve is one that has greater (or added) emphasis on ball velocity than on spin. Thus, a flat serve is one that is hit with the strings NOT brushing across the ball as much as in a true spin serve.

There are two simple phrases that create a clear mental image for most players in hitting both a flat serve and a spin serve. It deals with what the strings are doing to the ball.

For a flat serve the phrase is "at the ball". For a spin serve the phrase is "across the ball". In other words, bring the strings directly to the back of the ball, flattening out against it for a flat serve. For a spin serve, move the strings across the ball (in whatever direction is dictated by the type of spin desired).

However, it should be noted that when accomplished players attempt a "flat" serve, they still apply a great amount of spin to the ball. As the ball is hit with greater velocity, gravity has less impact on the downward arc of the ball into the service box. A player would have to be nearly 9 feet tall to be able to actually hit a perfectly flat ball with no downward arc over the net and into the service box!

To give you an idea of just how much spin is actually hit by pros hitting a so-called flat serve, look at this comparison of Pete Sampras' first and second serves:

PETE SAMPRAS FIRST SERVE SPEED AND ROTATION

	Serve Speed	Spin Range	Average RPM's
Pete Sampras	120mph	2100-4260rpm	2699rpm

PETE SAMPRAS' SECOND SERVE SPEED AND ROTATION

	Serve Speed	Spin Range	Average RPM's
Pete Sampras	85mph	3900-5357rpm	4623rpm

Tables from John Yandell's "Advanced Tennis Research Project"

From these tables, you can see that even Pete's first serve at 120 mph contains a tremendous amount of spin.

Here are some additional examples of spin and ball velocity among some of the world's top tennis players:

Name	Avg. MPH	Spin Range	Avg. RPM
Greg Rusedski	118	1222 – 4025	2549
Andre Agassi	102	1200 – 4284	2449
Andy Roddick	121	1324 – 2914	1865
Marat Safin	120	1249 – 2497	1782

Tables from John Yandell's "Advanced Tennis Research Project"

HOW TO HIT A "FLAT SERVE"

There are many ways to make the strings hit the ball fairly flat, including several grips that can accommodate this action. However, most grips other than the Continental grip have limiting factors. Thus, the motion described earlier in this chapter will be essentially the same with a couple of minor changes.

Change #1: Conceptually, just the mental picture of the racket flattening out against the ball instead of brushing up can produce the desired flat serve with greater ball speed.

Change #2: Toss the ball more towards the net. If the player stays sideways and attacks the ball, the racket will naturally flatten out against the ball. Also, by leaning in and still hitting across the ball, you will attain a "heavier" ball, one that still has good spin but with much more velocity. Of course, this action is more difficult. Beware of the tendency to open up your shoulders when you toss more into the court. Try to remember to lean in over your tossing shoulder as you begin the contact phase.

Change #3: You can rotate your grip subtly towards the Eastern forehand grip. If you keep everything else the same, this slight change will automatically flatten the ball on your serve. However, if you rotate all the way to the Eastern forehand grip, you will lose racket speed through a shorter swing distance.

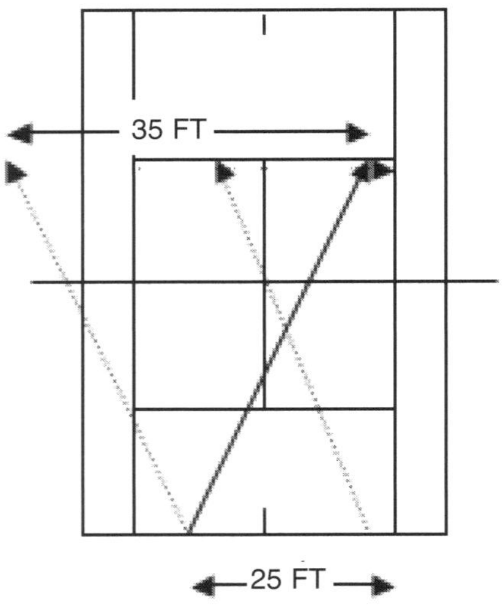

Diagram 4
If the same serve is hit while serving from the deuce court as served from the ad court, players must account for both the change in the players position (along the baseline) as well as the change in the target's direction.

Common Faults on Serving

Once the motion of the serve has been mastered, there are a couple of faults that players sometimes do unconsciously.

NOT CHANGING BODY POSITION ON THE AD AND DEUCE SIDE (DIAGRAM 4)

When a player learns to direct the ball, the aiming sequence is dependent on the player's position at contact.

For example, if a player serves a slice serve from the deuce court and positions his feet a certain way, he will need to change his position in relation to the court if he hopes to slice the same serve into the ad court. However, players often line up at the base line on both the ad and deuce courts essentially in the same position relative to the court. Thus, when a right-hander serves from the ad court without adjusting their aim (through their initial body position), they end up pushing the ball and flattening it out in an attempt to direct the ball towards the right-hand service box. Players must understand that not only is the intended direction changed from the deuce to ad courts, the position of the player (in relation to the baseline) is changed as well. An example of this is when a player serves from near the alley in doubles on the deuce side. When they move to the ad court to serve, if they are serving from near that alley as well, they have moved approximately 25 feet! If when serving to the deuce court and aiming towards the middle of the box, the serve from the ad side will need to be directed approximately 35 feet further to the right to get the SAME serve in on the ad court! Unfortunately, players stand in the same position relative to the baseline on both sides! If a player doesn't make a change in the body position between these two sides, a major stroke change must be enacted to get the ball to land into the ad court.

Beginners have a notorious habit of not making this adjustment. When a beginner or even an intermediate player learns to slice the ball on the deuce court, they inevitably hit the serve from the ad court too far to the left because of this issue of not making the correct adjustments. These players end up hitting the ad court serves flat in order to correct the directional change caused by both their position on the add court and the change in the target's position.

Because we have moved some 25 feet from one side to the other in serving from the deuce court to the ad, players often fail to calculate how much difference in aiming they need to compensate for this change. (This is especially true if serving a similar serve on each side of the court). It is common for players to line their feet up along the base line the same way no matter from where they are serving. While some advanced players can manipulate their upper body and swing pattern to compensate for this change, most make a definite adjustment between the two serving sides with their feet as well.

Unconsciously, most beginning players compensate for the trajectory change by simply pronating their racket earlier (turning the racket face outward) to hit the ball towards the intended target on the ad side. However, this creates a much flatter serve and does not allow the player to use the same service motion (slice, topspin, or flat) as they did on the deuce side. Basically, it means that the player will end up having to learn to control two distinctively different swing patterns, one for each side. (This can actually be desirable if it is learned intentionally!)

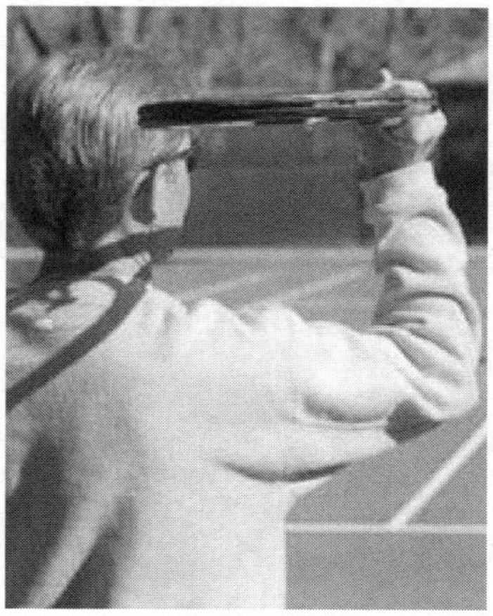

Figure 28
The "platter" serve, or serving with an Eastern forehand grip, is the worst grip for any player who wants to progress to higher levels of serving.

GRIP CHANGING IN MID-SWING

This is more common than most players and even tennis instructors realize! I have seen beginners to high-caliber players set up their serve with the desired Continental grip only to unconsciously switch grips in mid swing to something else (usually something near the Eastern forehand grip). While it is advantageous to hold the grip loosely, it is imperative that players NOT change the hand position on the grip during the swing.

This fault commonly occurs when a player wants to add power to their serve. The Eastern grip is a stronger FEELING grip. However, it prohibits maximum racket head speed and, thus, has less power than the Continental grip when used properly.

EASTERN FOREHAND GRIPS—SERVING PROBLEMS

In my opinion, the greatest fault or flaw that beginning servers can have is to serve with the Eastern forehand grip—intentionally or not! This grip can be seen as the root cause of many serving problems, primarily not being able to progress to more advanced serves. (Figure 28)

The Eastern forehand grip can be labeled as the most "simpleton" of grips any player could choose. If a player knew nothing about spin, racket head speed, or pronation, he or she would usually stand facing the net, holding the Eastern grip, and hitting the back of the ball flat on a line towards the target. A player can actually be very accurate with this grip and serve pattern until he or she chooses to hit a hard serve. Because this grip relies almost entirely on gravity to bring the ball down into the court, the chance of making an error with this serve becomes exponentially greater with any increase in speed.

Not only does this grip and swing pattern limit serve potential, it makes changing to the Advanced Foundation grip and swing pattern significantly more difficult. Players who incorporate the "Platter Serve' pattern do many things that are simply contradictive to that of any advanced serve pattern. Besides the grip, there are several issues that must be changed to make the complete transition to the Advanced Foundation. With the "Platter" Eastern forehand grip, players must:

- *Stand facing the net instead of side ways*
- *Contact is with the hand and elbow forward instead of behind the racket head.*
- *The arm, usually pulling down and pushing the racket forward generates less power.*
- *The racket tends to brush under the ball instead of across the back or side*

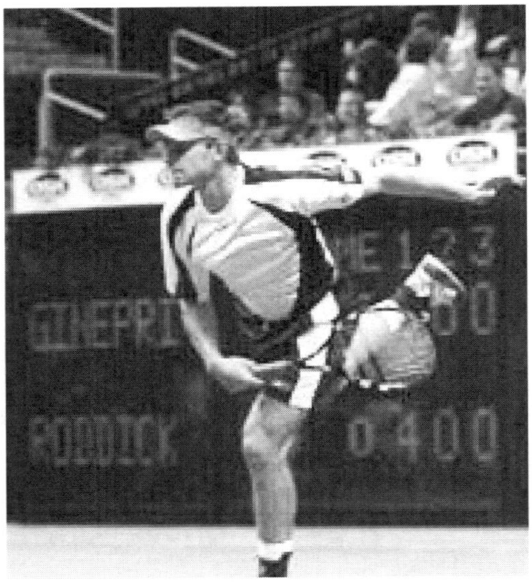

Figure 29
Today, almost all skilled servers push off and land on their front leg. (Left leg for right handed players.) Here, Taylor Dent executes the landing on the front foot with the extreme kick back of the right foot and leg.

STEPPING THROUGH WITH THE BACK LEG

Many traditionalists remember the legendary tennis greats Bill Tilden, Ellsworth Vines, Jack Kramer, and Pancho Gonzales, all serving while their back leg swung through at contact. These players would step with their back foot and end up on this foot after contact. Yet today, hardly a single professional player, men or women, use this footwork method.

Actually the rationale for the back foot stepping through on the serve once made perfect sense for these players. This was before a major rule change in the game that ended up forever altering the biomechanics of serving. In the 1940's and 1950's the rules required the server to keep one foot on the ground until after contact with the ball. This drastically limited the amount of knee bend or leg coil a player could use. Once the rules changed in the late 1950's, players began finding they could generate greater power through a forward and upward thrust prior to contact.

As I have described the counter-productive results of such footwork on the serve, you might want to review the "Footwork Notes" found on page 238. However, it is important to recognize this important concept. Amazingly, I have worked in clinics of so-called intermediate and advanced club players and have found that many of these players executed improper footwork on the serve. The loss of proper body rotation and the subsequent loss of racket head speed is one thing. Yet, the greatest hindrance associated with the back foot coming through too soon is the loss of shoulder position. When the back foot swings around, the hips follow and then the shoulders. (Unless the player consciously maintains the upper body sideways.) When serving, if the shoulders rotate prior to contact, the correct brushing of the ball will be impossible. This is why many players who do step through on the serve usually only hit flat serves. If the player were to slice the ball, the serve would land too far to the left (for right-handed servers). Thus, the player must pronate the forearm and flatten the ball just to get it to go in the general intended direction.

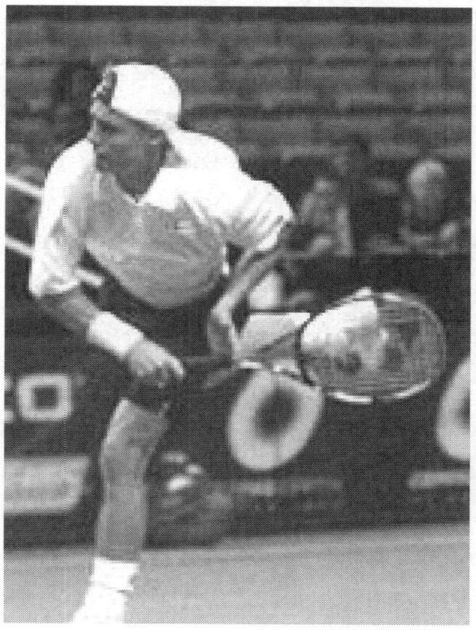

Figure 30
Note the similarities between Layton Hewitt's serve here and the others pictured in this section.

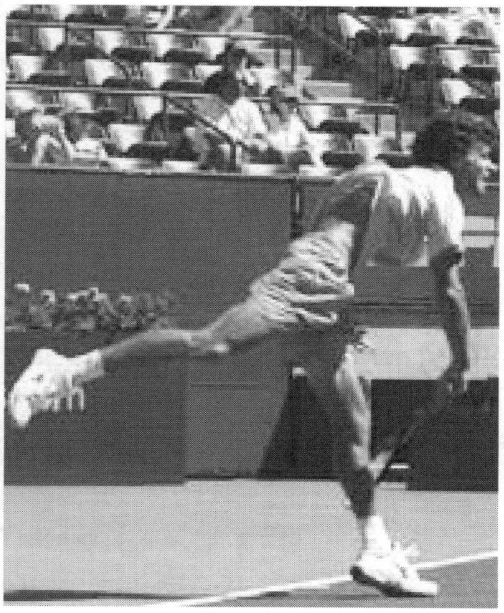

Figure 31
Gustavo Kurten kicks his back leg back and lands on his front, left leg, propelling him towards the net.

The greater issue is in learning the serve. Players who step through with their back leg tend to have difficulty advancing their serve within the progressive concepts presented throughout this chapter.

Practice Tool

To help you learn to serve by pushing off on your front foot and landing on it after contact, here is a technique to practice:

Balance and serve only standing on your front foot. (Left foot for right-handed servers.) Practice this slowly at first until you learn to balance. After a while, you will find you can serve just as fast, if not faster, than when you were standing on both feet. More importantly, you will learn how to coordinate your pushing off from this front foot and landing on it during the serve.

Serve Speed Deceleration (Pre bounce-post bounce)

Only recently the question "how much does a serve slow down by the time it reaches the returnee?" was answered. For decades, players, pros, and researchers only made guesses as to what actually happens to ball speed after the serve.

John Yandell of the Advanced Tennis Project made some compelling discoveries about this topic using high-speed video.

Using a shutter speed of 1000 frames a second, John filmed Pete Sampras and Andre Agassi in the final of the 2000 Sybase open. Through some exhaustive research using computers, John discovered the following information:

The most startling conclusion was that on the serve, the ball slows down radically over the course of its flight. On a 125 mph serve by Sampras, the ball loses around a third of its speed by the time it bounces, traveling only about 80 to 85 mph at the bounce.

But the computer showed that the bounce caused the ball to slow down even more dramatically. Just after the bounce, the ball slows down to about 65 mph, and in the split second before Agassi hits the return, the ball can slow down to 40 mph or less!

And what about the return? If you think Agassi can return the ball faster than it comes to him, you're right. The speed of his returns averaged 60-65 mph, up to 25 mph faster than the ball was traveling when he hit it.

It should be interesting to note that even a 125-mile per hour serve is not traveling even half that speed at contact by the returning player. Depending on how far back the returning player is standing, this speed can be considerably slower.

Moving from Beginner to Advanced Form

The issue of improving one's serve within the Advanced Foundation does not require radical change between the "introductory" and advanced methodology. Transitional learning involves almost mandatory change from the simple form of an Eastern forehand grip and the resulting frying pan or "waiter's" position, to the specific form recognized as skilled. However, the linear method of the Advanced Foundation provides for evolutionary changes by the individual as desire and player development occurs.

These evolutionary changes include:

- *Deeper knee bend*
- *Greater rotation of the upper body during the toss*
- *Slight alterations in the grip to effect more spin for individual style or desired result.*
- *Experimenting with various contact angles and toss positions*
- *Leaning in for greater power*
- *Increasing racket head speed through loose and relaxed body and arm positions*

These evolutionary changes usually come automatically for most players as they simply gain the natural control and expertise that comes from practicing the Advanced Foundation. As in any sport, players naturally want to create greater effect within the skill attempted. Tennis players who learn to play tennis within the Advanced Foundation are free to look for these patterns of play without forfeiting the principles that have already been established.

Conclusion

The serve is potentially every player's greatest weapon. (Or, at least it should be!) A player needs only a bucket of balls and a court to practice. The server has control of the ball before the serve and dictates when the serve will occur as well as control of where the ball will be at contact. The serve is a critical point of any player's game since it is the first ball put in play in any rally. Thus, a player with a good serve automatically puts their opponent at a disadvantage. Likewise, a player with a weak serve usually will start most points off on the defense.

A variety of spin, angle of trajectory, pace, and placement all can contribute to an effective serve. Take the time to study and practice all the elements of serving. Having a great serve provides a high degree of confidence in any player.

CHAPTER 12

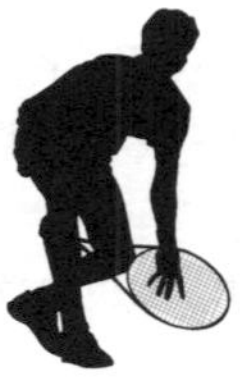

The Advanced Foundation
The Overhead

Introduction

The overhead is one of the most curious tennis strokes. The reason I say this is that, for some, the overhead is anticipated with almost salivary glee. For others, attempting the overhead is fraught with dread and trepidation. And for still others, hitting an overhead is simply not an option; these players opt to take any high ball and either let it bounce and run it down, or let it drop in order to volley the ball instead. Certainly, player strategies can almost eliminate the need for an overhead. There are those players who simply refuse to come to the net. When forced to move towards the net, these players, following a shot near the net, retreat, scurrying back to the baseline as fast as possible. It seems as if the net were radioactive or some sinister monster!

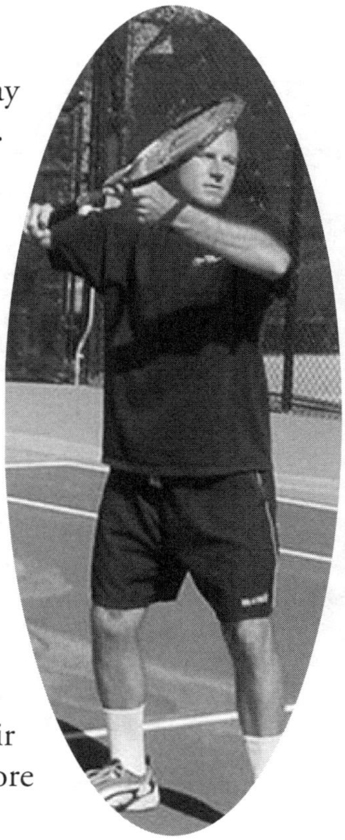

Figure 1
Overheads are either anticipated with confidence or avoided at all cost!

It can't be argued that those players who do develop a good net game will want to simultaneously develop their overhead as well. Certainly, if a player possesses a potent overhead, opponents will either attempt to hit lobs deeper and closer to the baseline (and subsequently hit more errors), or simply attempt passing shots instead. In either case, by having a good overhead you can press your opponent into making more errors by limiting their shot selection or increasing the chance of them missing through forcing a more difficult shot.

Women and girls as a whole have more difficulty developing and hitting offensive overheads. I state this subjective comment on simple realities: more males are introduced to similar over-head movements than females. The overhead and the serve are both dependent on upper body strength and control as well as proper rhythm and mechanics. Boys tend to play more sports associated with similar movements to the serve and overhead through actions associated with throwing overhand. Baseball and football both have overhand throwing components associated with their sports. However, girls who have participated in similar sports such as softball, volleyball, or badminton, tend to

The Overhead is like an exclamation point at the end of a sentence. It can have a significant psychological impact on everyone on the court.

!

learn just as fast as boys in hitting overheads. Since these sports also utilize similar overhand motions, the crossover learning from these sports tend to help a great deal when attempting the overhead stroke.

It is important to know that everyone is capable of learning, practicing, and achieving successful overheads! Learning some key position points associated with the overhead and practicing them using rhythmic swing patterns will help all players quickly acquire skillful and successful overheads.

Overview

The overhead is similar to the serve in more ways than it is not. It is important to be familiar with these similarities as well as understand that there are points that do, indeed, differ. I will address these various characteristics throughout this chapter. However, this is a good place to address some critical advantages in having a good overhead.

Overheads are what I often call "momentum shifts" (more on momentum shifts in Chapter 13 on Mental Tennis). An overhead hit with authority and conviction can literally demoralize an opponent or opposing doubles team. Likewise, if a player has an overhead shot present itself and they hit it out or in the net, this is a two-point shift; instead of winning a sure point, they lose it. Depending on the game score (or tiebreaker score), this can have significant meaning to the outcome of a set or the momentum of the match. For example, if a team is up 40 – 30 and they miss an easy overhead, instead of outright winning that game they are back even at deuce. The consequence of this miss is further embellished by what happens in the next point. (As I will discuss in Chapter 13 on mental tennis, shifts in momentum are usually established more by the results of the next point following such an event.)

The overhead is like an exclamation point at the end of a sentence. When a point is won with an overhead, it often has much greater impact than a simple volley winner or an unforced error. It can have a significant psychological impact on everyone on the court!

While the stroke mechanics of the overhead closely resemble those of the serve, there are specific differences that must be understood if a player hopes to master the overhead.

Differences between the Serve and the Overhead

1. *Logistically, the overhead is seldom hit from as far back as the baseline. (There are exceptions to this, especially at high levels of play.) Thus, the necessary trajectory needed to clear the net and get the ball in the opponent's court can be different.*

2. *The overhead does not have to land in the service box. With the difference stated above, the trajectory is not specifically determined by the location of the service boxes.*

3. Because of these two differences, spin is not as necessary of a component on the overhead. Since we can hit the overhead into the whole court (instead of just the service boxes), we don't need to apply as much spin on an overhead. The player will usually pronate the racket earlier on overheads to promote this flattening action on the ball.

4. Often, on a good lob we are forced to hit the overhead leaning back and even reaching backward as opposed to having the opportunity to lean into it like a serve. This requires very specific footwork patterns and body positions that are different than the serve.

Similarities between the Serve and Overhead

1. The grip for the overhead is essentially the same as the service grip in the Advanced Foundation: the continental. The continental grip allows for greater racket head speed as well as greater angular diversity in terms of targeting. (Please see notes on the Eastern forehand on page 252.)

2. The basic sideways body position is essentially the same as a serve. Even as the player's weight will usually start on the back foot for a deeper overhead, the player should finish the overhead on the front foot (left foot for right-handed players).

3. The back leg should stay back, even "kick" back upon contact with the ball. This motion can easily be seen among all good servers. (See Figure 2)

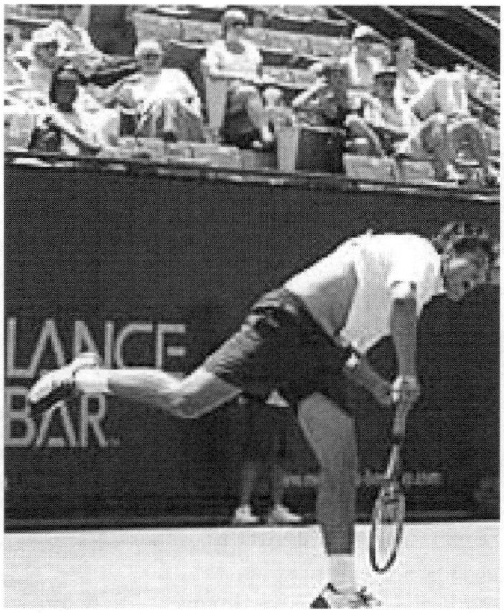

Figure 2
The serve, similar to the overhead will usually feature the back leg kicking back at contact and just after.

4. Pronation of the racket at contact is similar to that of a flat serve.

5. The follow-through components of both the serve and the overhead mirror each other. After contact, the arm relaxes and usually brings the racket across the body for the follow-through.

Basic Overhead Components

GRIP

Similar to that of the serve and of the volley, the player at the net should be holding a continental grip. This grip allows for the greatest racket head speed and potential angles for placement. (See Figure 3)

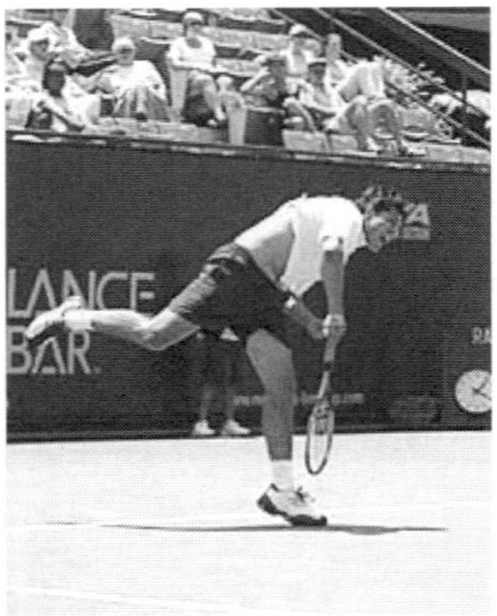

Figure 3
As players approach the net, a split-step followed by a balanced ready position is essential for proper overheads. The proper grip held here is the continental.

PREPARATION

The first overhead component is perhaps one of the most abused or unrecognized areas of importance on producing solid overheads. Typically, beginners and intermediate players prepare late for their overhead, creating a significant problem from the start. Often, players will see their opponents hit the lob and proceed to look up at the ball with their head. This moment of time looking up and evaluating the lob is time lost in preparing to move and hit the overhead. Most lobs can be hit with an overhead if the player reacts with the proper reactionary moves. Proper footwork and body movements are included in this preparation.

SPLIT-STEP

In order to prepare properly for an overhead, the player either approaching the net or stationed at the net must execute a proper split-step. This movement (discussed in Chapter 7 on Technique) allows for the player to be balanced at the onset of their opponent's shot. If a player is not properly balanced at this critical point, their center-of-gravity will be off-center, preventing them from being able to effectively move in certain positions. For example, if a player is still moving forward during and just after the opponent has hit the ball, they will not be able to respond to any shot hit away from them with reliability. Only balls hit right to them will be manageable. It is very easy to lob and pass those opponents who fail to split-step. (See Figures 5 & 6)

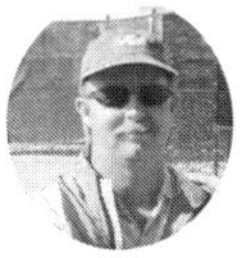

Author's Notes on the Eastern Forehand Grip for Overheads

Even though most beginners find holding the Eastern forehand grip easier to make contact for overheads, this grip is extremely debilitating in terms of progressing past a rudimentary level on the overhead. Similar to the negative effects this grip has on serving progression, the Eastern grip requires several changes in the player's position and stroke pattern in hitting the overhead from that of the recognized skilled Continental grip method. The Eastern grip promotes the "Platter" or "Waiter's" position (See Figure 4) where the player stands holding the racket over the shoulder in a palm-up posture. Once this stance is taken, the overhead has many limitations in addition to limited progressive improvement.

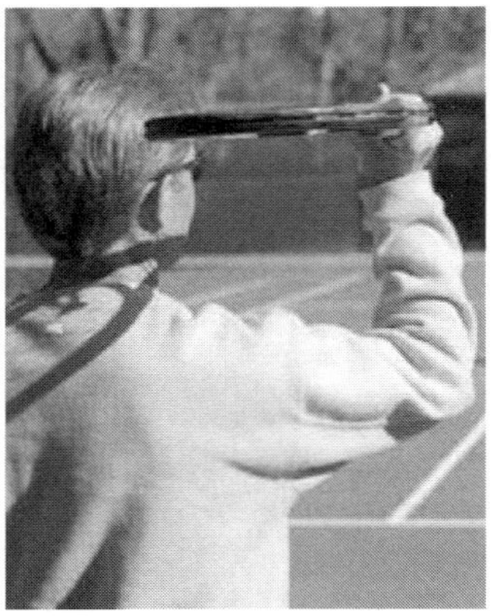

Figure 4
The Platter Position. Players using an Eastern forehand grip will usually end up in this position when trying to hit an overhead.

REACTION

Following a properly timed split-step, a player must react to the lob as early as possible. The proper reaction includes two specific moves: shoulder turn and racket preparation. These two moves will set the player into the best position to execute the best possible overhead.

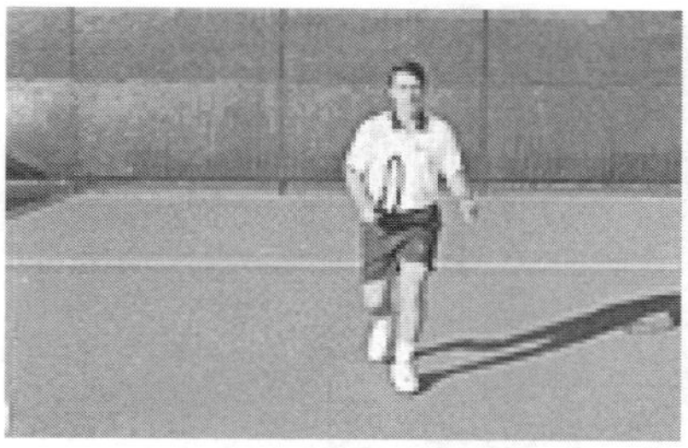

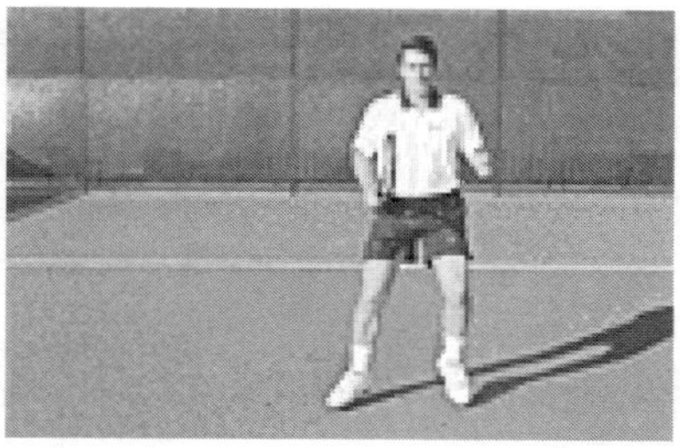

Figure 5 & 6 - The Split-Step
From any position on the court, a player in motion will want to pause, centering his body and his center of gravity allowing him to react from this balanced position to where his opponent will hit the ball.

SHOULDER TURN

When the lob is hit, the net player needs to turn the shoulders sideways immediately. For right-handers, this turn means to bring the right shoulder back while the left leading shoulder points towards the ball. The hips and feet should follow this shoulder rotation, setting the player sideways to the net. (See Figure 7)

RACKET PREPARATION

At the same time as the shoulder turn, the player should raise the hitting arm. The player's hitting elbow raising and moving back behind the player should initiate this preparation. The off-hand also starts to rise, sometimes briefly cradling the racket at the throat. (See Figure 7)

CONTINUATION OF THE BACKSWING

As the player moves into position for the overhead, the racket continues to rise over and behind the head while the off-hand points towards the ball. (See Figure 8)

During this backswing, if the lob is deep, the player will usually shift their body weight to the back leg and shuffle back in this position to get under the lob.

Pointing at the Ball

Some pros teach to point the elbow of the off-arm at the ball. This move is mentioned to help players turn their shoulders more sideways. This is not a bad bit of advice. However, I have found that if a player simply points at the ball with the off-hand, while turning and going back for the lob, their body will be in correct alignment for hitting the overhead. (See Figure 8)

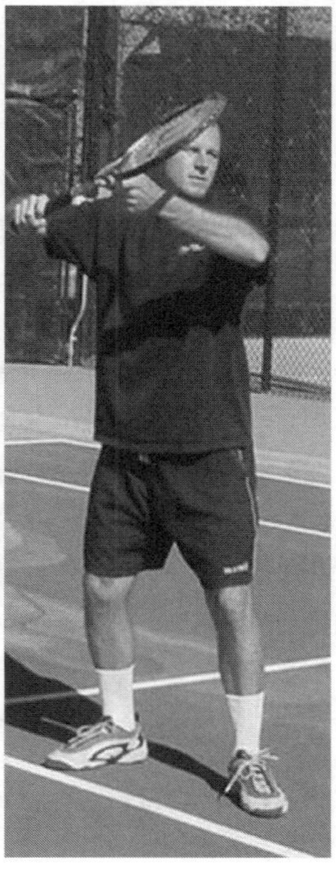

Figure 7
Immediate shoulder turn and racket preparation are critical components of preparing for the overhead.

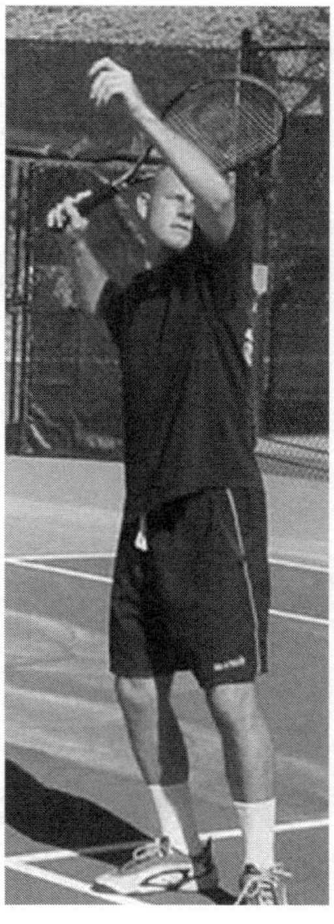

Figure 8
As the player moves back for the lob, the racket is brought back further and the off-hand points towards the ball.

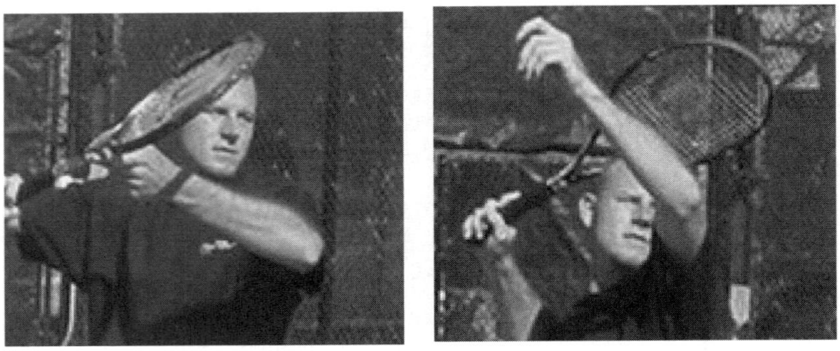

Figures 9 & 10
The "Comb back" move: the top edge of the racket remains pointed at the opposite court as the racket sweeps back over the head in a short motion.

Using the continental grip, the player's hand should hold the racket with the hitting side of the strings pointed slightly down. Although, this position can vary slightly from skilled player to skilled player, the main issue is that all players should not hold the racket with the hitting surface facing up towards the sky. This "platter" or "Waiter's" grip or racket position (because it resembles a waiter holding a tray or platter over their shoulder on the palm of their hand!) will sabotage the correct action the player will need to hit the overhead well. (See Figure 4)

I recommend a short backswing on lobs with the racket never pointing towards the back fence on the take-back. Using what I call a "comb back" backswing (since it resembles someone combing their hair back with their racket) helps keep players from pointing their racket head backwards. This helps prevent the palm from coming up under the racket. (Compare Figures 9 and 10 for this sequence.) Once players develop this short backswing pattern, many will customize it to meet their particular feeling and timing.

ACTION OF CONTACT

The next sequence of moves is complex. Once the key position points are recognized, the movements must be done in sequential rhythm.

Four identifiable movements occur at the same time during the contact phase: (Figure 11)

1. *The shoulders rotate slightly towards the net.*
2. *The pointing off-hand moves down towards the chest.*
3. *The hitting elbow moves forward toward the net.*
4. *The racket head drops behind the player.*

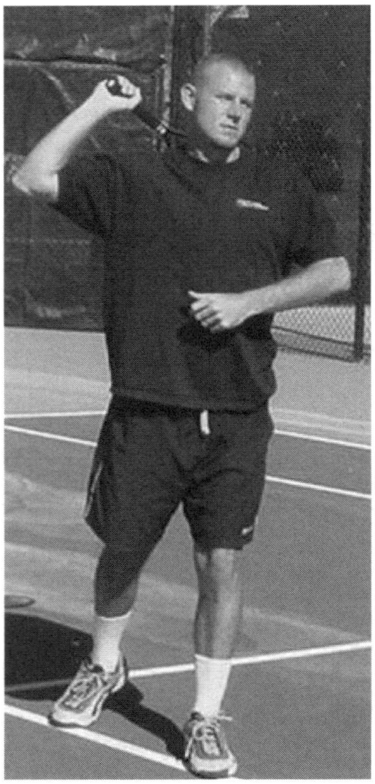

Notice that the hitting elbow remains up. One of the most common problems among players having difficulty hitting an overhead well is that they drop this elbow prior to contact.

The upper body rotation is minimal. (Figure 12) At this point, many beginners tend to rotate their upper body all the way around so they are facing the net. The cause of this over-rotation usually is due to the use of an Eastern forehand grip for the overhead. (This is because the Eastern grip requires the player to face the net at contact.)

As the racket drops down and back, this upper body rotation will actually swing the racket out behind the right shoulder.

Figure 11 – 4 Actions to Contact:
- The shoulders rotate half way
- Off-hand / arm to chest
- Hitting elbow moves forward
- Racket head collapses behind player

CONTACT

As the racket moves up towards contact, the top edge of the racket should be pointing up towards the sky. As the racket moves further towards the ball, the racket rotates out, bringing the face of the racket towards the ball. (Figure 13) Think of giving the ball a "high five" with the strings of the racket. This will give you the proper forearm movement to flatten the strings of your racket against the back of the ball. This rotation of the racket from an edge-on position prior to contact to a flattening out of the strings on the ball is called forearm pronation.

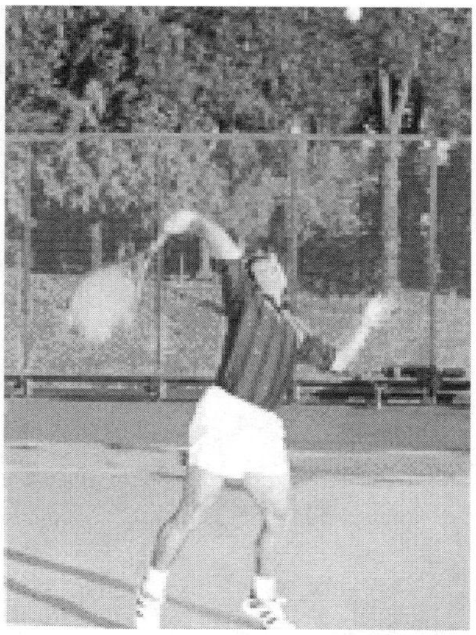

Figure 12
While there is shoulder rotation to the ball, the amount of turn is minimal. Here the players is commencing with his forward swing yet is still sideways to the net.

Angle of Contact

Your desire to hit your overhead to the left, right, deep or sharp angle will be dependent on the racket angle at contact. To hit the ball more to the right, a right-handed player will want to pronate slightly earlier. This will bring the strings to the ball at an angle. Hit the ball more on the right side and the ball will go to the left. By hitting down, more on the top half of the ball, the ball will land short. And finally, hitting more directly behind the ball will send the ball further. Practice the timing of each of these directional overheads within the stroke mechanics discussed here, and you will be well on your way to hitting effective overheads anywhere in the court you wish.

Another element of directional control is the position of the shoulders at the backswing and contact points. If a right-handed player wanted to hit the ball to the right (in what we call a "reverse overhead"), the player can turn their shoulders more to the right at set up for the overhead. Staying more in this position will allow the player to hit the overhead more to the right without having to pronate as early.

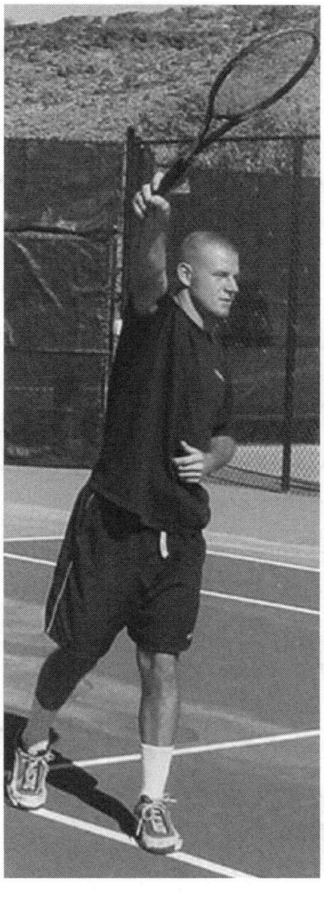

Figure 13
At contact, the racket flattens out against the ball.

Figure 14
Here, Pete Sampras allows his racket head to continue over and through the stroke while his hitting elbow remains high.

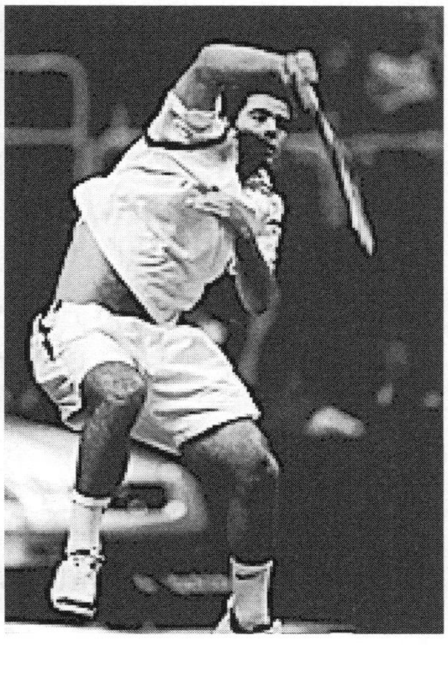

POST CONTACT

One of the key position points of the overhead is right after contact. The elbow will remain high while the racket continues its path through the ball and the racket head leads down towards the ground. (Figure 14)

A common mistake among many when attempting overheads is to drop the elbow during contact. Actually, these players are pulling the elbow down in an attempt to hit the ball harder. Unfortunately, this slows the racket speed and prevents the racket from

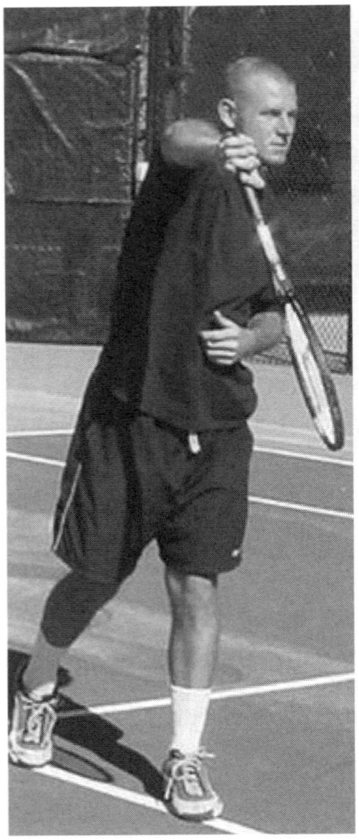

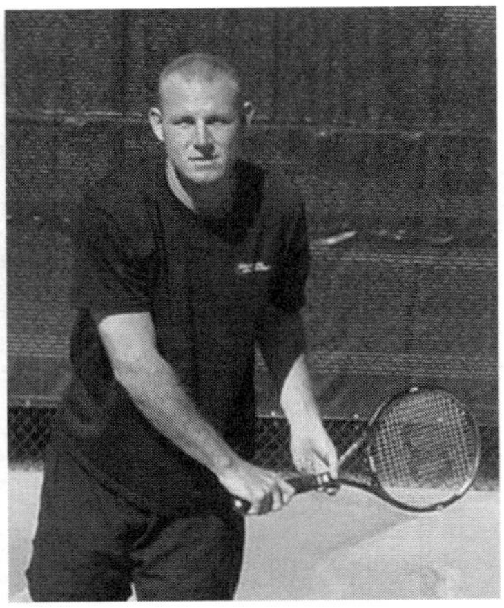

Figure 15
As the racket continues down after contact, the hitting arm relaxes. The shoulders then complete their rotation. The back foot remains

Figure 16
As the follow-through completes, the arm moves across the body much like the follow-through of the serve

pronating properly. In fact, players who do indeed swing with their arm in this fashion create faster racket head speed long after the ball has left the swing. This is because a player who pulls the elbow and arm down to hit the ball will have to lay back the racket to make necessary contact with the ball to send it forward. This arm movement is characterized the most in players who attempt overheads with the Eastern forehand grip. Use of the continental grip will allow the racket to pronate and finish over the hand as you can see in Figures 13 - 15.

The action of the arm coming through the ball will bring the shoulders around to face the net. The inertia of the swing will accomplish this. Players who intentionally rotate the shoulders during the swing will, indeed, over rotate too early. This will result in one of two things happening. With no instantaneous correction, the player will pull the ball wide. If the attempt is slow, the player will rotate the grip or wrist and push the ball forward in an attempt to not pull the ball wide.

FOLLOW THROUGH

As with the serve, the follow-through is to the player's left with a loose, relaxed, natural slowing down of the racket. Even as pronation sends the racket head to the player's right, the arm relaxes after this is completed and simply drops the racket and arm down across the body. (Figures 15 & 16)

Back Leg Problems

Think of your overhead as a forehand. As with the forehand groundstroke and volley, the back leg should not swing around during contact. With both these shots, the back leg might swing around in a "Brake Step" move after a pause of this leg during contact. However, as mentioned in both chapters on these forehand strokes, the back leg should stay back during contact. (Figure 15) This is true for the overhead as well. Players who swing their leg around during contact will over-rotate the hips and shoulders. It is critical for players to train themselves to keep this leg back.

As the player completes the overhead, the racket will cross in front of the body just as it does following a serve. (Figure 16)

Advanced Overhead Patterns

As players master the overhead, other overhead situations require slight modifications of the foundation learned here.

SCISSORS KICK OVERHEAD

When a lob is hit medium height and deeper, a player won't have time to move their feet as much as they would on higher overheads. This requires the player to "Challenge the overhead" and immediately jump up and back while making the standard overhead arm movements.

The "scissors kick" is a term that describes the leg action in this fast move.

1. The Turn: The player will immediately turn their shoulders and lean back on their back foot. For right-handed players, this would be the right foot. The racket immediately moves up behind the head. Some players will begin the push back with their left foot as seen in Figure 17. The key is to get sideways as early as possible.

2. The Jump: The player will push off from either his right or left foot (depending on balance). Jumping up and back, the player will continue the arm movements of the overhead. (Figure 18)

3. The Scissors Kick: As the overhead is hit, the back right leg immediately kicks forward and the previously front leg, the left, steps back to catch the player as they land on the ground. (Figure 19)

Figure 18

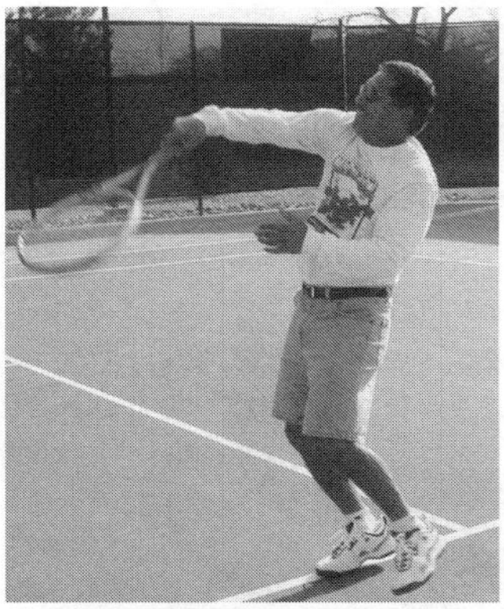

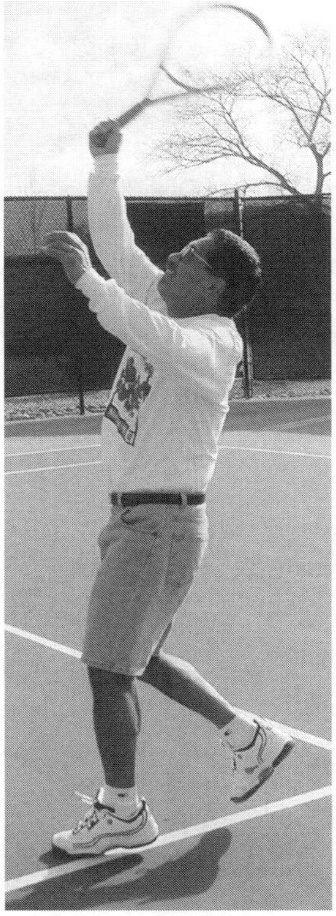

Figure 17

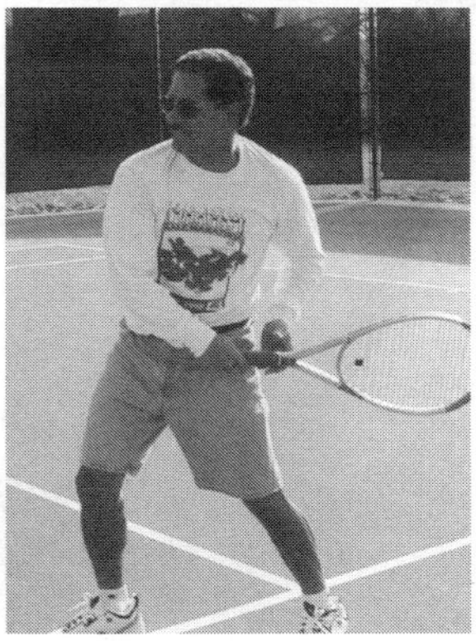

Figure 19

The Scissors Kick

When forced to lean back for a deep, quickly hit lob, the player will push off with either the right or left foot. However, the left foot must start in front of the right foot, just as described in this chapter. (Figure 17) As the player continues to swing, the left foot moves back to "catch" (Figure 18) the player as they continue to fall back after contact. (Figure 19) This body rotation, called "angular momentum," demonstrates that even as a player is moving backwards, a powerful shot can be hit forwards due to the body's rotation used in conjunction with a proper arm swing.

JUMP OVERHEAD

Once in a while when we are positioned at the net, a player at mid court will volley or half-volley a ball to us high and quick. While we could simply go up and volley this high shot back, a more offensive option would be to hit a quick overhead back at our opponent. This type of overhead does not provide us with ample time to turn or step back or even lean back (as in the scissors kick overhead). A jump overhead is exactly that—a jump straight up followed by a quick overhead stroke. (Figures 20 & 21)

This overhead requires a very short backswing with the racket dropping back only about two-thirds of the distance it normally would.

Contact is made almost exclusively with the arm with almost no shoulder rotation. The racket comes up and flattens the ball with the same pronation used to hit the regular overhead.

THE BACKHAND OVERHEAD

One of the hardest shots in tennis is the backhand overhead. This shot is basically a high backhand volley swung with a full drop or

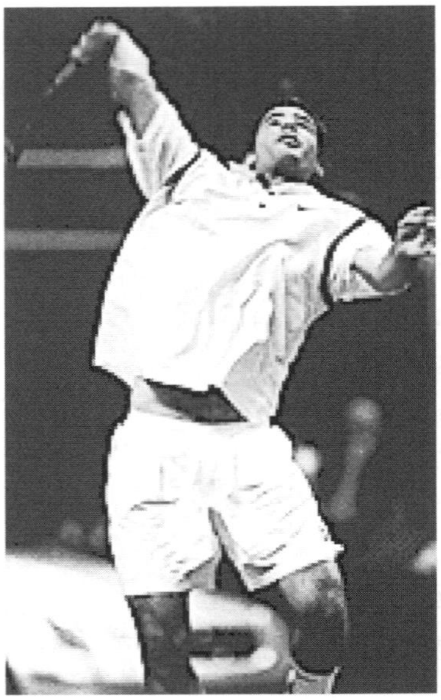
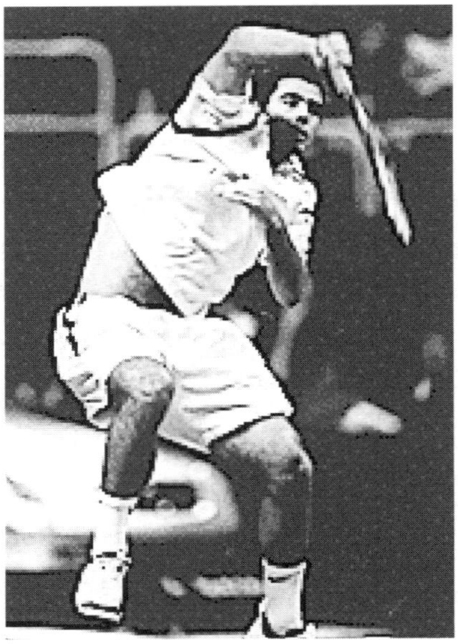

Figures 20 & 21 - The "Jump Overhead"
Here, Sampras goes straight up with his racket in an abbreviated backswing. The body has little time to coil. Instead, the racket makes a quick rotation over the head, pronating the racket to the ball. Note again the high elbow position after contact.

collapse of the racket on the backswing followed by a snap of the arm back through the ball. This is not a comfortable move by most players and must be hit and practiced thoroughly before players can come close to aiming the shot.

The backhand overhead is almost impossible to hit with any grip other than a continental. This shot is a clear indication of an "advanced" net player! The reason for this is that some players can get away with using the Eastern forehand and backhand grips against other mediocre players. However, only those players who have mastered the Advanced Foundation volley grip, the continental, can even attempt the backhand overhead.

In hitting this shot, the player must turn immediately to their left (as a right-handed player) and stand sideways to the net. Often, pros and skilled players can actually be seen turning almost completely with their backs to the net.

The arm raises up as if to hit a high backhand volley. However, the play will drop the racket head down, almost to the point that the butt-cap of the racket is pointing straight up. This move is followed immediately by the arm rotating up with the racket flattening out against the ball.

If there ever were a true "wrist snap" in tennis, the backhand overhead is the shot. This is because, generally speaking, the backhand overhead consists of the arm almost stopping completely in a straight, horizontal position over the head while the racket literally snaps over and through the ball. Players who swing with their arm will not gain any racket head speed and end up pushing the ball.

Conclusion

The overhead should be a weapon by all that play tennis. Unlike the serve, the overhead can be hit virtually anywhere in the court. Also, unlike the serve, the overhead is usually hit from well inside the baseline and closer to the net. Since the overhead stroke is indeed similar to the serve, these two aspects of aiming should provide for extreme confidence in going after each overhead with an aggressive effort.

Practice and dedication to the technique described in this chapter will insure proper development, increased potency, and improved confidence in your overhead.

Section 3

Strategies of Playing

In this, our third section, we will discuss the application of the strokes you are learning. The Strategies of Playing can be thought of as playing a chess match. Learning how the different pieces move, learning what the best opening moves are, learning what moves will be helpful several moves later, and how to close out a player on the run are all elements of chess that deal with strategy. The strategies used in playing chess are analogous to the strategies used in playing tennis. Once we understand "how to move the ball around," the next step is to determine which "moves" will be beneficial to the ultimate outcome of each point, and eventually the outcome of the match.

Obviously, this simple analogy falls far short in describing all the complexities of playing tennis…especially at high levels of skill. There are strategies for each level of play. They differ based on our opponent's level, our own level, and our personality including our own mental strengths and weaknesses. In addition, strategies for doubles are different from those strategies of singles play. Also, while one strategy might have triumphant results against one player, that same strategy might not work well against another. Thus, possessing the ability to change specific strategies as needed are as much a part of Tennis Mastery as the skills related to hitting a ball are.

But the Strategies of Playing go beyond the strategic elements of the game itself. This section also deals with the psychological aspects of individual play. This "mental" portion deals with emotions, reactions, mental preparations, and many other psychological conditions that are part of our individual psyche.

As players become more skilled, the strategies of the game become of greater influence and importance. Yet, no matter your current level, the more you become familiar with this aspect of the game, the more you are one step ahead!

CHAPTER 13

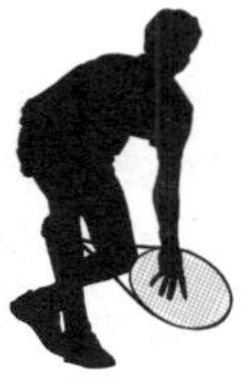

Mental Tennis within the Advanced Foundation

Mental Tennis can take on many definitions in how it relates to player performance on a tennis court. Many people associate "Mental Toughness" as being the all-encompassing phrase used to define an accomplished tennis player. This broad term has, indeed, been written about in tennis texts for decades. However, Mental Toughness is just a part of the overall "Mental" picture. Mental Tennis includes more. It includes both on and off-court preparation and understanding; it includes mental toughness training, and it includes something that can't be gained in practice: Competitive Experience.

Many players fail to recognize these associations. Thus, many of these individuals fail to study and, ultimately, are unaware of how they can and should train for the Mental aspects of tennis.

Mental Toughness is derived from the overall preparedness that a player understands as being a necessary part of Mental Tennis. In my opinion, Mental Toughness is a resulting factor, one that a player gains through his or her determination in reaching Tennis Mastery. Reaching Mental Toughness can be achieved through the actual practice of key component parts, such as those you will learn about in this chapter. Some of the preparatory portions can only be achieved through various types of key experiences. Key experiences include situations that occur only in match-play competition…experiences that force a player to encounter *real* pressure, or situations where pressure is substantially increased. This is why tournament tennis is an absolute requirement for players seeking to develop overall Mental Tennis as well as Mental Toughness. I will talk more about tournament tennis later in this chapter.

Confidence as it applies to Mental Tennis

Confidence is, perhaps, one of the most important ingredients to becoming a mentally sound tennis player. The true belief that you can and will succeed (in both shot manufacturing during competitive match-play and in the overall belief you will prevail in competition) is essential to solid Mental Tennis. Thus, becoming a master of the mental side of tennis does indeed include having sincere confidence in oneself. In fact, I can't recall a single player of the three thousand-plus I have taught who could perform well, especially under pressure, who lacked sincere confidence. Certainly, players described as reserved, tentative, or cautious, have seldom gone on to play successful competitive tennis at any competitive level.

This sincere confidence comes from a combination of two things:

Knowing you are well trained

This aspect is directly related to the Advanced Foundation. By training within a pattern of stroke, technique and strategies (ones that are known to be proper and progressive), a player goes into competition with a true sense of confidence. Players who possess inferior strokes, have to find ways to avoid or conceal such weaknesses. These players often have a false bravado of confidence that quickly crumbles in competition.

Knowing you are well prepared

This confidence is related to both your mental as well as physical conditions. Your mental condition is determined by your experience in competitive exercises as well as the depth of your "tennis knowledge." This tennis knowledge includes your understanding of strategies as well as a general understanding of shot selections and their potential outcomes.

Physical conditions include physical strength, endurance, quickness, and physical fortitude. (Fortitude relates to how well we play under the pressure of competition. This includes how well we play when we are ahead in a match and how well we play when we find ourselves behind.)

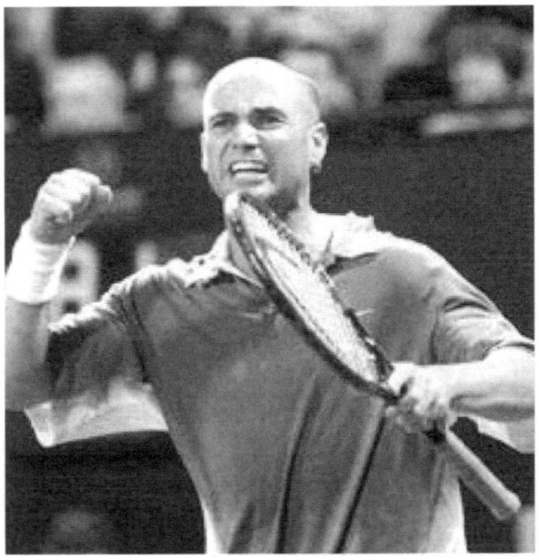

Figure 1
Mental toughness comes from a sincere fighting spirit. Virtually all champions possess this spirit as well as a sense of confidence that comes from knowing they are both well prepared and well trained.

Players who are well trained and well prepared generally have a sincere confidence that comes from within their physical being. Those players who lack either quality usually attempt to display some false sense of confidence. Such false confidence is usually exposed as the pressure of competition becomes more intense. As I will mention later, this false confidence usually leads a player to resort to other, more destructive mechanisms. These are designed to protect a player's ego.

COCKY VERSUS ARROGANT

I have used the term "cocky" to describe this sincere sense of confidence in many lectures. A player who is "cocky" does not appear to mind a missed shot, as he or she KNOWS they will still hit winners when needed, make incredible shots later in the match, and, most importantly, will prevail when the match concludes. Depending on personalities, the exposition of this cocky attitude can be expressed in a variety of ways. From simple facial expressions to fist-pumping, whole body movements to vocal commands, most competitive players have a unique way of expressing their confidence depending on each player's personality. The most stoic was Bjorn Borg whose cockiness was expressed almost completely by a silent fortitude and eyes that glared defiance. In contrast, during that same era, Jimmy Connors expressed an almost "bulldog" fighting spirit that made his somewhat diminutive stature seem Goliath-like. Observations more recently of top players today include the fast-paced play of Andre Agassi who re-emerged as one of the world's all-time tennis greats through the confidence of conditioning. Agassi, at the age of 30, used the assurance of being in terrific shape and parlayed this confidence in becoming number one in the world after plunging to a career low ranking of 144. When watching Agassi play, one can't ignore his penchant for fast play, especially on changeovers. His brisk walk with head held high, eyes wide and expressive, and shoulders back with the demeanor of the proverbial conqueror—whether he is ahead in a match or behind—demonstrates his particular brand of cockiness. This is a far cry from his earlier years of rebellious and contemptuous behavior both on and off the court.

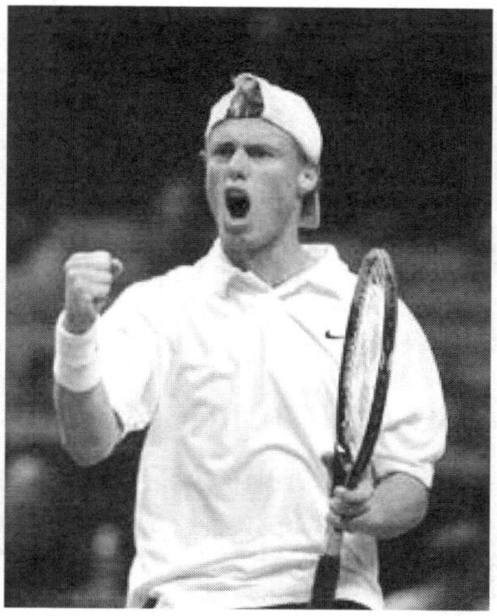

Figure 2
Most all players have a unique way of expressing their confidence through such actions as fist pumps to vocal expressions.

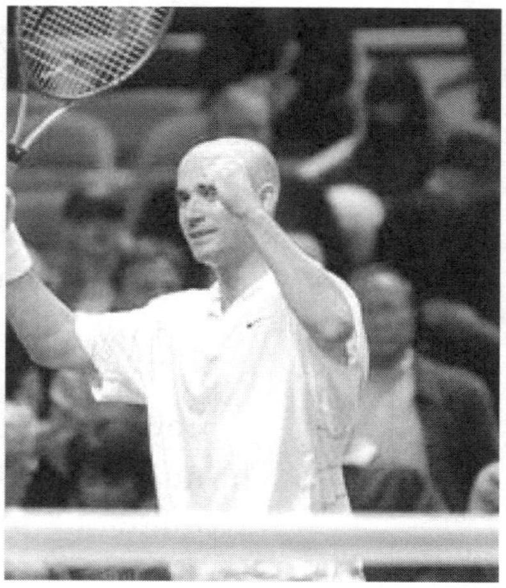

Figure 3
Andre Agassi showed the world how to reemerge and become a true champion.

In talking about this cocky attitude, I try to distinguish it from an "arrogant" attitude. Arrogance, in my opinion, is a player who—among other things—talks trash both on and off the court. An arrogant attitude can be associated with cockiness as much as it can be associated with confidence. (Or overconfidence!) However, I sometimes associate arrogance with ignorance. A player who is arrogant will oftentimes fail to be a prepared player, both mentally as well as mechanically. This is because arrogance does not tend to promote readiness. A sports psychologist that I heard recently labeled arrogance as "confidence unfounded" which I believe sums up this concept quite well.

A classic example of this difference can be illustrated through a match played back in 1987. That year, I had a team of mostly Asian boys at my school in Southern California. We were very good as we were ranked third in the CIF Southern Section of California. However, we were about to play a team from the wealthy community of Palm Desert, California in a first-round match of the CIF playoffs. The Palm Desert team was coached by a young man who either didn't know how high we were ranked, or thought too highly of his team to worry about the match. The Palm Desert team was composed of mostly large white guys who towered over my group of mostly Vietnamese players, none of whom were ranked at that time individually. However, as a team we were extremely deep.

The Palm Desert team exited their nicely furnished team bus with laughter and snide remarks whispered amongst themselves when they noticed our team's size and lack of

> It was interesting to witness the immediate crumbling of such Goliath-like players under the weight of my team's confident and, yes, even cocky play
> !

blond hair! It was actually embarrassing for me to witness their arrogant attitudes (which bordered on racism) that preceded the match.

The Palm Desert team members all had the latest Fila tennis clothes and several expensive rackets, all helping to promote an arrogant appearance.

Needless to say, my team looked like the proverbial underdog at the onset of the match!

At the conclusion of the match, things looked altogether different. Our team soundly beat Palm Desert by the score of 14 - 4 with most of the sets being a 6 – 0 or a 6 – 1 in our favor. The Palm Desert players now resembled whipped dogs, scampering speechlessly to their bus with their tails between their legs.

Were the Palm Desert boys arrogant at the beginning of the match? Absolutely. Were they cocky after loosing the early games of each of their matches? No. It was interesting to witness the immediate crumbling of such Goliath-like players under the weight of my team's confident and, yes, even cocky play. My players never responded to the derogatory statements made by the Palm Desert players throughout the match. In fact, my players played almost oblivious in regards to their opponents' attitudes while simply hitting winners and high-fiving teammates or shouting praise to each other through the course of the match.

Mental Toughness

There are many definitions for mental toughness as it applies to tennis. Some might say it is the resistance to choking. Others might define it as solid concentration or not easily distracted. These would certainly be in the right ballpark.

However, mental toughness is much more than what those definitions might infer. Through years of coaching and observing thousands of players, young and old, I prefer the following definition:

MENTAL TOUGHNESS IS A CONDITIONED AND POSITIVE RESPONSE TO ADVERSITY.

If you look at any competitive match, or set that has something riding on it, these matches and sets all offer adversity. Whether it is the match itself or the points within the match, potential conflict rides on every stroke. Certainly, there are variables that add or detract from the severity of pressure each match or point contains. Match variables could include whether or not an opponent is recognized as a threat, what the match means for the player or for their team if it is a team match. If it is a tournament, variables include the round in which the match is being played, seeded players, next round opponents, and others. Pressure point variables include what the game or set score is, points that are played in tiebreakers, points played after "momentum shift" points (more on Momentum Shifts later!); certainly game and match points carry significant pressure. Because of these variables, Mental Toughness can be used to describe how well a player reacts and responds to such variables.

It is always interesting to watch how players play under many of the diverse scenarios mentioned above. Some players play great even when nothing is riding on the outcome of the match. However, give the match some extrinsic reward and these same players crumble from the moment the first serve is struck. An excellent example of this behavior can often be witnessed when players put some monetary value on the outcome of a match. I seldom encourage betting on the outcome of matches. However, when money is sometimes the reward—no matter how much or how little—the real mental character of each performer is often revealed! (Golfing is notorious for this practice! Those of you who have played golf and played perhaps a simple betting game such as skins can relate to this pressure! A three foot putt can feel short or long depending on how much is riding on a make or a miss!)

When you play a singles or doubles match at some time, put a little wager on the match to test this theory. It can be as innocuous as having the losers buy the winners a soda or sandwich at the end of the match. Note how the character of each player changes compared to playing a simple social match. It can be a noticeable difference, or it might be so subtle that little change is detected. However, this little test can reveal a great deal about players and their state of mental toughness!

The truly mentally secure players are often the ones seen as not being affected by the added pressure of a bet. Some players might actually play more focused and intensely. Some might literally fall apart at the seams. This kind of pressure is most revealing.

However, there are other kinds of pressure that tennis players encounter from different situations. Sometimes, the worst kind of pressure is encountered when you are about to play someone whom you know you should beat. (And especially a player whom the audience knows you should beat!) This type of match sets up expectations which sometimes makes a player focus on the aspect of winning instead of playing each shot. When this happens, players often find themselves lost in the emotional and expanded confidence that is dominant in such a match. All of a sudden, the underdog scores a few points, and self-doubt and the fear of choking can take root in the player who is expected to win.

Since these pressure scenarios are common in tennis, learning how to deal with them is of the utmost importance. Within these next few pages, you will find several "tools" in helping you prepare in the handling of pressure, as well as actually dealing with the pressure when it does come.

Part I
How to Condition the Response

"MENTAL TOUGHNESS IS A CONDITIONED AND POSITIVE RESPONSE TO ADVERSITY."

A Conditioned, Positive Response: This means that it can be learned. I have not seen a single player who was not capable of developing Mental Toughness.

I have witnessed players who were not successful at developing Mental Toughness; some of these players were members of my own teams who had developed phenomenal strokes, incredible serves, lightning fast feet and terrific agility. We have all seen this type of player…the one who can drill with the best players, hit 100 mile-per-hour serves, and hit targets with ground strokes off the ball machine…

But they can't win a match.

What is this player missing that other players, those with perhaps even less natural ability, have?

You know the answer: Mental Toughness.

So how do you learn Mental Toughness…(now that you know it can be learned)?

You start with how you practice.

Let me ask a question. Do you currently create adversity and overcome it in every practice shot? No? Well, most people don't either. How can you add this element to your practice? These practice tips have been discussed in detail in Chapter 6 on Practice Philosophies. However, while we are on the subject of Mental Toughness, it serves you well to understand how these practice tips will contribute to this aspect of your mental game.

The practice techniques discussed in Chapter 6 that help build mental toughness include counting consecutive shots and the use of targets. All the areas of practice should be thought of as "mentally conditioning" your mind. They not only help you increase your stroke production, they also will make you a more mentally tough player. But this is just part of your mental toughness training.

Learning mental toughness is not like reading a book and memorizing some deeply affecting phrase. Mental toughness is actually a "result" of the hard work and playing experiences done within the overall progression of learning the game. In fact, mental toughness is generally a "response" that is seldom planned or expected. Most players who are mentally tough seldom talk about it, seldom think about it, and seldom play specifically addressing it. However, while in practice, most champions do indeed train for it. By working mentally tough drills, by setting up competitive situations and environments, and by improving the mind through reading and mental discoveries, a player will indeed improve his or her mental toughness as it applies to tennis.

Part II
How to take the response into competition

The ability to add mental toughness aspects to your practice will undoubtedly translate into a more mentally tough match player. But there is more.

As you become better prepared for your matches, you will find it difficult to accept defeat. My favorite coaching phrase is: "The harder you work, the harder it is to fail." Certainly, any hard work you perform will make the goals of that hard work that much more valuable to you. However, don't confuse the simple concept of "hard work" as being the gist of the lesson. Otherwise, you might find yourself discovering another concept: futility! Working hard on faulty form will only make changing that form more difficult when you realize that the faulty form is limiting you. Tennis mechanics at every level must be clearly understood so that you will be working "hard" on the very form that will give you the best results.

Once you have put in the hard work, the next step is implementation of proper form and strategy in competition. How often do we see tennis players working on specific shots or strokes in practice only to completely abandon those things in competition! It is no wonder that one of the first books on the mind in competition was a book dealing with the mental side of tennis!

In 1972, Timothy Gallwey's The Inner Game of Tennis was a revolutionary revelation in dealing with sports psychology. So popular was Gallwey's book and approach that over 700,000 books were sold around the world! I highly recommend that tennis players today pick up a copy of his book if not already in possession of it.

In Gallwey's book, he describes "Self 1" and "Self 2". Self 1 is our controlling voice, the critic. Self 2 is the self who performs. Gallwey says, "The more you trust self 2, the better you will play." When we let Self 1 dominate our actions (and our minds) in competition, we open ourselves to all the variables that tend to destroy our mental toughness. Those variables include:

- **Tanking:** *This is when a player simply "gives up". This is the "excuse maker", the whiner, and the complainer. Players resort to tanking to absolve themselves of the pain that accompanies losing. Players who tank matches don't hurt as much when they lose because tanking protects their ego. The tanker has a built-in excuse: "I didn't win because I didn't try." We can face our friends and peers with this false reasoning. The phrase, "I could have won if I really wanted to" is a common statement made by a tanker. While tanking protects the ego, it prevents a player from winning and, in a real sense, it can prevent a player from becoming a champion.*

- **Anger:** *This is when a player allows his or her emotions to control them. Showing anger, like tanking, is an emotional response designed to protect the ego. Anger provides a player with the excuse, "I didn't win because I was so mad." Anger also projects the false image of a player who is trying. Instead of focusing their energy on the match, the angry player focuses on how he is observed and perceived by others.*

- **Choking:** *This is the emotion that all competitors hate. It is a physiological response to fear and doubt. When a player doubts himself, the results are painful to experience and to watch! Everything seems to move too fast, players can't think straight, and there is a feeling of anxiety. When fear consumes us, the simple seems hard; the logical becomes illogical; the present seems like the past. In one sense, however, choking is a far* *better response than anger and tanking because even while we are choking, we are trying. Choking is more of an innate response to competition than a conscious choice. Although anger and tanking are sometimes chosen avenues for many, choking is almost never an elected response.*

When players gain confidence, their ability to play in "the moment" increases. Highly skilled players learn through a variety of experiences to play tennis without focusing on these detrimental tendencies. Those experiences usually include both a practice foundation based on the principles I have introduced in this book, and playing experiences that are gained through a variety of competitive environments. A player simply can't accelerate through lessons to obtain the aspect of actual playing experience. All players will have varying degrees of success in gaining the necessary mental aspects to playing under pressure. Some players might be ahead of the mental game through having some previous sporting experiences. Others can have a predisposition for becoming mentally tough while others have to work at it for a long period of time. I have found that the mental capacity of players, those who can play tough when the pressure is on, is more an inbred trait than the athleticism necessary to simply learn tennis strokes. More players have overcome limited natural physical conditions faster and easier than players who have to overcome limitations related to the mental game!

There is an excellent axiom that I read in the book "Zen in the Martial Arts" by Joe Hymas that is related to this issue of playing in the moment:

"Seize the Moment: You must learn to live in the present, not in the future or the past. Zen teaches that life must be seized at the moment. By living in the present you are in full contact with yourself and your environment, your energy is not dissipated and is always available."

Tennis players who play competitive matches with any part of their mind focused on the outcome of any match will not play within their "competitive moment." Examples of situations that will take players out of their "competitive moment" are:

- Worrying about what the results of the current match may mean
- Still thinking about a great shot hit
- Still thinking about a bad shot hit
- Thinking about your next match while still playing within another match
- Worrying about what will happen if they lose this game/point/set
- Thinking about how great they are playing
- Thinking that they are going to win the match: Thinking that they should easily win or lose a match before it begins and during it
- Fuming about a bad call made earlier in the match
- Thinking about the lucky shot your opponent hit any time after the fact

The most common example of these listed is when a player serves an ace. I don't know what the statistics are, but it is very common for a player to double fault on the subsequent point following an ace. The reason is simple. The server is conscious of the ace and believes he or she can do it again. The lingering memory of the ace is still strong in the mind of the server. Instead of focusing on what exactly the server needs to do on the next serve, the memory of the ace is still the predominant mental thought. Thus, the server following an ace does not focus on specifically what he or she wants to do on the next serve. If the first serve is missed, the player often focuses on not wanting to double fault following such a great serve (the ace) on the previous point. Again, the player is not focused on where they want to hit the serve, they are thinking about the potential outcome if they make or miss the serve.

Dealing with Fear

Fear is perhaps the most powerful emotion that can affect us on a tennis court. Fear of losing, fear of winning, fear of looking bad, or fear of the unknown can all have a direct effect on our ability to play well. Most athletes know that they perform at their best when they are loose, focused, and aggressive. Fear can sabotage these three key elements and make a person play tense, distracted and apprehensive.

Jeff Greenwald expresses this concept of fear in his program "**Fearless Tennis**":

> *Everyone talks about self-talk, that it needs to be positive, upbeat. Sure, that can help. But more powerful yet is the ability to come on court truly ready to play absolutely fearless tennis. I believe every one of us, somewhere in our lives, has been a fighter, has toughed it out through a difficult situation -- or maybe we just want to be tough. The trick is, on the court, not to be victimized by the first and automatic thought that may come into your head -- "Oh, god, he's ranked, or seeded, or misses nothing in warm-up. I'm gonna get creamed!" Go down that train track and you know where you're going to get off -- at the Big "L" stop, embarrassed and angry at yourself. Instead, let the second thought surface: "Wait a minute. I can do this. I belong here. I'm just going to go out and enjoy the hell out of it." Amazing how you can play when you feel that way.*

Dealing with the Ego

Notice that the three negative response variables, (tanking, anger, and choking) center on the player's ego. When a player is concerned with his ego, tanking and anger are the first to show their ugly head! I have used a phrase for years as a general statement to developing better mental tennis:

> *"When we play and practice not to satisfy our ego but to satisfy our goals, we allow the best tennis to emerge."*

Think about this phrase. If we are concerned with our egos, we are concerned with what others think about us. If, however, we are concerned with our goals, we are then focused on things related to our development as a tennis player. If they lose a match, ego-centered players will look for excuses. Goal-centered players will look for ways to learn from the loss and improve.

The ego can sometimes be used to help reach goals. When we want to prove something because of our ego, we then almost subconsciously recognize the value of goals. Coaches can use the ego of his or her team to accomplish this. I will discuss this in detail in a moment.

Players trained in elementary stroke patterns (that are not recognized as skilled or progressive) and recognizing that they need a mental change are often victimized by their own ego. Let me give you a scenario:

Julie, who is 35 years old, is a 3.5 player. (10 years at 3.5!) She has finally broken down and received accurate tennis instruction on her serve/volley/backhand. (You can choose!) She has worked in practice on her new stroke and knows what she should do to hit the ball correctly within the parameters of the new technique. However, when she gets in a match, she goes right back to hitting her old, inferior strokes.

Why?

Julie felt that if she tried her new strokes there would be a perception of failure: If she used her old strokes, she believed she could at least compete at the 3.5 level in which she was used to playing. So, Julie let her ego dictate what she did in the competition. Instead of forgoing the ego and making or missing with her new strokes in match play (and improving each shot in the process!), she took the ego-easy way out!

Sadly, as she continues repeating this scenario throughout her playing days, she will, of course, continue to play at the 3.5 level essentially forever.

INTENTION DRIVEN VERSUS RESULTS DRIVEN PRACTICE AND COMPETITIVE PLAY

For any shot in tennis the object of the shot has little to do with the outcome of the match, yet a great deal to do with the eventual outcome of any particular point. Thus, a player who is focused on the ramifications of winning or losing is focused on the results or outcome of a match. This type of focal attention prevents a player from focusing on the more immediate and more important type of attention: intent.

When you hit any ball in a match or in practice, the shot should have a specific intention. That is, a mental focus of what specifically you want to do with the ball. Intentions can be as simple as getting the ball over the net for beginners. Or, intentions can involve very complex shot-making skills. Examples of these complex shots can be a sharp angle passing shot on the run that involves hitting a reverse forehand with significant topspin but hit with minimal ball velocity. Skilled players through extensive experience and practice, group these complexities into a single mindset. As players advance, this grouping of more complex actions becomes a single intention. Beginners using the Advanced Foundation may have to make conscious connections within any given intention. They may only be able to concentrate on the racket path. Or, they may be ready to engage the proper footwork with the reverse forehand finish. Regardless of the level of experience, each player must have a clear intention of what shot is desired. Too many players allow the ball and their perceived lack of time to dictate the shot...namely just trying to get the ball back.

This intention takes the mind away from the potential outcome and places it where it should be: on making the shot. When practicing, always ask yourself, "What is my intention?" once your coach, partner, or opponent has hit the ball.

This concentrated mental thought soon becomes a subconsciously trained reaction through practice. This kind of mental tennis is often viewed as "playing in the zone." By consciously focusing on your intention, you actually design the rally shot by shot. Obviously, your intention must match your ability as well as your opponent's shot. For example, a beginner's intention should not be to hit an inside-out, open-stance topspin shot at full speed! However, a beginner who is developing within the Advanced Foundation better be thinking about hitting a specific shot, such as a topspin or a slice, as well as a general placement of the shot. Without the intention clear in the player's head, the player will resort to those patterns which are more natural—but more detrimental to the player's advancement.

The more a player practices the intention focus, the more it becomes the way the player will play in competition. Highly skilled players can falter in match play because they lose this focus on intent. They become focused on other issues that have nothing to do with hitting successful shots. Thus, all players must remember this aspect of mental tennis. When the intention is clear, fear, anger, and ego will seldom control a player's emotional condition.

Tournament Tennis

As I mentioned earlier in this chapter, playing tournament tennis is an absolute must for any player wanting to master tennis. The reason for this is that there is no other method that replicates the pressure and importance of playing tennis. In most tournaments if you lose a match, you're done. (Or, at the very least, you are in the back draw or consolation!) This kind of pressure is hard to emulate in practice. The closest I have come to matching this pressure is through team challenge matches. Challenges present a similar pressure due to the fact that if a player loses their challenge, it usually costs them a position on their team ladder. Challenges among high school teams, those that determine whether the winner will play varsity or junior varsity, are especially pressure-packed!

In addition to the pressure created by playing tournament tennis, players who attend a variety of tournaments gain the advantage of observing many other players competing. A classic example of this importance can be illustrated through a situation that occurred when I first moved to Arizona and took over the coaching of one of the top-ranked juniors in the state.

Justin was ranked number 4 in the 16's of the southwest division of USTA. Although Justin had played in most of the tournaments within Arizona, he had never ventured outside of his USTA section. During his junior year I took Justin to California to play some of my former players that I had coached prior to my move to Arizona. While in California I had Justin play a kid named Robert. When a sweaty Justin returned from his match, I asked him how it went.

"That kid is tough! He beat me 6 - 1" Justin said between breaths. "Was he your number one kid?" he asked.

"Yes," I said with a pause to let Justin have a moment of solace before I dropped the hammer on his ego. "He is number one on JUNIOR VARSITY," I said. There were actually 9 other players above Robert on the ladder.

Justin learned a most valuable lesson at that moment. Even as good as Justin was in his USTA section, there were players—by the hundreds—who could not just beat him, but beat him badly. Justin returned to Arizona with a new mindset. He now had a much better grasp of what he must do to be a better tennis player. It wasn't that Robert or any of the other player opponents of Justin in California were that much better than Justin. In fact, Justin had all the shots they had. Yet, in the mental tennis department, Justin was more or less a beginner. In reality, the players in California had hundreds, if not thousands, of players who were competitive, all living in their own backyards. Justin was one of only a couple dozen truly competitive players that lived in Arizona. The players who recognized this discrepancy were the ones who traveled to all the competitive parts of the country to gain such competitive experience.

Improvement Roller Coaster

For almost every individual on this planet, improvement in anything is seldom a steady, progressive state that can be measured in equal, incremental steps. If anything, improvement in most skill-related sports occurs in consistent inconsistencies! Tennis is no exception to this statement. In fact, tennis improvement is probably one of the most inconsistent of sports in which players can expect to see some essence of steady improvement. One day a player can be playing so well they can't believe they can possibly lose. On another day, (and sometimes on the very next playing date!), often players can experience their worst performance ever. The variance between these highs and lows is usually controlled through a player's mental toughness. In other words, players who are mentally tough don't seesaw as drastically between these two playing descriptions. The most mentally tough players also don't stay down very long. And finally, the mentally tough player does not allow bad days to affect them as long or as deeply as a mentally weak player does.

CYCLE OF IMPROVEMENT

Improvement must be NOT recognized in a subjective acknowledgement of indication, but in qualitative and quantitative measurements. These values for improvement include:

- *Hitting more consistently*
- *Hitting with more angles, more consistently*
- *Hitting with more variety, more consistently*
- *Hitting harder, more consistently*

It may be obvious, but this issue of continued improvement can be measured primarily by a player's ability to utilize consistent and reliable swing patterns. If there are flaws in a swing pattern, in form, in footwork, in balance, or in coordination, the ability for a player to hit "more consistently" in each of these areas I just mentioned will be diminished. Thus, it will be critical for every player to work towards this quality.

In tennis, the way we perceive improvement is often referred to as a "roller coaster" as this analogy quite aptly describes the issue of how most tennis players experience improvement. These "Cycles of Improvement" are founded on the concept that I call "consideration."

CONSIDERATIONS

Consider that when a new stroke is first attempted, the body must coordinate many unfamiliar or uncomfortable patterns. Any player who has been playing tennis for any period of time will recognize that change is difficult. One of the objectives of this book is to eliminate, or at the very least, diminish the need for making changes. Of course, if a player has been playing tennis prior to reading this book, then change is inevitable! So, assuming that change is needed, almost every single player will go through a challenging period: trying to keep from doing what is comfortable—yet wrong—and attempting that which is right, however difficult and uncomfortable. Not only are these changes difficult and uncomfortable...they will be relatively unsuccessful for some period of time!

This pattern of adjustment will be an ongoing experience. The good news is that as players come nearer their Advanced Foundation, both the difficulty and the frustration will diminish.

Yet, all players must consider that improvement and perception of success will rise and fall like our proverbial roller coaster. Some days you will find tennis easy and flowing, other days it will feel forced and unfamiliar. This is common, even for advanced players. Beginners often look at advanced players and think, "Wow, these guys are so good, how can THEY have a bad day playing?" Yet, even for advanced players the PERCEPTION of how they are playing—to themselves—can reach peaks and valleys similar to those experienced by any other level of player. Remember, that as players become more proficient, the EXPECTATIONS rise for those individuals. No longer are advanced players simply satisfied in getting their serve in or hitting the ball over the net! These players now aspire to do more with the ball. This means a greater chance of failure. This failure can be diminished or eliminated if the player has developed proper strokes as they develop. (Which is another reason why the Advanced Foundation is so very important.)

General Playing Strategies: Playing Smart Tennis

As we have mentioned, hitting strategies will change as a player progresses and improves. Likewise, playing strategies — or a player's "game plan" — can change dramatically as a player's skill advances. Typically, the hierarchy of playing strategies evolves into more complex and defined methodologies (as they apply to the targeting of each shot) as a player's hitting ability progresses. Obviously, our playing strategies will change not only when our own abilities increase, but also when our opponent's abilities improve! If an opponent can't get a ball over the net, then the only strategy we should be concerned with would be to "get the ball in play." However, when opponents meet or exceed certain playing strategies, we must adopt a more effective strategy based on our own abilities and limitations.

A simple example of this development as it might apply to groundstrokes is as follows:

Eventually, the odds will favor the player who is both persistent and consistent !

Beginning Playing Strategies

- *Hit the ball*
- *Hit the ball over the net*
- *Hit the ball over the net and into the opponent's court*

Intermediate Playing Strategies

- *Hit the ball more consistently in opponent's court*
- *Direct the ball to opponent's weakness*
- *Hit the ball with intentional slice or topspin*
- *Hit the ball with greater depth*

Advanced Playing Strategies

- *Hit shots with a variety of depth and angles*
- *Hit shots with a greater variety and quantity of spin*
- *Hit with disguise*
- *Hit behind opponents. (Hitting shots to the same spot as your previous shot)*
- *Hit winners from the baseline*
- *Hit with power*

It should be obvious that the first concept to evolve in terms of a specific playing strategy involves directing the tennis ball. Whether it is hitting to an opponent's weakness, hitting deeper shots, hitting the open court, hitting angles, hitting drop shots, hitting behind opponents, or hitting winners, the ability of a player to hit each of these shots depends on their ability to command direction on his or her shots. Notice, too, that power is the last item identified on this list. The reason for this should also be obvious: power reduces a player's ability to consistently direct their shots. The player who focuses on a strategy that centers on power is the player who will so often find themselves on the losing side of many a match. There are many reasons for this outcome.

It is inevitable that players who use more power than they can control will eventually make a mistake. Opponents, who can effectively get to the shots hit by these power hitters and simply block the ball back into play, will make their opponent hit the ball more often. By getting the ball back in this fashion a player can prolong each rally, increasing the likelihood that the power-hitter will eventually miss. Most players who exhibit this patience and work to keep the ball in play will be rewarded with more points won than lost. Players who have mastered the strategy of patience acknowledge that the power-player will indeed win some points with such power. It is a lot like the golf phrase: "Drive for show, putt for dough". Yet, in the long run, the number of misses will almost always outnumber the winners. Eventually, the odds will favor the player who is both persistent and consistent!

Obviously, if a player has both control and power, then we have a player who has mastered the game at a very high level of skill. The question is how do we get to this level of skill?

The answer to this question is provided in the second section of this book, the Strategies of Hitting. By developing strokes that are based on the Advanced Foundation as described in this book, players will make progressive improvements in both stroke consistency and power development. Through application of the methodologies taught in this book, players will evolve more powerful strokes while maintaining form associated with the highest percentage of consistency. Certainly, when players start applying more power to their strokes, any incorrect form will magnify the errors created by the same faulty form.

When a player plays a match, in most cases, the pressures of making each shot will be quite different than the pressure of hitting shots during practice drills. The pressure of what a point means in a match is far different than the pressure of a rally or a ball hit in practice! When each shot has weight, whether it is from the standpoint of winning or losing a rally, or winning or losing a match, the player will feel that weight in the form of pressure. Drills and practice rallies seldom offer any of the same pressures as a rally in a match. If power is the last element of players' strategy, it should also be the LEAST sought-after playing-strategy a player should consider during a competitive match. Keeping the ball in play is an absolute must for every player who hopes to not only win more matches, but to develop the ability to apply power when it is indeed necessary. Players who try to hit too hard too early end up having to back off; typically they end up hitting shots considerably weaker than usual because of falling behind in attempting to hit too hard too soon. This strategy of trying to hit too hard too early often produces a dinking mentality; a player becomes so afraid of losing points from initially hitting the ball too hard, they go to the other extreme: dinking the ball.

However, in terms of progressive development, players must be cognizant of a very important principle: In trying to keep the ball in play, players must attempt to accomplish this strategy by using strokes and form closely related to those described in this book (strokes that are accepted methods for progressive improvement). That is, players should hit using the best form they can within stroke speeds that will insure the highest degree of success. We call this

PLAYING WITHIN ONESELF

This is an important concept. Too often, players attempt to hit shots that are low percentage for their skill level. Like addicted gamblers, some players, because they successfully executed one of these low-percentage shots once, think they can hit it again. Unfortunately, the reality of the matter is that the few times they were successful in making low-percentage shots, it was more a matter of luck than skill. Even though it is important to push oneself to try higher levels of skill-related shots during both practice as well as competitive opportunities, it is important to try them within the bounds of proper form. Players who sacrifice balance, form, and footwork in favor of raw power will seldom, if ever, be able to develop consistent mechanics to the degree that consistent power can be achieved. It is this discipline that often hinders a 3.5 player from advancing to the 4.0 level even if the 3.5 level player possesses a proper advanced foundation.

There is a balance that players who must strive to attain while playing matches if they want to continue to improve. Hitting shots that are associated with proper strokes and progressive improvement must be attempted as often as possible during competition. However, while in actual competition, there is a recognition that players will want to play shots offering the greatest opportunity to win. The problem lies when a player changes from attempts related to proper form to attempts that simply get the ball over the net. For the most part, it is this strategy that limits player advancement as it relates to competition. Until a player accepts the fact that they will make errors even when they attempt correct form, they will continually revert back to elementary tennis strokes with which the player feels comfortable and confident. This example is clearly evident when watching players who are trying to change from a rudimentary stroke method to a more advanced; these players often revert back to the comfortable patterns of play that are usually the very mechanics the player is trying to change!

Many players attempt proper form and will end up often making fewer mistakes than with the faulty form that they might be trying to change. However, because the proper form might feel uncomfortable (and essentially less confident), the player actually feels the proper form was less successful! For example, a player who has dinked his second serve his whole career finally learns how to hit a competitive spin serve. In attempting to use the spin serve, the player double faults on occasion. To avoid this embarrassment, the player reverts back to his "safe" dink serve. Yet, the player still double faults almost as much (and sometimes more!) as when he was using the new spin serve! Because of the "comfort" level of using the dink serve, the double faults while dinking the serve are less unpleasant, and thus easier to accept.

It becomes very evident that when players continue to revert back to "safe strokes," those that are comfortable, familiar, and confidant (within the player's limited playing abilities), they will never advance to the better players they are striving to become!

DON'T SET YOURSELF UP TO FAIL...BY WHAT YOU SAY!

One of the most common mental breakdowns doesn't even occur on the court. Players can sabotage their on-court success by not what they do, but by what they SAY off the court.What I am talking about is the over-confident words spoken by a player about how well they are going to play… or about how badly they are going to beat a player or team. We often call this "trash talk" and we see it especially at the junior levels.

Trash talk is, more often then not, a sign of weakness. Players who have to tell others how good they are seldom live up to their boast. (And most people know it!) In addition, it sets up a player who engages in trash-talk to almost always fail. Here's how.

By stating that something is going to happen—or more specifically, by stating how you are going to annihilate some opponent before you start—you set a standard for how that match should proceed. If at any point in that match your opponent wins a couple points, a game, or even a set, you have already failed, even though you haven't yet lost the match. This sets up a situation that is basically "nothing to lose" for your opponent, and "everything to lose" for our arrogant player.

While I have seen this exact situation cost a match for many a player, a match, the most dramatic example of this came when I was coaching a high school doubles team in the finals of our league championships in Arizona.

My players, Max and Richard, were both seniors. Neither player was ranked high in the southwest region, and neither one was really what one would consider gifted athletes. In fact, one of the boys had a propensity for extreme nerves while the other was quite seasoned in pressure play and had often performed quite heroically. In the finals, they had truly met their match in the final round against a team from a school near Scottsdale called Saguaro High School. The team they were playing was the previous year's state champions in doubles and had gone through the tournament without dropping a game in any set. In all honesty, they were head and shoulders the better team.

As the two teams headed to center court walking through the spectators, one of the Saguaro opponents spoke loud enough for everyone to hear, especially my doubles team.

"John, looks like another 6 – 0, 6 – 0 match," the one boy said. The other boy, not quite as brazen, did however, issue a confident grin and a short laugh.

The match proceeded with the Saguaro team dispatching the first set as predicted, 6 – 0. The second set had the same ominous feel as the Saguaro team was up 2 – 0 and their big left-handed server was up next. (I don't think we had gotten more than a point off his tough, left-handed kick serve.) Amazingly, my players hit a couple of nice low slice returns at the server's feet and ended up getting a couple of easy volleys that we put away convincingly. A few points later, we ended up breaking the kid's serve on a simple unforced error by one of their players.

All of a sudden, their prediction was wrong. It was no longer going to be a 6 – 0, 6 – 0 match. In fact, we ended up holding serve making it two-all. Everyone watching could feel the momentum swing. The Saguaro team from that point on was playing NOT to lose another game… and in the process played tentative points. We ended up winning not only that set 7 – 6 (and 7 – 5 in the tiebreaker!) but we won the third set 6 –2 as well.

I know deep down, that the Saguaro team not only should have won that match, but also should have repeated as State Champions. They were that good. However, they ended up losing in the second round of the state tournament and were never heard from again.

How much that one little prediction cost this team such possible rewards was quite a discovery. It would be impossible to say for sure that that single statement was the core of their demise. However, the statement lingered in the minds of all involved, I believe, and indeed had a significant baring on the outcome of the match. Of course, there were many points that had to be made for the event to unfold the way it did. But I feel certain that this fateful match was inevitable due to the few spoken words by our opponents. I vowed to make sure that every player of mine knows that true story and never makes the same mistake.

Momentum Shifts

Momentum Shift is an important concept to understand. The more you understand it, the more you can take advantage of certain points that can result in these momentum shifts. Also, through this knowledge, you will know when to really buckle down and play tough!

A momentum shift is actually several points played in a specific order at specific periods during a match. The shift can be simply a change in momentum by a player or players through the course of identifiable points. There are several examples that are clear Momentum Shifts in a match:

1. THE LUCKY SHOT

Depending on the score of a match, the intensity of a match, and the importance of a match, the "lucky shot" can create a significant momentum shift in a match.

Usually the lucky shot itself (a framed winner, a behind the back winner, a freaky net cord shot, etc.) is not enough for a momentum shift. However, when a team or player wins the point immediately following the lucky shot, (and if the next point results in winning a game), then the momentum can shift. The psychology of this is as follows: A player is losing and hits the lucky shot. It happened at deuce when the player was down 3 – 0 in the set. Instead of losing the point and now about to lose another game, he is now up in the game with the advantage. If he wins the next point and wins the game, instead of being down 0 –4, he is down 1 – 3. This is a big difference…especially if the game won was a service break. Should the losing player win his serve, he is right back in the game instead of being on the brink of a blow out.

Players on the receiving end of this lucky shot must not dwell on it at all. They must shake it off and resume playing just as competitively as before the lucky shot occurred.

2. THE LONG RALLY

A long rally, in a similar match as I described in the "lucky shot" scenario, can have similar effects. A long rally can be both physically and mentally draining. If the player behind wins an extremely long rally, and then wins the next point after it, the player who was ahead can feel like he literally can't catch his breath. Winning the point immediately after such a rally is very important. Also, like our "lucky shot" example, the score of the match can add weight to such a long rally.

3. THE INTIMIDATING PUT-AWAY

This shot, the big put-away (usually an overhead or a decisive volley), can be psychologically important in a match. This is especially true for doubles, especially if you hit the net man! If a team that is behind belts an overhead or a crisp volley through the opponent's net man, the emotional lift can be strong. Often, when a player hits such a shot at or near the net man, the net man will turn and lecture his partner for setting him up. This creates a bit of disharmony in the team and opens the door for increasing friction depending on what happens soon after such a shot. Usually, the players become too careful in their shot-making so that they don't make the same mistake again. Such a strategy of being too careful can make the momentum shift complete.

Conclusion

Mental tennis includes many facets of the game. From the way you practice to the way you respond to adversity, mental tennis is an important aspect to your success in competition. If you train and prepare within the Advanced Foundation, you will be well on your way to establishing sincere confidence in your game. Such confidence not only improves your chances of winning on the court, but when you play with such confidence, playing tennis becomes extraordinarily fun!

CHAPTER 14

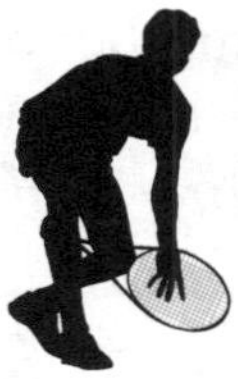

Singles Strategies within the Advanced Foundation

Introduction to Singles Strategies

The game of singles provides a terrific forum for individual style and personality. Unlike doubles, where play is much more directed and dictated by circumstance and position, singles can encompass a great deal of variety, even at the higher levels of play.

Historically, at the pro level, the singles game has gone though a series of favored strategies often based on the evolutionary strengths that the general pro population favors. Some of these various strategies could be summed up by these generalities:

1) Serve and Volley
2) Baseline Bravery
3) Chip and Charge
4) Fighting Fatigue
5) Baseline Bombs
6) All-court Athletes
7) Serve and sit down

While these phrases are written somewhat tongue-in-cheek, they accurately describe the many singles' strategies that have been perpetuated over the course of professional play. The following is a general premise of each strategy, including a partial listing of pros that could be considered practitioners of each:

1) **Serve and Volley:** The intentional act of serving and coming to the net.

Players: *Pete Sampras, Taylor Dent, Tim Henmen, Patrick Rafter, Martina Navratilova, Stefan Edberg, and Stan Smith (and a majori ty of professional men who played between the 1950's and the 1970's!)*

2) **Baseline Bravery**: Players who stay back at the baseline and rally almost exclusively with the patience of a Zen master.
Players: *Chris Evert, Tracy Austin, Steffi Graf, Monica Seles, Ivan Lendl, Michael Change, Bjorn Borg.*

3) **Chip and Charge**: After any number of groundstrokes, these players look for every opportunity to slice short balls and come to the net.
Players: *Billie Jean King, Jack Kramer, Ken Rosewall, John McEnroe, Ilie Nastase, and many of the professional men playing between the 1950's and the 1970's!*

4) **Fighting Fatigue**: Die hard players who are physically determined to hit as many balls as it takes and run down every shot possible.
Players: *Michael Change, Bjorn Borg, Jimmy Connors, Jim Courier, Chris Evert, Boris Becker, and Steffi Graf.*

5) **Baseline Bombs**: Aggressive baseline players who pound topspin ground strokes with laser-guided precision.
Players: *Venus and Serena Williams, Lindsay Davenport, Andre Agassi, Jennifer Capriati, Ivan Lendl, Rod Laver and Andy Roddick.*

6) **All-court Athletes**: These players are known for their ability to play any style of game as needed including baseline play, net-attacking play, power and finesse, etc.
Players: *Rodger Federer, Tony Trabert, Rod Laver, Arthur Ashe, Andy Roddick, Andre Agassi, Martina Hingis, and Justine Hinin-Hardenne.*

7) **Serve and sit down**: Big, BIG, BIG serves!
Players: *Goran Ivanisevic, Bill Tilden, Pancho Gonzalez, Andy Roddick, Greg Rusedski, and Pete Sampras*

Obviously, many of these champions are listed in more than one of these categories. There are many others that could easily be included that I did not choose. However, it is interesting to examine how many of these players carved their singles' game from many of these fairly specific strategies.

What constitutes a "Strategy"?

Certainly the most rudimentary strategy, singles or doubles, would be to "get the ball over the net"; not exactly the most prolific of game plans! However, once a player begins to develop strokes and can control the ball through the repeatable use of those strokes, he or she can then begin to emulate specific strategies. Without this control, any strategy will be basically worthless since the directional control would be unattainable.

SINGLES STRATEGIES

Once we are able to control our shots, then the issue of specifically what shots—and where (strategically) those shots are hit, becomes our next area of interest.

BASIC STRATEGIES

Generally, there are two basic singles strategies in tennis. They are:

A. Attacking Strategies
B. Retrieving Strategies

It is probably obvious that attacking strategies are offensive in nature while retrieving strategies are defensive. Although competitive tennis usually includes a bit of both, most players attempt to play within one or the other as their principle strategy. In both strategies there are shots and placements that are more effective than others. However, even understanding this, there are exceptions to each "rule".

Perhaps the most notable exception to every rule is this: If your opponent has a glaring weakness, exploit it. For example, if your opponent has a weak backhand, it is usually going to be in your favor to hit most of your shots to your opponent's backhand! Forget going down-the-line on approach shots or hitting crosscourt shots in rallies; hit as often as you can to your opponent's weakest shot!

If all things are equal regarding your opponent's strengths and weaknesses, then there are specific strategies to learn and apply while playing singles. Whether you are favoring an attacking strategy or a retrieving one, there are some basic rules of rallying that all players must understand. There will be times in which an attacking player will have to stay back and hit shots that resemble a retrieving strategy until they get a shot at which they can attack and come to the net. As you can see, often an attacking player must play an "all-court" game. Likewise, many retrieving players will be forced to move towards the net and play an attacking game. This usually occurs when an opponent has hit a drop shot or even just a short ball; the retrieving player won't be in a position to retreat back to the baseline in time to defend his court after their shot.

Retrieving Strategies

When playing from the baseline, there are strategies that offer greater percentages of potential success. They are based on three Basic Strategic Principles.

1) Strategies that increase the percentages of hitting your own shots successfully
2) Strategies that create lower percentages for your opponent to hit their shots successfully

If these first two strategies are essentially equal to both you and your opponent, then:

3) Creating opportunities to win the point through a series of shots that lead to an outright winner is your third and most advanced strategy. This strategy can be labeled as an "Aggressive" retrieving strategy.

THE "CROSSCOURT RETRIEVING STRATEGY"

Generally, intermediate to advanced players should keep the majority of baseline shots crosscourt. The reasons are as follows

- *Crosscourt strokes take the ball over the middle of the the lowest part of the net.*

These first three crosscourt rationales refer to the first of our "Basic Strategic Principles"; namely increasing the percentages of our own shots which are hit successfully.

- *Crosscourt strokes take into account the largest amount of court space. Hitting crosscourt provides for approximately 3 more feet of court length than hitting down-the-line. (The hypotenuse of a right-angle triangle is longer than the side of the triangle.)*

These next three crosscourt strategies generally deal with our second "Basic Strategic Principle"; namely, attempting to lower the percentages for your opponent to hit a successful shot.

- *For most intermediate players, hitting a ball crosscourt is easier to control with proper form than hitting down-the-line.*
- *Strategically, a down-the-line shot gives your opponent several options in which to attack you. (More on this concept later.)*
- *Crosscourt shots move the ball away from the center point of the court. This means that through the use of crosscourt groundstrokes, you can move your opponent further away from the middle of the court. As a result, they will have further to run to get back to a ready position that is centered on their side of the court. (Down-the-line groundstrokes tend to move the ball parallel with the sidelines making the distance your opponent must move to get to the ball less than a similarly struck crosscourt.)*
- *Repeated crosscourt strokes generally produce rallies that created multiple opportunites for hitting behind your opponent. (We will talk about this strategy in a moment.)*

Next time you watch a professional tennis match, count the number of crosscourt shots hit in a match. Even at the professional level, these players still hit approximately 60 to 80 percent of their groundstrokes crosscourt, depending on the surface. (Court surfaces will affect the speed of the ball after the bounce. Courts such as clay and "Har-Tru" will produce a slower speed of the ball after the bounce than 'faster' courts such as grass or hard courts—made of concrete or asphalt.) Faster courts can sometimes make a down-the-line shot effective in some situations other than approach shots and out-right winners.

Generally, retrieving strategies involve playing a baseline game that focuses on patience. Since it is difficult to hit outright winners from the baseline, hitting balls hard in attempting such a strategy seldom produces winning points. However, players who develop proper form for consistent power will create openings and opportunities for winners and forced errors by their opponent from the baseline. Certainly, more power will force opponents to cover more court in less time. This will put more pressure on them to either attempt better shots, or they will become more out-of-position as a rally progresses. Both of these scenarios will force opponents to hit lower percentage shots… the ultimate objective of a retrieving playing strategy!

Crosscourt strategies involve a baseline player hitting crosscourt on virtually all groundstrokes. As mentioned, crosscourt shots offer several advantages. A player, when given a crosscourt shot, will automatically hit behind their opponent by hitting a cross-court shot in response. Anytime you can hit behind your opponent, you create a unique advantage: your opponent, who just came from the corner you are hitting to (to cover the open court), must change direction to return back to the corner he or she just came from! Because this requires more energy than simply moving in the same direction they are heading (as if to cover a down-the-line by you), over the course of a point, subsequent shots of this nature tend to wear down your opponent. Sooner or later your opponent will hit a weak shot, one that you can hit to the open court for a winner, or that you can once again hit behind them with more offensive pace. Either way, they will have difficulty retrieving your shot. (As you can see, even in this "retrieving" style of play, you can create offensive opportunities through patience and shot selections.)

Attacking Strategies

Attacking strategies center around two distinct patterns of play:

A) Serve and Volley
B) Approach and Volley

Both of these strategies are dependent on a player's ability to get to the net…and then do something while at the net! Thus, these players will want to have effective serves and approach shots in which they can follow in behind and approach the net. In addition, attacking players must possess crisp, offensive volleys to finish off the point. In addition, a solid overhead is a must for the attacking player. (Here again, an advanced foundation in each stroke is imperative to successful strategies.) It is also an advantage for an attacking player to develop drop volleys and angle volleys. While it is more often advantageous to hit your volleys deep and firm, a short angle volley or drop volley can be increasingly advantageous. For example, if a player has pushed an opponent deep into his court, hitting another deep volley will not necessarily be as effective a shot as a drop volley. (This is one distinctive area of the net game that clearly separates the 3.5 level player and those at the 4.0 level and above. The reason for this is that many 3.5 level players use the Eastern forehand and backhand volley grips. As mentioned in Chapter 8 on volleys, this grip precludes most players from developing a significant angle volley as well as drop volley.)

Effective serves and approach shots are not based solely on power. In fact, certain approach shots are limited due to the physical laws of motion. For example, slice approach shots can only be hit so hard until they can't possibly land in the court. (Please review the slice groundstrokes in Chapter 9 and 10.) Thus, no matter how good you are, the slice can't be hit beyond a certain range of pace. In this case, placement and depth become paramount.

Attacking players tend to favor fast surfaced courts, such as grass and hard courts. These surfaces keep approach shots low and makes returning a serve more difficult.

Players favoring net-attacking strategies include Pete Sampras, Tim Henman and Patrick Rafter. In the past, many of the men's champions chose the attacking strategy. Stefan Edberg, Ken Rosewall, Rod Laver, Pancho Gonzales and Roy Emerson were champions of the past with attacking strategies. One of the best known and most effective attacking players was John McEnroe. McEnroe didn't hit as hard as many of the past or present attacking players; however, his timing, anticipation, and knowledge of court geometry was superb. He used cunning instincts to win a significant number of matches and tournaments in his career. Women did not favor an over all attacking style of play until the late 1960's and early 1970's. Billy Jean King was one of the first who favored attacking the net. In addition, past champions like Martina Navratilova, Gabriela Sabatini, and Virginia Wade ventured to the net quite often. The "modern" women's game now features many players who often finish points off at the net. These women tend to combine an attacking strategy with an effective and penetrating ground game, forcing opponents into hitting shots that they can attack. Venus and Serena Williams, Lindsay Davenport, Justine Henin, and others are the current generation of aggressive women players seen on tour.

APPROACH SHOTS

Even as slice strokes have limitations in terms of power and pace, there are many advantages to using a slice stroke as an attacking shot. Here are some of the advantages offered by hitting a slice:

- *A slice is generally an easier stroke to hit while moving towards the net; the slice lends itself to be hit while moving forward during the shot itself.*
- *The slice tends to make the ball stay lower after the bounce.*
- *The slice is generally easier to hit down the line.*
- *It is easier to disguise a drop shot while using a slice as an approach shot.*

WHEN TO APPROACH

Typically, attacking a short ball hit by your opponent is the best opportunity to hit your approach shot. Thus, your ability to play an effective retrieving game while waiting for these opportunities is important. Too often, intermediate players become impatient and attempt to approach the net on shots that are not appropriate. These players often hit a shot from behind the baseline and then try to race to the net. Several potentially negative results can come out of such an approach:

- *From starting in such a defensive position, the attacking player usually will not be able to advance as close as desired. This will usually result in the player hitting a first volley from a much deeper position.*
- *Your opponent will have more time to move to cover the approach shot due to the shot coming from a deep position on your side.*
- *It is more difficult to hit a deep, penetrating shot effectively and consistently from such a deep position.*

In addition to these problems, typically a player will try to rush the net faster to make up for the distance he needs to travel. Thus, the player is not only often out of position, they are also usually out of balance when attempting to volley. Players who tend to rush headfirst to the net with minimal balance and a late, or a non-existent split-step, often are passed with even the slowest of passing shots.

Anytime a player approaches the net, your opponent can attempt four possible shots:

1) *Pass you down-the-line*
2) *Pass you crosscourt*
3) *Hit it right at you*
4) *Lob*

Your ability to limit the effectiveness or opportunity for any of these shots to be accomplished by an opponent will offer greater opportunities for you, the attacker, to finish each point off with a relatively easy winner.

WHERE TO HIT THE APPROACH SHOT

Geometrically, down-the-line approach shots offer the best offensive potential for the attacker and the least opportunity for the defensive player to pass. However, with understanding, both crosscourt and down-the-middle approach shots can be effective alternatives under many circumstances.

Down-the-Line Approach

When a player gets a short ball, hitting this shot down-the-line as an approach shot is usually the primary choice. While down-the-line involves two problematic issues, (having less court to hit into and hitting over the higher part of the net), it offers several strategic advantages:

- *Hitting down-the-line takes away some of the angle that your opponent might use against you in attempting to pass.*

- *Hitting down-the-line allows the attacker to stay on the same side of the court as his approach shot, an advantage when covering the net.*
- *Down-the-line approaches tend to provide more opportunity to hit an open-court volley winner off of an opponent's attempted pass.*

By making your approach shot deep, low, and with a reasonable amount of pace, you limit your opponent's ability to execute any potential response with effectiveness. And, if your opponent has a weakness on groundstrokes, you certainly increase the probability that you will get an easy shot at the net to put your opponent away.

Crosscourt Approach

The greatest problem that exists if an approach shot is hit crosscourt is the opening your opponent has to hit their passing shot down the line. This is due to the attacker's general inability to cover the side of the court on which they approached. The most effective passing shots occur when the distance between the opponent's contact point on the pass and the point on the court behind the attacker is the shortest. Thus, down-the-line is the shortest line of flight that the ball needs to take to get past the net player. Going crosscourt on a pass has the ball traveling in the air longer before it reaches the net, giving the net player a fraction of time longer to react and reach the volley.

Attacking players must understand that there are also some advantages for your opponent in hitting a crosscourt passing shot. The first advantage is that the pass will travel near the middle point of the net…the lowest part of the net. Also, as a general rule, crosscourt shots are easier to hit under pressure than down-the-line. However, in order to hit an effective crosscourt passing shot, the opponent must hit with a considerable amount of topspin, because going crosscourt on the pass reduces the amount of depth in which the ball can land inside the court. (See Diagram #1 below.) A down-the-line pass has the entire length of the court in which the ball can land. (Of course, the down-the-line passing shot has less diagonal error room!) As an attacker, you must consider that your opponent has this option.

Down-the-middle Approach Shot

A third choice in hitting approach shots is simply hitting the ball down the middle of the court. This is not a bad strategy as it offers several advantages. First, approaching down the middle allows the attacker to hit the approach shot over the lower, center portion of the net. These extra inches can give an attacking player a little more error room and, perhaps, allow the player to hit a more powerful approach. Hitting down the middle often is usually a shot that is hit towards your opponent's body, as opposed to the side of the opponent. Many opponents will actually hit better when they are given the opportunity to move towards a ball as opposed to moving out of the way of one hit right at them. Perhaps the most important advantage to hitting down the middle is the reduction of possible angles afforded to one's opponent. Take a look at these two diagrams depicting possible angles that an opponent can pass. (Diagrams 1 & 2)

While approach shots down the middle have advantages, there are inherent disadvantages associated with this strategy as well. The two primary disadvantages are:

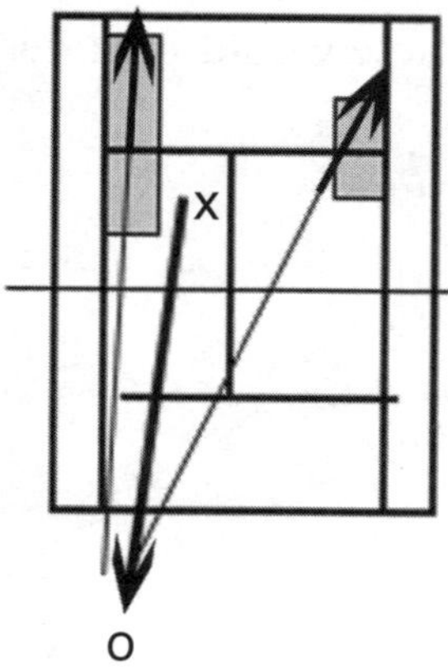

DIAGRAM 1

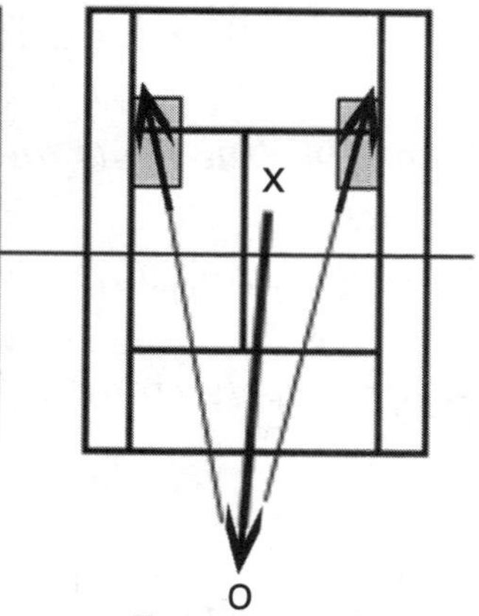

DIAGRAM 2

Approach Shots and Potential Passing Shots

Diagram 1: Approach Shot down the line: Attacker **X** hits down-the-line (▬▬▬) Potential passes (______) by opponent **O** are back down-the-line or crosscourt. The crosscourt response does offer error room over a lower part of the net, yet less court in which to land the shot (as depicted by the shaded boxes). The down-the-line pass provides a larger landing area but the passing shot must go over the higher part of the net.

Diagram 2: Approach shot down the middle: potential passing shots are over higher parts of the net and provide smaller court areas in which to pass.

1) that the attacking player has less open court in which to volley the subsequent potential winner and, 2) the attacking player has two equal halves of the net to cover for the potential passing shot. The latter issue makes anticipation a bit more difficult. Approaching down-the-line (and even crosscourt) moves the opponent to one side of the court in chasing down the approach shot. This opens the court up for a potential winning volley—provided that the attacking player is able to get to the volley and then execute it successfully!

As you can tell, there are many possible scenarios for both the attacking player as well as the defensive player. As you gain experience, you will learn what shots work best for you and what works well against a variety of opponents. It is important to know what options are available to your opponent so that you won't just be guessing while at the net.

"MAKING" YOUR OPPONENT HIT A SPECIFIC SHOT

Advanced players can improve the likelihood of knowing what shots their opponent will hit after an approach shot. By favoring one side of the court slightly, your opponent will sense an opening which they can exploit. However, if you know this, (especially because you intentionally left a little opening for your opponent), you can anticipate the shot hit and "poach" to the part of the court you left open.

By possessing certain strengths or weapons, you can also eliminate options your opponent might consider. For example, if you have demonstrated early in the match (or through reputation) that you possess a killer overhead, then your opponent might not elect to ever give you a lob. Players who have great mobility and solid overheads can play closer to the net in anticipation of one of the passing shots their opponent might choose instead of lobbing. By being able to play closer to the net, the attacking player can cut off potential passes with less distance to cover.

Retrieving Strategies against Attacking Strategies

Obviously, if you review the attacking strategies just covered, you can readily see your options as a retrieving player when playing against such an attacking style. The options the attacking player has while at the net are designed to counter some of the options a retrieving player has to defend such an attack. The best advice to offer a retrieving player is to make sure you have all the defending shots. These would include:

- *Being able to hit low, topspin, down-the-line shots on both the backhand and forehand sides*
- *Being able to hit topspin, sharp-angle crosscourt passing shots*
- *Being able to lob effectively, both offensively (topspin) and defensively (slice or block)*
- *Being able to hit hard shots right at a net player*

Foot speed and anticipation are also items which defensive players need to work on to give themselves as much of an advantage as when playing attacking shots. Traditionally, retrieving players have always been relatively fast players. Some of the best retrievers in the game included Michael Chang, Bjorn Borg, Arantxa Sanchez-Vicario and Chris Evert; all possessed terrific foot speed and anticipation skills.

AGGRESSIVE RETRIEVER

A style of retrieving that has become notable in recent years is the aggressive retriever. These players possess more aggressive groundstrokes, yet don't necessarily attempt to attack the net even when opportunities are sometimes presented. Players who play this distinctive style of game include Andre Agassi and Monica Seles. These retrievers set up points by pressuring opponents from the baseline with angles and depth, opening up the court and waiting for the opportunity to take advantage of such openings with powerful topspin groundstroke winners.

ALL-COURT PLAYERS

Today's modern game seems to be moving towards players who favor an "all-court" strategy of play. These players have all the shots; attacking groundstrokes, effective approach shots, spectacular overheads, touch and finesse, and lightning-quick finishing volleys. Players who have executed such strategies include Pete Sampras, Roger Federer, Andy Roddick and Taylor Dent on the men's tour. Many women are also adopting this all-court strategy with great success. They include Venus and Serena Williams, Martina Hingis, Kim Clijsters and Justine Henin-Hardenne.

Advanced Singles Strategies

Players who have mastered all shots have some additional playing strategies they should consider. When a player can hit any shot from anywhere on the court and direct that shot anywhere desired, then they have even more options to employ.

DELAYED ENTRY

John McEnroe mastered this strategy in winning many of his championships in the 1970's and 1980's.

Delayed entry or delayed approach is exactly that: coming to the net later than an intentional approach shot. It can be described as an unexpected approach shot.

When a player takes a short ball and comes to the net, the opponent knows exactly what is happening. He knows he is going to have to execute a passing shot or a lob. This affords a defensive opponent a bit of an advanced warning as to what he is going to do with this shot.

However, if a player hits a reasonable groundstroke crosscourt, the opponent is seldom expecting his opponent to follow that shot to the net. Typically, the opponent is just thinking of lofting a deep groundstroke back into the court off of such a casual shot. Certainly, for the attacking player coming in, such a non-threatening shot can be far less difficult than defending an intentional passing shot. The difficulty is getting to the net without the opponent having time to renegotiate their shot to take into account the player coming to the net. This is when the delayed entry is handy.

If you have mastered the volley from all parts of the court, especially being able to hit deep volleys from the middle part of your court, you can then experiment with this delayed entry strategy.

The idea is to hit a normal groundstroke, usually crosscourt, and usually deep. While your opponent is moving back to retrieve this deep shot, you quietly move into the middle of no-man's land, the area between the service line and the baseline, favoring the side of the court to which you hit your groundstroke. This movement should be done just as your opponent has begun his backswing. At this point, few opponents can accurately make a significant change in their swing.

Make a split-step in this no-man's land point and then move to intercept your opponent's shot. You should have a fairly easy ball (since your opponent is not attempting to pass you), and you should have a fair amount of open court in which to hit an offensive volley. (This is because your opponent will not have as much time to react to you now volleying the ball instead of waiting for another groundstroke.) Considering that you are coming in on a ball at mid court, usually taken out of the air, you create less time for your opponent to cover your volley.

DROP SHOT APPROACH

This strategy depends on a player's ability to deliver an effective drop shot and then have good volley skills for a quick volley.

The Drop Shot Approach is hit essentially as you would when having a short ball where you would normally hit a deep, attacking approach shot. Typically, opponents will be anticipating a deep, offensive approach shot when they hit a short shot. This moment of anticipation creates the opportunity to hit the opposite, a drop shot. If the drop shot is done well, the opponent will be in trouble from the start. They will need to quickly move towards the net and end up having to hit up, in most cases, once they get to the ball. The problem for many players who hit good drop shots is that they end up staying back and watching their opponent try and get the drop. This gives the opponent pretty much the whole court in which to push the ball up and over the net.

However, if the player who hit the drop shot moves into the net, the opponent will have to try and maneuver the ball in such a way that they won't hit the ball to their opponent now up at the net. This requires a much more skilled shot. So, right off the bat, by coming into the net following a drop shot, you force your opponent to hit a more difficult and lower percentage shot than if you had just stayed back.

Also, by coming to the net, you will be in position to hit virtually any shot into the open court. (Since your opponent has had to come to the net to retrieve your drop shot, you have over 95% of the court left open behind and to the side of your opponent.)

It is important to approach the net following your drop shot on the side of the court nearest your drop shot. Force your opponent to try and hit crosscourt. All you will have to do is block any shot he hits into the open court.

I sometimes call this a "hard-easy" shot. This is because sometimes you will have to make a quick reaction or have to really reach to get the volley from your opponent who is trying to take your drop shot and do something with it. (That's the hard part!) However, if you can simply hold your racket firm and not swing, it is a relatively easy shot to hit as a winner since you have so much open court.

FUDGING

If you watch the pros play singles, you will often see a player hit a crosscourt backhand and not return to the middle of the court. They will often stay off-center, favoring their backhand side. This is called "fudging," and it is done for several reasons:

- *They are baiting their opponent to hit-down-the line, a lower percentage shot.*
- *They are baiting their opponent to hit to their forehand (down-the-line).*
- *If their opponent hits the ball crosscourt, the player can hit a forehand inside-out, a simple crosscourt backhand, or a potential winner down the line with an "inside-in" forehand.*

This is a fairly recent strategy, probably because players have begun hitting such offensive inside-out forehands.

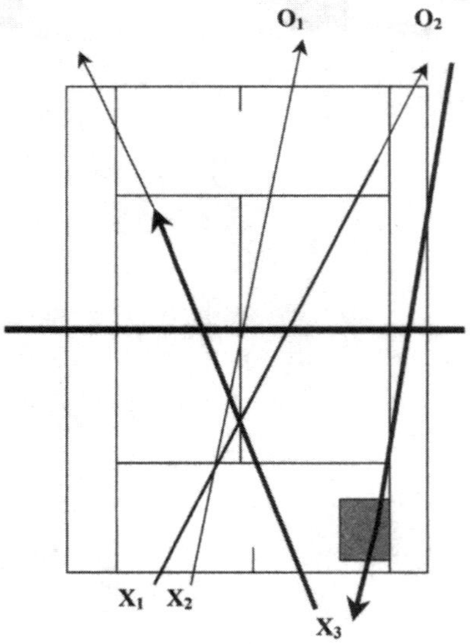

FUDGING

If X_2 hits too much down the middle, he must stay more towards the middle of his court. However if X1 hits a significant angle crosscourt, he can fudge over to his left. The reason is that in order for O_2 to hit down the line from such an angle, he has a very tiny landing zone in which to hit a good shot. (Shaded Box) Even if O2 hits a decent down-the-line shot, the ball will be moving towards the middle of X's court. This will not only make it fairly easy for X to run down, but also provides for a good angle crosscourt in which X_3 can hit for a winner or, at the very least, an offensive shot.

Game Plans

Game plans utilize specific strategies against specific opponents. Virtually every player has some elements that could be considered strengths and others that would be considered weaknesses. It is the well-rounded player who can vary his game plan to attack an opponent's weakness. Where strategies are generally match characteristics, game plans usually evolve during a match by each player.

If you were playing a person who has a terrible backhand with minimal control and consistency, your game plan would be to simply exploit the backhand. Tennis champions study opponents when possible and define a game plan to attack such weaknesses. The following are examples of game plans designed to work against a variety of opponent's strategies.

AGAINST THE MOONBALLER/DINKER:

Players who like to stay back and rally until the end of time usually dislike being at the net. If you don't want to stay out and push balls back and forth, you must take this player out of their comfort zone. Drop shots are most effective against such players. These drop shots don't always have to be perfect. Just bringing a player to the net and either making them run back to the baseline or hit an overhead or volley can be enough. One of my favorite plays against such a player is to hit a drop shot and come to the net myself. Any decent drop shot will force your opponent to hit up to you when they get to the ball. Drop shots hit to the side of the court will open up your opponent's court for a fairly easy winner.

AGAINST POWER PLAYERS

Let the big hitters hit their winners. Unless these players are really on their game, they will have more errors than winners. Furthermore, if you can shorten your strokes and either block or slice such hard hit balls back a few times in every rally, the power hitters will eventually miss. Drop shots again work well against such players as do hitting slower paced balls deep into their court.

AGAINST PLAYERS WHO HAVE A SINGLE STRONG SIDE. (SUCH AS A GREAT FOREHAND OR BACKHAND.)

While common sense would tell you to keep the ball away from such a shot, there are many times that you will want to hit the ball specifically to a player's weapon. For example, if a player has a great forehand, in order to get the ball to their backhand you will need to open up the backhand side of their court. Getting first serves out wide to their forehand can open up an opponent's backhand. When players only try to get the ball to the weakness, such players are often camping out on that side of the court, making it more difficult to squeeze the ball into the court on that side. When this happens, you will have to work the ball out wide to their strength and hope to get a ball that is playable to their weakness.

AGAINST STRONG WESTERN-GRIP FOREHAND PLAYERS

The western or semi-western grip has become the preferred grip among many top-level players. The western grips provide greater topspin and potential power from the baseline. However, they also have an Achilles heel. Western grips don't do well on low balls. It is very hard to get the racket open enough on low balls with the western grips to lift topspin shots over the net. This has created the need for players to reinvent an historical classic shot: the slice. An excellent strategy against western grip players is to take balls hit by your opponent that are near the middle portion of your court and hit a hard, slice backhand towards your opponent's forehand corner. This ball will do two things: a) the ball will tend to curve out away from the center of your opponent's court and b) the ball will stay very low off the bounce. These two effects make it difficult for players who favor western grips to hit an offensive shot. Players can follow such a slice towards the net and hope for an easy volley, or they can stay back and expect a short ball to attack with the next shot. The harder the ball is sliced, the more the ball will stay low and fade away from the opponent. (Please see Chapter 9 on the backhand for more on the slice backhand.)

Conclusion

Simply put, Singles Strategies can run the gamut of possibilities. Depending on a player's personality, strengths and weaknesses, and stroke preferences, any number of strategies can be favored. Certainly, the ability to change strategies based on our opponent's strengths and weaknesses is a blessing to all players. Most current top players possess the ability to effectively change their particular game plan in relative increments to counter their opponent's game. However, it is often advisable to stay within strategies with which you are most comfortable and confident. Play to make those strategies work against every possible opponent. Certainly, many strategies have become hallmarks for individuals and have often become the strategies which others have come to emulate. My best advice to you is to watch as much professional tennis as possible, pick players who you feel play a style and strategy which you imagine yourself playing. Then, imitate these players as best you can within a strategy that exemplifies your own personality, strengths and weaknesses.

Finally, there are numerous books written on singles strategies. These go into great detail of "what if's" and general singles theory. I could not begin to address all of the circumstantial shot selections that could occur in any given match. As one can imagine, as the quality of play increases, the dynamics of circumstantial strategies change. In this chapter I have offered the two main types of singles strategies as an overview. As you play more singles, you will learn that many atypical nuances—those that are NOT covered in these books mentioned can and will occur! By following the foundation of singles play described in this book, you will have a good understanding of how to deal with most of these occurrences with effective responses.

CHAPTER 15

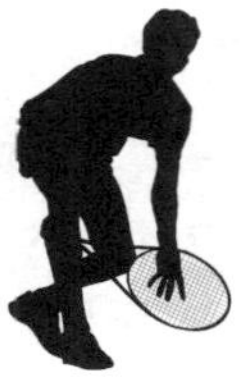

Doubles Strategies within the Advanced Foundation

Introduction to Doubles Strategies

Amazingly, even though more than 80% of the general tennis-playing public in the United States plays mainly doubles, over 90% of televised tennis is singles play! It is no wonder that a vast majority of amateur players don't play doubles nearly as well as they could or should! Seldom do these players get a chance to see high-level doubles in action. Yet, good doubles play is extraordinarily dependent on key strategies, and, sometimes dependent on specific player positions and movements decided by events that frequently change during a rapid exchange of shots.

The central strategy in doubles is quite simple, however: hit shots that your opponents can't return. Or, even more simply stated, "make em' miss!"

However, similar to singles play, as a player develops shots and strokes that are more deliberate, consistent, effective, and diversified, the strategies of doubles play becomes more defined and complex. Unlike singles, where just getting the ball over the net can be sufficient to beat a multitude of players, in doubles such a strategy can often be fatal! With a net man located just steps off the net, a shot in singles that would normally be a safe, routine shot can be rejected with authority by a doubles net player.

Often, players who possess less dominant stroke mechanics can still be dominant in doubles against players possessing much more refined strokes. This is usually a result of such players acquiring experience and knowledge in these key doubles strategies. Thus, it is paramount for players to learn not only an advanced stroke foundation as presented in this book, but they should also learn strategies associated with playing effective doubles.

There are many nuances and strategies related to good doubles play that I will address in short segments I call "Doubles Rationale." These will help introduce "exceptions to the rules" or advantageous situations that might not follow the basic advanced foundation described. In addition, I will address the most common faults, positioning errors, and poor shot selections that the vast majority of players execute while playing doubles.

Doubles Foundation

Like developing strokes where learning proper grips and footwork leads to developing proper swing mechanics, advanced doubles play has a foundation based on player positions, movements, and, of course, proper stroke execution. In fact, the issue of player positions alone (or lack of knowing just what this entails!) is one of the factors distinguishing a typical 3.0 level player from a 4.0. Again, as we have mentioned, player progression is not necessarily dependent on player athleticism, desire, or even playing opportunities. It is, however, very dependent on the quality of information available to the player.

This is such an important topic that there are entire books dedicated to doubles play. I recommend that you check out the reference pages at the end of this book and look for several of these texts dedicated to the fine art of doubles play. In the meantime, enjoy this in-depth discussion on the "Advanced Foundation" of doubles play. Your study from this resource alone will be sufficient for you to gain advanced doubles play.

Doubles Positions

There are very distinct positions for every player in doubles. Each position has specific objectives—both defensively and offensively—based on a multitude of doubles situations. Understanding these positions and their corresponding intentions will be a major step in your progression as a doubles player.

It has amazed me in nearly three decades of teaching tennis that so many people don't have a clue as to where they should be positioned prior to the serve nor where they should correspondingly be at various junctures during a rally. Time and time again, players will lose points, not necessarily due to stroke mistakes or weak shots, but simply because they didn't know where they should have been positioned during a particular point. Likewise, players often give up excellent opportunities to end points with easy shots because they again weren't in the right position. And inevitably, players will often lose points they should have won because they hit the ball beautifully, but they hit it in the wrong direction based on proper doubles strategies!

As you can see, all three of these scenarios are not necessarily dependent on shot-making abilities, only on the knowledge (or lack of knowledge) of player positions or the directions of where certain balls should be hit.

PLAYER POSITIONS PRIOR TO THE SERVE

There is no excuse for not standing in the right place prior to the serve—nothing is happening to force you to make a quick position change! Obviously, you know exactly what is going to happen…a serve will be made with an attempt to land the ball in the service box. Certainly, we don't know if the serve is going to be fast or slow, deep or short, flat or with spin, or to the receiver's forehand or backhand. Because we don't know the efficacy of the serve, this is one of the reasons we have specific positions for each player prior to the serve.

Offensive Team: The Serving Team

I don't care how good or bad your serve is, you are the offensive team when your team is serving. The reason for this statement is simple: the serving team knows the serve can't be poached or attacked by the net player on the receiving team. Unlike any doubles rally where the ball is hit back to our partner, we know the net person can't attack the ball coming from our partner on the serve. This is why the net person of the serving team plays up at the net and the partner of the returning player plays a defensive position on the service line instead of closer to the net. Because the returning player's partner does not know for sure just what kind of return will be made (nor does he know if the serving team's net person will be poaching), he or she MUST be in a defensive position when their partner is returning serve.Please see the two diagrams below.

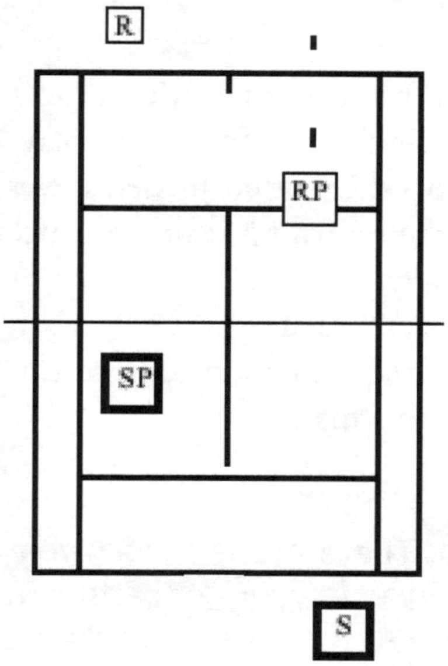

Positions when serving to the deuce court

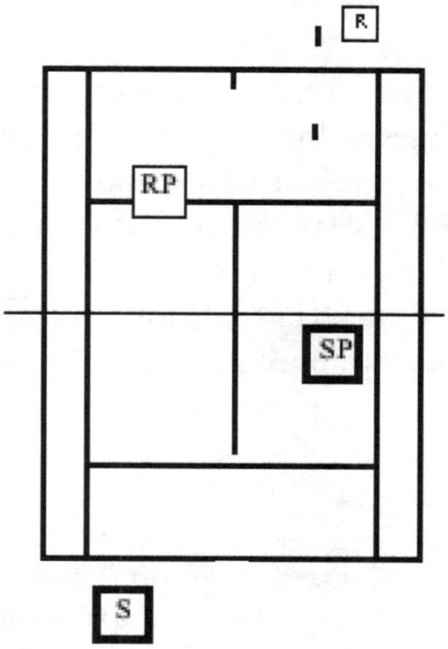

Positions when serving the ad court

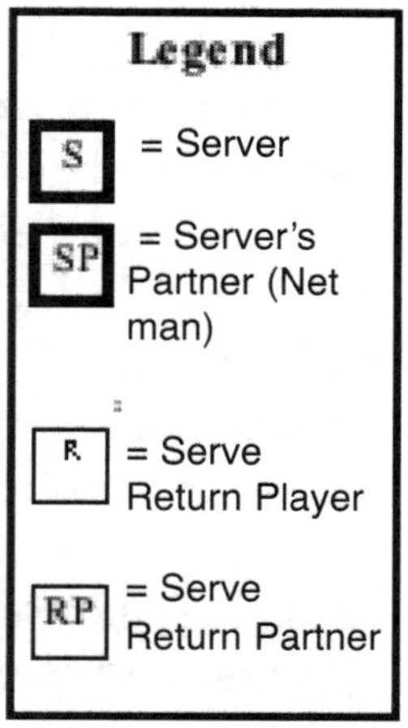

THERE ARE VERY SPECIFIC REASONS AND RATIONALE FOR EACH OF THESE PLAYERS'S POSITIONS AS THEY RELATE TO DOUBLES PLAY.

SERVER S

The server in doubles has the primary role of getting the serve in. Obviously, if the server can't get the ball in play, all the players might as well sit down on the bench during the serve and have some refreshments! (Please refer back to Chapter 11 on the Serve for this lesson!) In this section on doubles play, we are going to assume that the serve will land in the correct service box. However, depending on the quality of the serve—among other things—each player's subsequent role and position will change dramatically. We will address these various changes as we address each player's position during a point.

Notice the server is serving from near the alley. This position can be manipulated in terms of various serving locales along the baseline. The rules allow the server to stand anywhere between the center service mark (the small line located at the center point of the base line) and the imaginary extension of the doubles sideline. Certainly, players will create subtle service variances by adjusting this position for different serves.

Doubles Rationale
By standing out further near the doubles sideline for the serve, the server creates greater angular opportunity for his or her serve. However, advanced players must understand that this same severe angle on the serve creates equally severe angle-opportunities for the serve return player. Logically, servers will want to be ready to cover such a return if they serve out wide.

More important than possessing power, the server should be concerned with attacking any known weaknesses by the returning player on their first serve. Too often, players attempt a big ace on their first serve and then have to follow these often-missed serves with a weaker, defensive serve. Such ineffectual serves give the returning team a chance to become the attacking team. Instead, servers should generally try to serve to a player's weakness, (usually the backhand side for most beginner to intermediate players, or right into the body of more advanced players). This gives the server's partner a chance to utilize his or her offensive position at the net in a more productive manner.

Doubles Rationale
The first serve is a critical aspect in successful doubles. There are two main reasons for this. First of all, by getting the first serve in, you involve your net partner in a much more offensive role. Second serves that are weaker than a first serve set up a defensive mentality for net partners. Returning players can tee-off on such weak second serves hitting shots that are often aimed right at the net man.
Second, a second serve provides a bit more confidence for the returning player. The returning team knows that either the serve will be in or they simply win the point on the double fault. On first serves, there is a sense of uncertainty for the returning player: "Will it be this one or the next one?" Psychologically, the first serve landing in can be more effective than having an equally effective second serve.

We will address the role of the server and what happens after the serve is in play later when we begin to discuss positions dependent upon situations during a point.

SERVING PARTNER SP "THE NET MAN"

The net man is positioned at the net for very specific reasons. First and foremost, the net man is in a position of offense since the opponent's net person can't intercept the serve. As a net man, we KNOW the ball is going to be returned by the back person (the returning player) on the other team. Depending on the quality of the serve, the net man is either going to intercept the return (on an effective serve) or protect his alley and himself if the serve is very weak (and if the opponent's are very good!).

Where to stand specifically at the net is also dependent on the quality of the server as well as the intentions of the net person themselves. Here are some scenarios to consider based on possible positions of the net man.

1) NET MAN PLAYS CLOSER TO THE ALLEY. (USUALLY ABOUT A STEP FROM THE SINGLES SIDE LINE)

1st Rationale: If the serve is consistently weak, the net player might want to protect the alley more consciously. For the returning player going down the line, his option may appear more difficult (due to the net man being closer to the ally) forcing him to hit crosscourt.

2nd Rationale: Among more advanced players, by visually making the return down the line look less advantageous (by standing closer to the alley), the net man can focus more on poaching and anticipating the crosscourt return. As I will mention again later; if the net man stands more towards the middle of the court, then the returning player will have the opportunity to take advantage of a larger opening down-the-line. By offering two distinct options for the returning player to hit to, the net person is literally frozen. They usually have to protect the alley so much that even close balls returned crosscourt, within normal reach of the net person, are not attempted by them. They can't react to such a shot due to their protection of the potential down-the-alley shot.

3rd Rationale: Some instructors believe that standing more towards the middle of the court makes the returning player's crosscourt return more difficult. While this is true by a marginal measure, there are a couple of reasons why this rationale has faults. First of all, standing a couple of steps towards the middle doesn't produce a substantial fear in the mind of most returning players. There is still a considerable amount of space afforded to the returning player due to the space the alley adds to the court when hitting crosscourt. Most intermediate to advanced players will have no trouble hitting returns away from the net player who is playing a step or two closer to the middle. Likewise, due to the greater possibility of the returning player hitting down the line, a net player who takes such a position will again be frozen in trying to anticipate just what shot the returning player might hit.

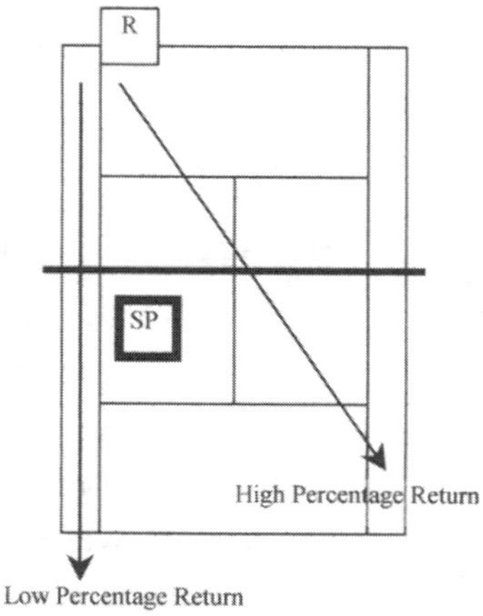

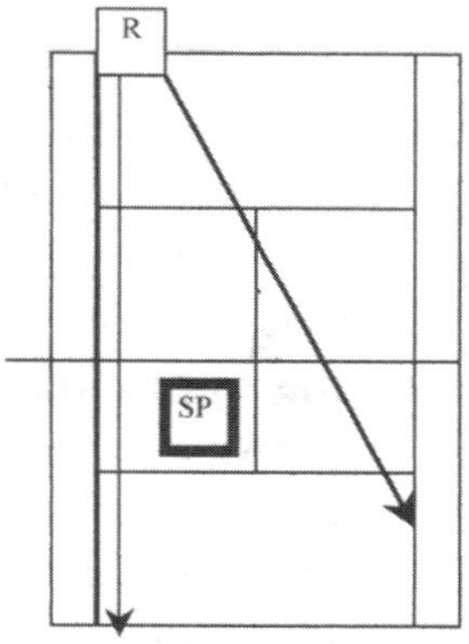

DIAGRAM 1

By the net man setting up more towards the middle, the return player has two options—Down-the-line and Crosscourt. The net man will now have to protect his own alley limiting his chance to poach the return.

2) NET PLAYER STANDING MORE TOWARDS THE CENTER

1st Rationale: As I have mentioned, there are disadvantages to this position for the net player. However, there is one exception to this logic. That is, if a net person is actually "baiting" the returning player to hit down-the-alley, then the net player would want to stand more towards the center of the court. The actual down-the-line return of serve is a relatively a low percentage shot. Not only is there only a small space between the net player and the doubles side line for which to aim, but this return has to cross the net at the highest part of the net! I teach players to occasionally stand more towards the center of the court when playing the net with this one strategy in mind: I call the strategy a "reverse poach". The idea is to bait the returning player into thinking that the down-the-alley shot is open enough to try. Just as the returning player looks down to make contact on the return, the net person starts to poach back towards the alley in anticipation of the very down-the-alley shot they baited. Since a normal poach usually has the player moving towards the middle or their partner's side of the net to intercept a ball, this poach has the net player literally moving back to the alley. Hence the name "reverse poach."

3) Net player playing very close to the net

1st Rationale: Certainly this position can be intimidating to some beginner or even intermediate return-of-serve players. Often, returning players become so conscious of the net player they literally hit the ball right to them as opposed to hitting the open parts of the court rendered by such a position. I don't recommend this position to most net players, however. By playing so close to the net, you invite your opponent to lob you. With such a large open area to hit the lob, most good players will have no trouble hitting an effective, offensive lob. Yet, on the other hand, this can be a terrific strategy in certain circumstances. First, if you have a great overhead, you will have a way to force the lob. If you are quick with your hands and feet, you can cover most lobs since these are slow moving shots. The problem arises when beginners and intermediate players try to play close to the net. Their first reaction to a lob is to look up. Instead of immediately turning and reacting with his or her racket and feet, the player watching the ball rise wastes too much time to get back and under the ball for the overhead.

Another problem with this close-in net position occurs when players have inferior volley skills. Usually, players who use an Eastern forehand/backhand grip for their volleys can't change grips in time to react to a quick shot at the body. In fact, I usually recommend to players who are playing against opponents using Eastern grips at the net to simply hit the ball at the net man (aiming for the backhand side of the net man near his body). More times than not, the net player will react with the wrong grip and hit the ball a mile out or into the bottom of the net.

4) Net player playing back, deeper off the net

1st Rationale: Playing back off the net provides many players a sense of time when playing the net. And this is true. Players DO have relatively more time to react to balls. Older players often like to play several steps back from the "normal" net position for this very reason.

2nd Rationale: This position allows a player to cover lobs more easily since they are already slightly back in relation to other net positions. This can be a great strategy when playing opponents who like to lob often. Whenever you limit your opponent's options, you can more effectively anticipate the options that are left to them. In this case, if you take away the lob, you can poach a bit more aggressively towards the open, crosscourt return.

Poaching

The idea of poaching (anticipating a shot by your opponents to the open part of your court and moving to intercept this anticipated shot just prior to or during your opponent's swing) is usually an advanced strategy. Confidence in poaching is usually accomplished more through playing experience than through practice. However, players can improve their poaching abilities through game-situation drills. The most important part of poaching is recognition of what shots are most likely going to be hit by your opponent. If they can identify when their opponent is in trouble or has only certain shot options, aggressive players can start to move to these places even before the opponents have made contact with their shot.

Beginners must first recognize that it is perfectly OK to move to your partner's side of the court if, by doing so, you can make a better shot than your partner due to your position. Too often, beginners feel it is "rude" or poor partnership to invade their partner's side of the court! There is nothing rude or un-sportsmanlike in poaching! (Sometimes when one player simply "hogs" the court, it can be not only detrimental to effective doubles play, but socially inappropriate as well.)

There are times when a player should poach. If I am a net player, and either my partner or myself have hit a truly effective shot creating trouble for our opponents, I should realize that a weak shot is forthcoming. I can assume that if my opponents are indeed in trouble, they a) are not going to hit a very offensive shot, and b) they probably are going to try to avoid hitting the ball to the net man. In both these cases, as the net person, I should be ready to intercept ANY ball that is hit by this opponent who is in trouble! If my partner has hit a great serve, any return should be considered mine under the same logic.

There are other situations when poaching should be considered. I will address these when we talk about other positions and situations in doubles points.

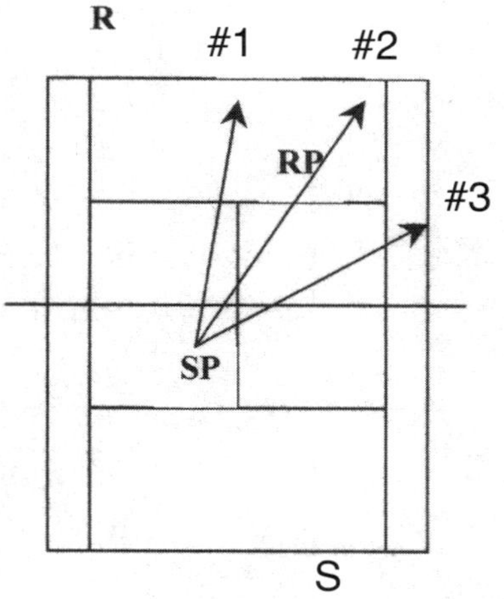

DIAGRAM 2

The Server's Partner (SP-the "Net Player") has three options on a high volley:
#1 Down the middle;
#2 Through the Net Player (RP)
#3 Wide of the Net Player

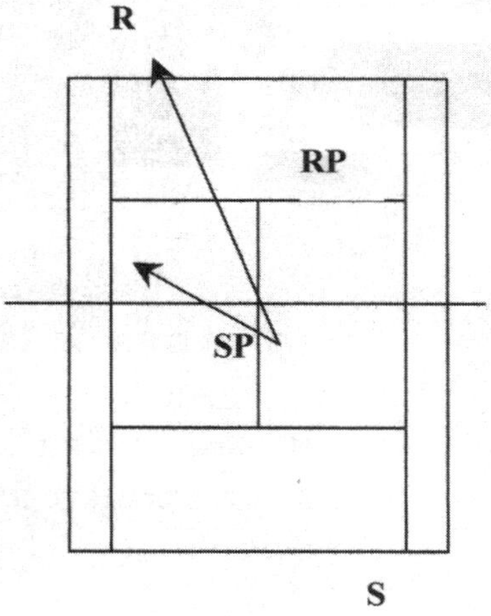

DIAGRAM 3

Poaching on a low return
The Server's Partner (SP) poaches on the return. However, the return is hit soft and low. SP can take this soft ball and angle volley off a winner from such a ball.

WHERE SHOULD THE POACHED VOLLEY GO?

One of the most misunderstood concepts in poaching is where to hit the ball once you have anticipated an easy volley. Too often, the poaching player (or any net player who receives a volley) doesn't choose the best option with the ball. There are three main responses when a player gets a ball close to the net. These responses are based on the ball's position at contact when the person volleying the ball is near the net.

1. A reachable high volley poach: This ball should be hit THROUGH the net man's feet. (See Diagram 2, #2) Too often, in playing against teams who play one up and one back, the player who gets an easy volley will hit the ball more down the middle instead of through the net man. (Diagram 2 #1) A ball down the middle is usually easy for the back player to return. So, instead of winning an easy point with the put-away, the team that had the easy volley may have to run down a lob or another volley depending on what the back player on the other side can do with the ball. Often, a player will try to avoid the opposing net man and try to hit the ball towards the outside angle of the opponent. (Diagram 2, #3) This is the smallest part of the court in which to hit a ball. By trying to hit to this small area, the player with the high volley can often make a small mistake in aiming and end up hitting the ball wide. Hitting a high ball through the opposing net player is the highest percentage shot for winning the point.

Quite often, I hear players say, "I didn't want to hit my opponent." Some social matches and perhaps mixed doubles, a player who is skilled at hitting the volley should try not to blast the ball through the opposing net player when offered such a sitting duck. Most players can hit slightly away from the net player reducing the risk of actually hitting the player with the volley. However, most experienced competitive players know that this IS the proper shot (hitting through the net player) and most net players will acknowledge this shot with a "Nice Shot" response, even if they get hit.

2. A reachable soft low volley poach: In this case, because the player will have to hit the volley up in order to clear the net, it is definitely not advisable for the net player to hit this low volley up towards the opposing net man! If we hit up on the ball to get it over the net, chances are it will still be going up to some degree as it gets to the opposing net man. If you want to have the ball slammed down your throat, hit your low volleys to the net man!

Low volleys can be hit offensively, however. If, while poaching, the ball ends up too low to drive through the net man, you can angle the ball off to the opposite side of the court with a very short drop volley. (See Diagram 3) This shot is usually only possible when players learn to volley correctly using the continental grip. (Please refer to Chapter 7 on "Advanced Volley Techniques" for more information on this concept.)

3. A harder-hit, low, reachable poach: Sometimes, even when your partner has hit a solid serve or deep return, your opponent might get an offensively hit, low ball crosscourt. In many cases, this ball is just too low to try to go through the opposing net player. Also, it is hit too hard to try a soft, crosscourt angle volley. In this case, it is time to play percentage and conservative tennis! Instead of trying to force a winner off such a return, you will be far more successful in simply returning the ball back to the deep player and hope you get a better opportunity to hit an offensive volley. (Diagram 3)

RETURNING PLAYER R

The player returning the serve has the primary responsibility to return the serve safely and if, possible, effectively (away from the net person on the serving team). The position of the returning player is dictated by two general factors: where the server is standing when serving and the level or ability of the server to deliver an effective serve.

When a server moves out wide to serve (near the singles or doubles sideline), the returning player must respect the potential angle with which the server can take advantage and move out wider himself. (See Diagram 4) Likewise, if the server moves more near the center of the baseline to serve, the returning player should move more towards the center of his baseline. So often, intermediate players don't recognize the geometric angles offered to servers by their position. A simple slice serve can ace an unsuspecting returning player.

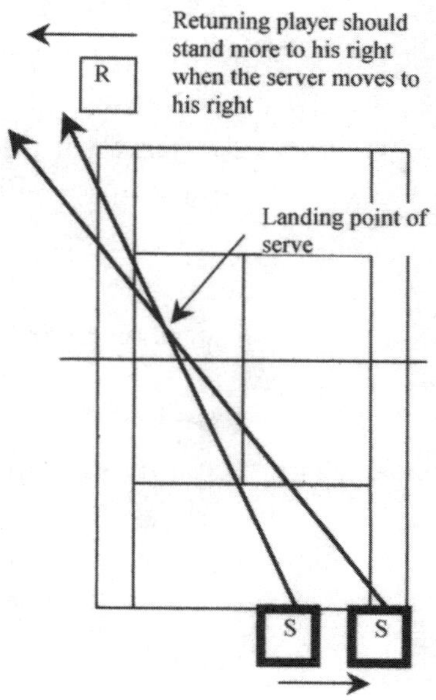

DIAGRAM 4
When the Server moves out closer to the doubles sideline to serve, the angle of a serve moving away from the Returning player is increased.

Returning Options

There are four main options that the returning player can consider:

- *Crosscourt*
- *Down-the-line*
- *Lob*
- *Drop shot crosscourt*

Understanding all the possible positions and related responses by the net man as described earlier in this chapter can help the returning player make decisions on which shots will be most effective. Obviously, playing experience—where trial and error will provide clues to the "when and where" of trying specific shots—is essential. However, if a player is not aware of options and possible results, then simply playing doubles will not necessarily lead to successful or skilled play. By knowing what is possible during points, acknowledging and recognizing how mistakes and good shots were possible, a player will enhance his or her ability to progress, and a player will learn to play better doubles.

Each of the possible responses made by the returning player has variation and ramifications. I will cover each of these briefly.

CROSSCOURT

The standard service return is crosscourt. Unless the net player on the serving team is poaching, the crosscourt return is the safest choice. (Even if the net player is poaching, a good low return will be difficult to handle.)

One additional responsibility for the returning player is regarding line calls on the serve The returning player has the best view of the ball when it lands near the sidelines of the service box. Therefore, it is this player's responsibility to call the serve wide if indeed the serve is wide. Often, players assume that it is the returning player's partner who should make this call. This is not correct. The defensive net player of the returning partner can not make an accurate call on balls that land near the center service line. Because the ball itself hides the inside portion of the court between the ball and the line, the partner of the returning player cannot accurately call this ball in or out. Because the returning player views the ball as it approaches, he or she can much more accurately see if the ball bounced wide, in, or on the line on the serve. However, the returning player's partner has the responsibility to call serves "out" that land long.

Down-the-line

The down-the-line shot can be a weapon or sheer suicide in different tennis matches. Namely, if a returning player feels the net man may be poaching, down-the-line on the serve (or during any rally), this can be a great shot. However, many players when hitting down the line overhit the ball, trying for too low of a percentage shot.

I do recommend early in every match for the returning player to hit specifically at least one ball down-the-line. This is to let the opposing net player know that the returning player can—and will—hit down-the-line at some point!

Lob

The lob off the return is often a very good shot. The best time to lob is if the server is right-handed and is serving to the deuce court. This lob, down-the-line, will be to the server's backhand when they run to cover this lob. One of the hardest shots for many intermediate players is in hitting an effective backhand shot off a higher bouncing ball, such as that from a lob.

Drop shot crosscourt

When playing teams that don't follow the serve to the net, a drop shot crosscourt is a great offensive shot. Since these players don't like to come to the net anyway, you can take them out of their comfort zone by hitting a decent drop shot. Also, if you play a team that hits lobs all day long, then bringing them to the net with a good drop will force them to hit something other than a lob! (Make sure to come in to the net following an effective drop shot! You will usually be rewarded with a fairly easy volley when you do!)

RETURNING TEAM'S NET PLAYER RP

The Defensive Net man

The partner of the returning player, the "defensive net man" must understand many concepts related to this position. There is basically only one place for this player to stand prior to the serve. (At the advanced levels, there are some strategic exceptions to this rule that I will discuss later.) The most advantageous position in which to stand is on the service line about midway between the singles sideline and the center service line. Though there are minimal options for this player to consider regarding position, this player must know and perform several specific tasks.

Initial Responsibilities and Actions for the Defensive Net Man

1. **Line calls**: This player is in the best position to make calls on serves as they relate to balls that land outside the service line. As mentioned, the return-of-serve player has responsibility for calling the sidelines on the serve. However, his partner, the defensive net man, has responsibility for calling serves "out" that land long of the service line.

2. **Focal Attention**: Immediately following a successful serve, the defensive net man's attention must be directed towards the serving team's net man. This is the only person that can literally hurt the receiving team immediately following the serve… especially if the serve is an effective one. Obviously, from what we have already discussed, the

serving team's net man is going to be looking to attack any return possible, especially when the serve is potent. As mentioned, the net man on the serving team will attempt to hit almost all put-away volleys through the net man on the receiving team. It is of paramount importance that the returning team's net man is watching every move made by the serving team's net man. With this close observation many shots that might otherwise be winners by the serving team's net man, could be thwarted through the reactions and expectation of the defensive net man. All too often, the defensive net man will turn and watch his partner return the serve only to turn back towards the net just in time to see the net man crushing a volley right at him! Instead, by watching the net man on the other side, the defensive net man will have a better indication of what is going to happen.

What happens after the return?

The strategies used (and understood) here reveal some of the cognitive differences between 3.0 players and those who progress past this level.

Most 3.0 players stay back after the serve and the returns. Most 4.0 and above players attack the net at every opportunity.

Amazingly, by staying back, players create greater confusion and difficulty for their team. In addition, players who stay back create substantially different patterns of play for their net partners than those who follow their serves and returns to the net.

I will address both strategies, coming in and staying back, in the next two sections of this chapter. There are times when players will have to play back, even though they might be attacking-type players. Likewise, there will be times players will be drawn into the net and have to play there, even though that may not be their preferred style of play.

Defensive Doubles: One-up and one-back

This formation is notorious among 3.0 and 3.5 doubles players, especially with women's teams. The obvious reason is a lack of volley and overhead confidence among these players. If you are going to attack the net, you are going to either hit volleys or overheads when you get there! There are even times when attacking players are forced to retreat to this one-up, one-back position. This most often occurs when one team effectively lobs a net-attacking team. If the lob can't be hit as an overhead, then one player will have to cover the lob by retreating back. When this occurs, all the same rules of strategy apply to this team as they would when a team plays this stratagem intentionally.

When two teams play each other with this formation of one up and one back, the team that understands the concepts that I will be presenting will be the team that can still dominate, even from this position.

THE PATTERN

I call the strategy of one up and one back a pattern as doubles players must understand they each have very specific patterns of movement based on who is hitting and what shot has been hit. The net player of any up-and-back team has extraordinarily important positions to play.

Remember that the serving team is in an offensive attitude immediately when the serve lands in. That is because only the back, returning player may hit the ball. The serve is the one-and-only shot that can't ever be poached! Once a serve has been successfully returned crosscourt away from the net man, the returning team is now in an offensive position. Because of this immediate transition from offense to defense, the net player of many serving teams fails to ascertain this change in circumstance.

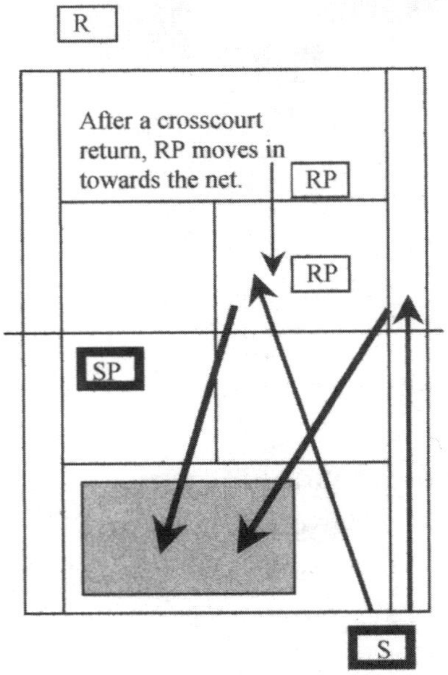

Diagram 5

After the return has been made crosscourt, if the net man of theserve fails to back up, there will be a large space for to hit an easy volley winner should RP get a chance to volley.

Role of the Serving Team's Net Man after the return. (Diagram 5)

Since the return has been made crosscourt, away from you, the net man, you now are on a momentary defensive mode. This transition to a defensive mode is because of two things:

1. *You don't know for sure what your partner will do with the ball. He may hit the ball intentionally, or otherwise, to the net man.*

2. *You don't know what the opposing team's net man will do. She may decide to poach on your partner's crosscourt shot.*

In either of these two situations, if you are still planted up close to the net as you were when your partner was serving, you are a sitting duck! In addition, by staying up close to the net, you leave a huge gap between you and your partner that would be big enough to drive a truck through! This gap makes for easy pickings if either of our two situations presented above happened. (Please see Diagram 5.)

As you can see, if the server S hits a ball either down-the-line or crosscourt within reach of the returning partner's net man RP the area in which this net player may hit the ball for a clean winner is substantial, (as represented by the shaded area).

In order to decrease this area, the net man SP must back up to cut off any easy potential volley to which the returning team's net man might have access. Certainly, if S hits a very poor shot right to RP then his partner SP may still have no chance of staying in the point. However, by simply rotating back to a defensive position (usually at the service line), SP will increase the difficulty for RP to have an outright winner (by his presence within this hitting area). As you become more advanced in your play, you will also increase your ability to react to these put-a-ways in such a manner that you end up volleying the ball to stay in the point longer.

There is a phrase in doubles that is very misleading. The phrase is "In doubles, always be moving forward." When one player stays back, this strategy makes that phrase inaccurate. Anytime a player must stay back to return a shot, his corresponding net man must retreat to this defensive position near the service line.

Now, if [S] hits a good crosscourt in response to the return, then his net man [SP] can move forward to resume an offensive position. In fact, there is plenty of time in which [SP] can move back into this forward, offensive position. This is because the ball will travel all the way back to the back player, giving the previously defensive player time to regain an offensive position.

Whenever a ball goes back to the back player, the net partner of that player MUST watch the opposing net player while assuming this defensive position. The actions of the offensive net player will reveal what is going to happen.

DOUBLES RATIONALE

When a ball is hit back to your partner who is staying back, you will be able to judge how defensive your stance needs to be. For example, if your opponents hit a very hard and deep shot to your partner, chances are he won't be making an offensive, controlled shot back. In this case, it is important to assume the worst and back up quickly and move perhaps even further back behind the service line to give yourself plenty of reaction time for a certain offensive shot by your opponent. Depending on the quality of your partner, you can often anticipate what they can or can't do with certain shots. This is why pros, when they are the returning net man of the returning player, are often seen standing closer than on the service line.

Obviously, this pattern of moving forward if your partner hits a good crosscourt, and moving back if the ball is hit past you back to your partner, is going to be repeated during a rally. (Hence the label "pattern" at the start of this section!) It is inevitable that one player is either going to eventually make a mistake and hit to the net player or the net player is going to go for the crosscourt shot and poach. In either case, the player that is prepared by moving back defensively as described in this section will still provide some chance of that team staying in the point.

COMMUNICATION

Between points, it is a good habit to chat with your partner. It can be discussing where the serve or return is going to be attempted, or if the net man will be poaching, or simply to pump each other up. (See Figure 1) This gives the team a chance to focus and to be clear on what to expect. Also, by talking, opponents will start imagining what the heck could be coming up!

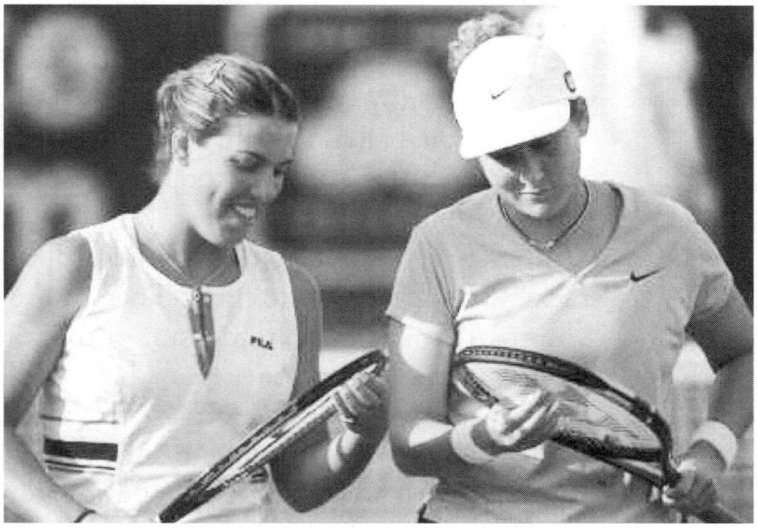

Figure 1
Between points, it is an excellent habit to talk to your partner. Discussing return or serve options, net play or just to pump each other up, talking is taking advantage of having a teammate.

Good Doubles

The ability to play doubles skillfully depends on several factors. The first of these is a good serve and return of serve. If either of these factors is weak, the team will be at a disadvantage right from the start. A good serve gives the serving team the offense right off. If a defensive return is made, either the net man or the server himself can move in and produce an offensive volley.

Having a good return of serve can negate the offensive position of the serving team and get the returning team in an offensive mode early in a point.

The next important skill is the volley. At high level doubles, some aspect of a volley almost always follows serves and returns. Such volleys can include high offensive volleys, low defensive volleys, half volleys and angle volleys. Limitations in any of these will again create problems throughout a match.

Finally, a good overhead is important. Being able to finish points off with overheads can send a powerful statement to any opponent. Inevitably, a doubles team will play a pair of players who lob all the time. Without the ability to hit offensive overheads, these lobs will frustrate the heck out of any team.

Lobs

Lobs are important and are especially effective against 3.0 to 4.0 doubles teams (teams that have not mastered offensive overheads). The lob can be offensive or defensive in nature. Offensive lobs can be hit as a service return or groundstroke over the net man, or hit off a volley against a team at the net.

Defensive lobs can be played to give yourself a chance to get back in the court. For example, if you are running down a shot out wide or deep in your court, throwing up a lob can buy you time to get back in the court. Of course, you may end up running down another shot if your opponents have a good overhead!

All players must learn to "challenge" each lob. That is, when a lob is hit over your head, you don't automatically say "yours" and let your partner run it down. Try to react and attempt to return every overhead. This is how we learn what is reachable and what isn't. 3.0 and 3.5 players are notorious for letting lobs go over their head and not challenging them. The reasons are simple: they are not confident; they don't know what their true limitations are.

LOB REACTIONS

When confronted with a lob, most beginners-to-intermediate players react by looking up at the ball as if evaluating whether they can reach it. By the time they figure out it could be hit, it is usually too late to get their racket up, their body sideways, and their feet shuffling.

The first reaction to any lob, regardless of height and depth, should be to get your racket up and prepare to hit it. Then, if the ball ends up far out of reach, yell "yours" to your partner and switch sides out of the way. Remember that a lob is hit relatively softly. If you and your partner know how to play doubles, your partner will have plenty of time to run down a good lob.

If your partner is the one being lobbed, you will have to prepare to cover the lob as if your partner was not going to be able to reach it.

After your split-step, turn and begin moving back behind your partner. At some point, you will be able to tell if your partner will be able to hit the ball, or will be unable to do anything with the lob. If your partner does hit the lob (as an overhead), you simply switch back to your side of the court and look for your opponent's shot. If your partner can't hit the lob, continue to retrieve the lob.

IF YOU GET LOBBED

Obviously, if you get lobbed with a ball that you simply can't reach, you must switch sides and cover your partner's side of the court (since they will be going behind you on your side of the court to retrieve the lob). Also, it is vital that you back up to at least the service line while your partner is running down the lob. From this position, you can play defensively if your partner hits a weak shot. Or, you can move back in towards the net if your partner hits a good, offensive shot. I see players switching from under a lob who stay close to the net...only to get pulverized when their partner ends up hitting a weak shot off the opponent's lob.

GENERALITIES

In doubles, there are some basic principles that players should know in order to limit the number of "stupid" shots hit, and to simply avoiding being in the wrong place at the wrong time. These include:

- *Don't hit to the net man unless you are hitting an offensive shot*
- *Don't hit to the net man on the first volley off a return or off a serve*
- *Don't move close to the net if the ball is hit deep to your partner*
- *Move with the ball sideways; if the ball is wide, you slide with it.*
- *Move with your partner if they move sideways.*

Conclusion

There are many situations in doubles that will arise as you play more and more doubles. I can't possibly address all the variables that can come up, as there are hundreds of situations that don't follow any pattern. However, the routines that I have suggested in this chapter are fairly foolproof. If you learn these positions and patterns of play, you will limit the chance of being out of position or hitting the wrong shot.

Watch as many doubles matches as you can and try to identify each player's position and movements in relation to the position of the ball.

Doubles is a thinking game with many complexities that are not necessarily as common in singles play. As players develop greater shot selection and effects, doubles becomes more and more interesting.

Finally, doubles has many additional facets that I could not possibly include in a book such as this. Please refer to the reference page at the end of this book for additional resources that can help further your understanding of doubles play.

CHAPTER 16

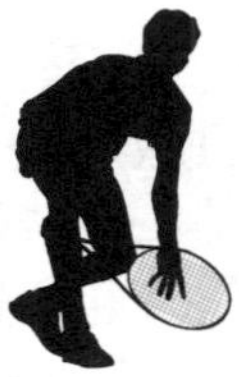

Understanding Tennis Equipment

Knowing how to skillfully play tennis opens up many new understandings about the game. One of these understandings involves tennis equipment...namely how the multitude of tennis paraphernalia—from strings, to rackets, to grips, to shoes—can help players reach peak levels of performance. While even beginners to intermediate players can feel a difference between various types of rackets or strings or grips, it isn't until a player has mastered the game that equipment can provide legitimate help. For example, recognizing that one racket feels different than another is not going to help change inferior stroke patterns. However, the subtle advantage of some equipment over others becomes more of an advantage when a player becomes proficient in the sport. Players who have mastered proper strokes are more in tune with the feel and touch they are afforded by various rackets, grips, and other equipment. Moreover, the appreciation for these subtle differences are magnified as skilled players gets better.

Because there are so many advances in tennis technology today, players often become confused and feel ignorant about the various choices available. (And rightly so!) Consider strings alone. There are multifilament, monofilament, and hybrid strings, gut, synthetic gut and polyester strings; Kevlar, multiwrap and rough strings are but a few of the general string types available. Some strings promote a soft feel, others a firm or "crisp" feel. Others are designed to help generate greater spin; others are designed to increase durability. Such terms as "dynamic elasticity", "resiliency", and "tensile strength" can further induce confusion.

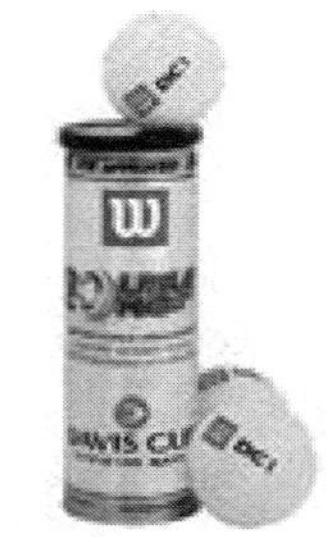

Figure 1
From rackets to shoes to balls to grips, there are a host of tennis related products that a player can choose from! Understanding the construction advantages and disadvantages of each product can help all players make educated decisions on what they should try.

I am confident that all players, regardless of their current tennis ability prior to picking up this book, will gain the skills necessary to appreciate such equipment differences through learning the Advanced Foundation that is presented within these pages. Thus, I will provide a solid "equipment foundation" that will provide you with greater knowledge of the very equipment you will ultimately use to play skilled tennis with!

GRIPS

The construction of tennis grips has changed right along with the advances made in racket design. Thirty years ago, the industry standard was high-grade leather products. The "Fairway Grip" was one of those trade names that skilled players recognized as the "Cadillac" of grips. However, even as the Fairway grip was soft and provided a natural tackiness upon its installation, it was susceptible to the elements causing it to quickly harden and become slick to many players.

More recently, synthetic grips have become the norm. Cushion grips with foam or a gel-like substance imbedded in rubber layers provides extreme comfort in a supple softness that also lasts longer than natural leather grips.

Overwraps are a thin disposable wrap that goes over the racket's existing grip. These have become extremely popular over the last ten years. These grips can range from super tacky to super absorption, depending on the needs of each player. Dirt, oils and moisture quickly deteriorate the qualities of these thin overwraps, hence their disposable nature. Depending on the player's profusion of sweat and oils from the hand, these overwraps can last from a few days to a few months. Players typically keep a few boxes of these in their tennis bag and can easily change the grip within a few minutes as needed.

One of the most neglected aspects of player's equipment is their grip. Too often, players let their grips deteriorate over time and don't recognize this deterioration since it happens slowly over weeks or months. Because we become accustom to our dilapidated grip, we seldom think about replacing it. I generally recommend players replacing their grips at least every other month for casual players, more often for tournament and competitive players. Obviously, if you use an overwrap that you are replacing regularly, the need to replace the thicker main grip will be less.

STRINGS

As I have mentioned, there is great diversity in tennis string. However, most synthetic strings (man-made) are constructed in one of three general configurations:

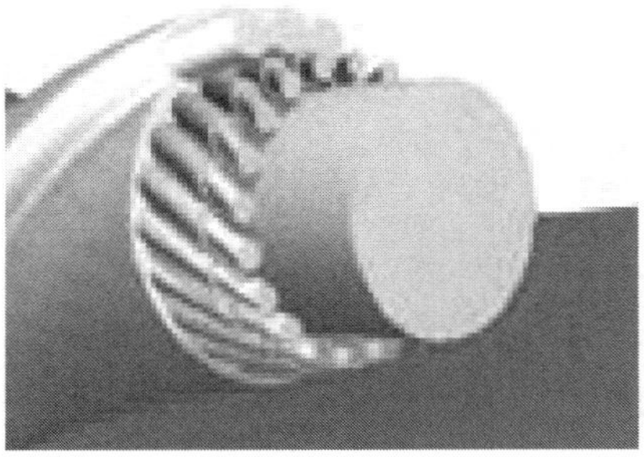

Figure 2
Monofilament Sting: A solid center core usually surrounded by one or more layers of microfilament strings.

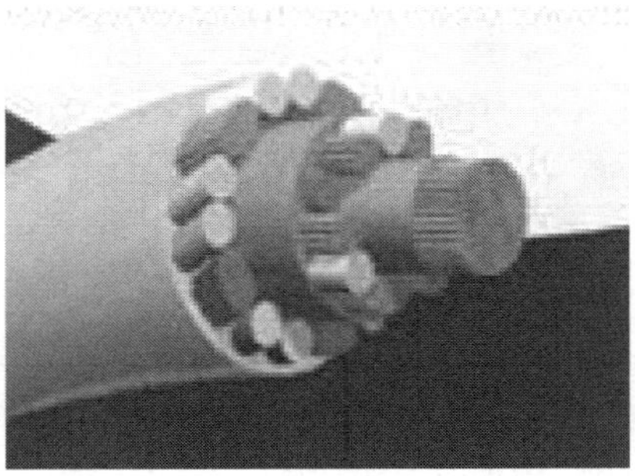

Figure 3
Multifilament String: Center core of multiple microfilaments surrounded by additional microfilament strands.

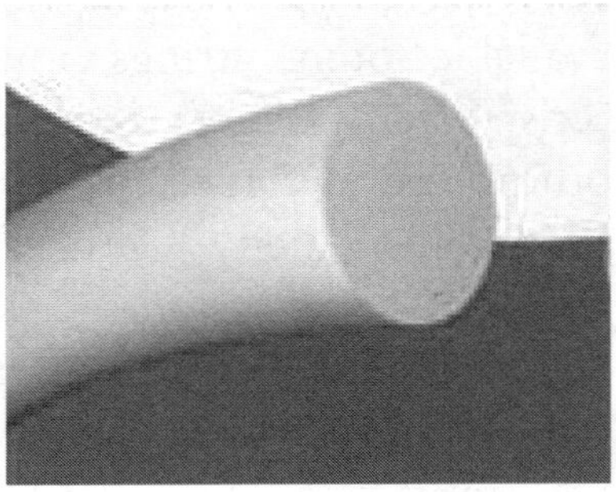

Figure 4
Solid String: Various materials make up a single, solid strand.

1. **Monofilament**: These strings have a solid center core usually wrapped with a few microfilament strings. (Figure 2)

2. **Multifilament**: These strings have a core of many microfilament thread-like strings. Most of these also have a wrapping of additional microfilament strings. (Fig. 3)

3. **Solid**: This string is simply a solid piece of string with no microfilaments surrounding it or making up the core. (Figure 4)

All these strings can have added coatings over the outside of the string or covering inside layers of the string to add durability. Also, some strings will have thick outer filaments creating a "rough" texture to the string, theoretically to add spin to the ball. (From greater friction between the ball and the string.)

Materials

Within each of these construction configurations, the actual material used for the parts of the string can vary greatly. Here are the general materials and their advantages in string construction:

4. **Nylon**: Various polymers and resins create a wide range of nylons that can be incorporated in strings.

5. **Polyester**: An extremely durable material with little resiliency. This string has exceptional durability at the cost of arguably poor playability

6. **Kevlar®**: A bulletproof material that is very stiff. Usually used in the main strings (up and down strings) of the racket, Kevlar, a brand name for the material, provides excellent durability for the frequently broken main strings. Cross strings are usually nylon for less stiffness.

7. **Natural Gut**: Made from the intestines of lamb, sheep, cow and other animals, this is still the preferred string among most pros for the superb playability and feel. Natural gut is very expensive, running upwards of $40 to $50 dollars or more for one string job. Most casual players can't take advantage of the increase in feel or playability due to their skill levels. For most players other than pros, it is more economical to use synthetic strings.

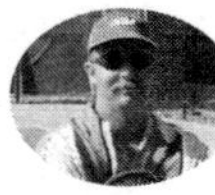

Stringing Note

When stringing a racket with Kevlar, the strings will feel tighter and stiffer than other strings. This is because Kevlar does not stretch much upon impact with the ball. Thus, players need to be aware that the tension of Kevlar might need to be lower than other types of strings due to this feature.

Advantages of Various String Construction

The best playing string for most players are multifilament strings. This is because the ultra thin microfilaments that make up the majority of this string have inherent qualities related to playability. These strings tend to be more resilient as well as provide a slightly softer feel to the players. Multifilament strings are usually the most expensive synthetic strings on the market.

Monofilament strings (usually called "synthetic gut") are considered a "mid range" string. These strings usually provide a firmer feel with average to above average overall playability. Depending on the outer wrappings, (which provide additional feel and softness), monofilament strings can play with some of the characteristics of multifilament strings. However, monofilament strings are generally lower priced providing an economic factor of affordability for many players.

Kevlar string is a hybrid sting that is somewhat of a monofilament string with various microfilament layers around it. Kevlar is a brand name for a type of fiber that is extraordinarily strong. Found in bulletproof vests, Kevlar resists breakage, cutting, and stretching. This string has almost no elasticity making it the firmest string on the market. Brand names that use Kevlar include Wilson's "Hammerlast" and Prince's "Pro-Blend" strings. Most Kevlar string sets include two sets of string: Kevlar for the up-and-down strings, (the "main strings" of the racket), and usually synthetic gut or other more resilient and elastic type string. (If the racket were completely strung with the Kevlar string, the string bed, upon impact with the ball, would be so stiff it would feel like hitting with a piece of steel!) Kevlar has extraordinary durability. However, this durability comes at the cost of feel and softness as well as elasticity found with most other strings. The overall cost of these Kevlar blended strings is not much more than most synthetic gut strings.

Polyester Strings are usually a solid piece of string that is usually more elastic than Kevlar but still has minimal resilient values. The durability is about the same as Kevlar but for most players, polyester has a "dead" feel. In other words, the player does not feel much of the ball upon contact and hears a dull thud with each hit.

Natural Gut is still the preferred string choice among most top ranked players. There is something about natural gut that has yet to be perfected or duplicated with synthetic strings. The feel and response of the ball off the strings is superb with gut. The durability is usually quite good for most gut strings. (However, players must avoid high humidity or any moisture on the strings. Water will dry out gut or cause the string to lose its elasticity and tension.) The down side to gut is the cost. As I mentioned, compared to the average cost of synthetic gut, (which runs anywhere between fifteen and twenty-five dollars a string job), gut will cost upward of fifty to sixty dollars each string job!

String Gauge (Thickness)

Tennis string is gauged by a series of numbers similar to that used in describing electrical wire; the higher the number, the thinner the string. A thick string obviously will last relatively longer than thin strings of the same construction. This durability comes at the sacrifice of playability. Thick strings don't have as much resiliency than thin strings resulting in less "feel" for most players. Thick strings are typically around a 15 gauge for tennis.

The vast majority of recreational players as well as many competitive players use 16-gauge string. This thickness tends to play much better than 15-gauge string yet has fairly good durability. (There is what is called a "light 15-gauge string that is in-between 15 and 16 gauge string.)

Many pros and other skilled players prefer 17-gauge string. This thinner string tends to play exceptionally well for those who a) can afford having to string their rackets a lot! And b) are skilled enough players who can recognize the attributes of thin string. 17-gauge string is far less durable than 15 and 16 gauge strings. For hard hitters, or those who hit with a lot of spin, 17 gauge can last as short as one or two good sets! Pros who use 17-gauge string can go through three to five rackets in a normal match! If cost is not an issue, (and the inconvience of having to string your rackets everyday!) than 17-gauge string might be fun for you to have put in your racket. But unless you are a 5.0 NTRP rated player, the playing attributes of 17-gauge string won't have much effect on your play!

TENSION INFORMATION

String tension has been a very misunderstood concept for decades. The problem is that for various types of players, different string tensions provide different playing qualities. For the average swing-speed player, the tighter the strings, the more control. The looser the strings, the faster the ball can leave the strings. However, there is a limit to both of these parameters. Too tight, the player won't feel the ball nor will the ball rebound from the strings with much force. Too loose, the strings won't contract upon impact any substantial degree producing less return force to the ball from the racket.

However, for players who exert great forces to the ball with faster and longer swing patterns, exceptions to these tension characteristics can occur. With a fast swing speed, the player can cause the ball to compress against the strings with more force thus stretching the strings upon impact substantially. Thus, if a player strings his or her racket tighter, the strings can indeed transfer this compression back to the ball with greater force than if the strings were strung with relatively less tension.

Most players develop an affinity for particular tensions. Some like extremely loose string, (usually those who hit a lot of underspin shots and lobs), and others like very tight strings. Most, however, play best with mid-range string tensions.

TENSION CONSEQUENCES

When players use very tight string tensions, there are some consequences that can come about. These should be considered when playing.

1. **Elbow and arm injuries**: When a racket is strung very tight, the impact stress of each hit is transferred more directly to the hand, elbow and arm.Vibration and the absorption of these stresses can lead to "tennis elbow" and other related injuries. Instead of the string "giving" with the shot, tight strings won't stretch as much or give as much. This means the ball's velocity will translate into impact stress to the racket and to the arm. In addition, miss-hits shots, or balls hit off-center, will be very hard on the arm with high tensions. This is because the tighter the strings, the more rigid the string bed. This will intensify the vibration and torque the player feels from miss-hitting shots.
2. **String longevity**: Tight strings tend to break much earlier than strings strung at more conventional tensions. The fact that the string is stretched out more in the frame means the ball will tend to increase this resiliency factor on each hit. The friction of the strings rubbing on each other with each hit will be aggravated more with tight strings, again causing premature wear.
3. **Racket Breakage**: Stringing some rackets beyond their manufacturer's specifications can increase the chance of the racket cracking or breaking prematurely. Rackets today are often constructed with ultra-light space age materials. While many of these materials are indeed stronger than many historical materials used in rackets, they are still very susceptible to over-stress caused when strung beyond their designed capabilities. Miss-hits on high-speed shots such as serves and overheads can lead to immediate frame failure of many rackets when strung too tight.

HOW OFTEN SHOULD I RESTRING MY RACKET?

This question is very misunderstood by most casual or recreational players. This is because they think if the string hasn't broken yet, they don't need to restring their racket.

While this is true in the simplistic sense that the racket can still be played with, (without broken strings), these players don't recognize the qualities and characteristics of string diminishes over time.

String loses both elasticity (the ability to stretch) and resiliency (the ability to return to original length) beginning the first day after being strung. The degree of this loss is dependent on several factors. These can include: the type of string used and how tight the original tension was; the amount of play the racket is exposed to as well as the general stroke patterns of the player, (topspin versus flat). Also, the overall air temperature or humidity will contribute in varying degrees to a loss of string characteristics.

As a general rule, rackets should be strung every three months, minimum. Because the loss of string characteristics and quality is slow and gradual, few players recognize the loss of these traits over time.

Why Strings Break

This may seem obvious, however, strings break as players improve in two areas: Pace and Spin.

While hitting harder, (pace) certainly places more stress on the strings, the bigger culprit in string breakage is spin. When a ball is hit with spin, the strings move across the ball creating friction of the main strings (the up and down strings) with the cross strings. These movements of the strings cause the cross strings to cut into the main strings. (Because the mains move back and forth across the cross strings on each hit.) This cutting into the strings is called "Grooving." Adding pace to topspin increases the action of the strings on each other and will cause earlier breaking of the strings. Typically, one of the sure signs of a 3.0 player and 4.0 and higher players is the time it takes for each to break strings! 3.0 players tend to dink balls, tend to ease up on second serves, hit much flatter when they do try to hit hard, and, overall don't hit as many hard balls in any given rally. 4.0 and above levels tend to increase their topspin exponentially compared to these lower levels and, because they can keep the ball in play better with spin, can indeed hit balls with greater pace.

As players improve, they will have to pay the price of increasing the number of times they will need to replace their strings! However, many players end up using some of the highly durable strings to reduce the number of string jobs they will have to have done! (Which is why so many good players today own their own stringing machines!) Advanced high school and college players—as well as the pros—can often go through a new set of strings in one or two days, depending on how much playing and practicing they do. It is not uncommon for top level players to have 3 to 6 rackets or more in their bag. During a tournament where players will end up playing several matches a day these performers can easily break strings (and even rackets!) several times over the course of the event. Also, string gauge will have a great deal to do with string longevity. Thin strings, usually 17 gauge or higher, will break considerably faster than heavier string gauges. (15 gauge is considered thick or heavy, 16 is the most popular gauge, 17 and even 18 gauge string plays very well but obviously breaks much quicker.)

Smart players will have several rackets, exactly the same in terms of grip, racket type, and string type and tension with them when they play. It would be difficult to switch to a completely different racket or one that is strung differently in the middle of a big match. Players can't switch rackets and ask to hit a few warm-up shots before resuming the match! Players must immediately resume play even after a racket needs replacing.

RACKET STRINGING PATTERNS

The majority of modern tennis rackets have a conventional string pattern that consists of main strings, (up and down strings), and cross strings. What varies between rackets is usually the number of strings that make up the string bed. In other words, the number of cross strings or main strings might be different between some rackets. There are two terms used to differentiate between the number of strings that go across or up and down in a racket: Open and Closed.

Open String Pattern

This pattern provides greater distance between strings by using less cross strings and/or main strings. Normally, an open string pattern will have 16 main strings and 19 to 20 cross strings. With larger spacing between strings, an open string pattern arguably allows the strings to "bite" into the ball more on some shots. Some players claim they feel greater spin is achieved with this string pattern. Another assertion is that fewer strings makes the string bed more "lively." This is reasonable since the fewer strings in the pattern, the greater the ability for the strings to stretch upon impact.

Closed String Pattern

A Closed string pattern is a denser pattern due to an increase in the number of main and cross strings. A closed pattern usually has 19 main strings and 20 to 21 cross strings. This pattern is also argued to produce more spin due to more strings in contact with the ball. The logic is that more strings create more friction and thus more spin. This certainly makes sense as well. However, a closed string pattern produces a stiffer string bed upon impact and an overall firmer feel.

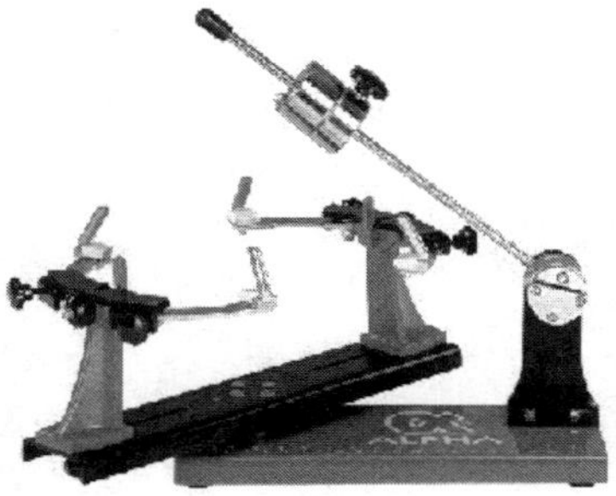

Figure 5
Simple Drop-weight stringing machine.

STRINGING MACHINES

This is an area that few players are knowledgeable about. When we have our rackets strung, we drop them off at the sports store and pick it up when it is ready. For the most part, few recreational players have ever seen a racket strung, let alone know that there is a difference between stringing machines. These differences can create a vast discrepancy between one stringing machine's tension accuracy and another.

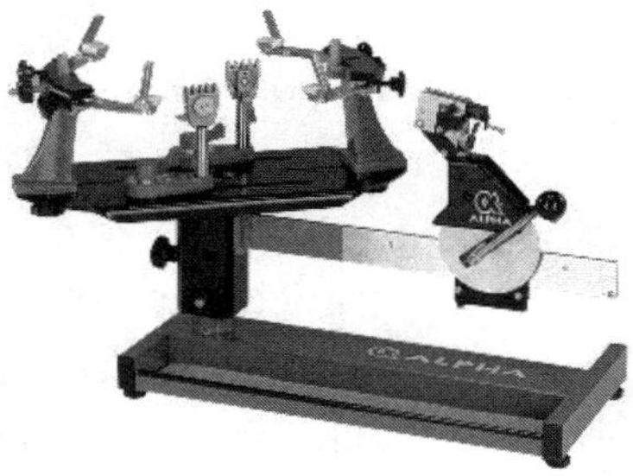

Figure 6
A "Crank Pull" Machine. Using a handle connected to a gear assembly, the string is pulled to a desired tension and then the crank locks out.

Type of Stringing Machines

1. **Drop Weight**: (Figure 5) These machines use a system of weights and clamps to pull the string tight. These are usually the least expensive machines to purchase. However, there are some drop-weight machines that are not cheap! The advantage to the drop weight machines is that they never need calibration. That is,

their pulling is always going to be the same as long as the force of gravity remains the same! Another positive feature of drop-weight machines is that they are "constant pull" machines. That is, the string is constantly pulled at the prescribed weight until the sting is clamped off and released off the tensioner.

2. **Crank Pull Machines**: (Figure 6) For the last few decades, these machines have been the standard among most tennis shops and private stringers. A crank-pull machine uses a gear assembly and spring-released locking mechanism to pull the string to the desired tension. These are generally easy to use and are fairly reasonably priced. The problem with these machines is that the spring loses some accuracy over time and must be calibrated and adjusted often, depending on use. Also, because the machine immediately locks out when the tension is reached, many strings will stretch slightly prior to being clamped off. Depending on the type of string, the finished tension of any particular racket could be off by several lbs of tension. (From the actual selected tension.)

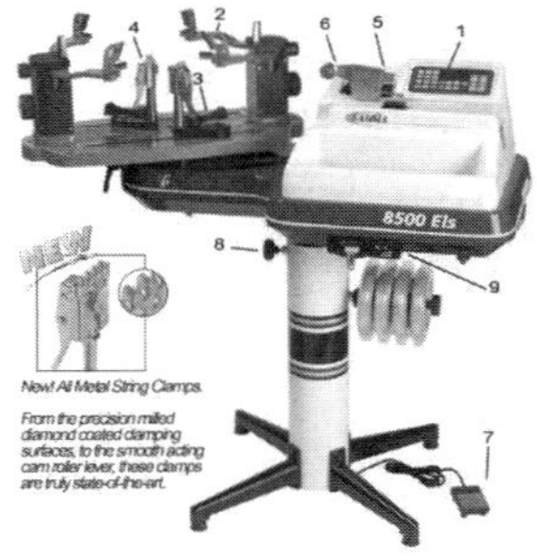

Figure 7
An electronic "constant pull" stringing machine.

3. **Constant Pull Machines**: (Figure 7) These are machines that use electronic motors or hydraulic motors to pull strings tight. These can be very accurate; some to within two-tenth's of a pound! In these more expensive machines, (some running up-wards of $5000 dollars!), the motors create a constant pull on the string at the desired tension. Like the Drop-Weight machines, this type of machine counters the loss of tension from strings stretching by constantly pulling the string at the desired tension until the string is clamped off.

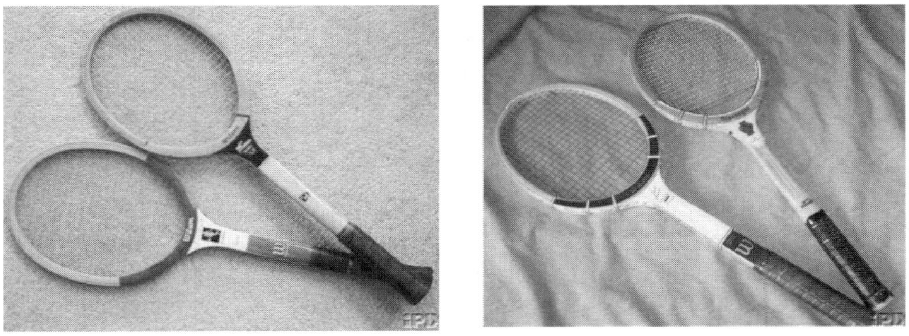

Figures 8 & 9
Wooden rackets dominated tennis for the first 100 years.

TENNIS RACKETS

Perhaps more than any other sport, tennis has seen considerable changes in the implements used to play its game. Tennis rackets have made spectacular advancements in both design and construction materials. Some attribute the changing of the modern game of tennis a result from these advancements in racket structure. It can be argued that those changes include more power offered to players compared to that of historic wooden frames provided. While it can't be argued that today's rackets do indeed exhibit more power, there are many other contributing factors that have nixed the historic game plans of the past in favor of a significantly different game played today.

Construction

Historically, for about the first hundred years, tennis rackets were made primarily of wood. Some later versions of the wood racket integrated additional laminates including fiberglass and plastics, or various other wood types. (Including maple, ash, pine, and even bamboo!) Metal rackets didn't make their appearance until the late 1950's. (Although, in the 1920's the Birmingham Aluminum Co. of Birmingham, England made a tennis racket entirely of metal and even with metal strings! The "Birmal" was ahead of its time featuring even a leather grip, something that wouldn't be commonplace until the 1930's.)

Initially, metal rackets were too heavy compared to the wood models of the day. It really wasn't until aluminum could be extruded into a racket shape and still made rigid enough to be swung without warping or breaking that metal rackets began to emerge. In the mid-1930's Dayton Steel Racquet Company made frames that were either entirely made of steel or had steel frames inserted into wooden handles. Strung with piano wire, these rackets, heavy as they were, became very popular and ideal for institutions and schools. (They were considered extremely durable—however very head heavy!)

One of the first truly commercially successful aluminum frames was the Spalding Smasher. This racket appeared in the late 1960's and was quite indestructible while being relatively light. In the early 1970's Jimmy Connors, former world number one singles player, made the Wilson T-2000 popular by its endorsement and use in winning all of his 10 Grand-slam titles and some 15 additional American major tournaments. The T-2000 was a steel racket with an interior wire mesh that held the strings in a suspended "trampoline" like netting. Prior to Connors making his marks with the "steelie" T-2000, (a nickname given to the racket when it first make its debut!), Billie Jean King won the U.S. Open title in 1967 using the racket.

A second shift in tennis design and construction came in the late 1970's when Prince Manufacturing, (a company known for making tennis ball machines), designed an oversized tennis racket. The Prince Classic was an aluminum frame with a green plastic insert at the throat. At 110 square inches, the hitting surface seemed enormous compared to the some 70 square inches most rackets were relegated to. It didn't take long for the oversized revolution to take place. By the mid-1980's, most racket manufacturers were finding themselves making large-head rackets.

Over the past twenty years, the last shift in racket design was in construction materials. Graphite became a household name in the early 1980's as manufacturers discovered new and ingenious ways to interlace graphite fibers with other materials to make rackets lighter and stiffer. One of the first graphite rackets to emerge was the C-6 developed by a company that tennis great Tony Trabert lent his name to. Prince Manufacturing took its big head rackets and started making the "Prince Graphite," a racket that really seemed to set the standard for oversized graphite rackets in the early to mid-1980's.

Today, there are so many new materials integrated in tennis rackets it seems you have to have a PhD in alchemy and physics to decipher all of them! Tungsten, magnesium, Kevlar, boron, and titanium are but a few of these new materials. I suppose it won't be long before someone claims to have Kryptonite in a racket! And, believe it or not, some companies are even putting WOOD in their rackets!

Certainly, many manufacturers would like you to believe that some space-age material imbedded in your racket will make you play like the next Pete Sampras. While making rackets lighter and stiffer have some playability qualities that can enhance a players performance, the key that all players must remember is that strokes, form, and technique, and the control of those issues is still the deciding factor in a player's ability and skill!

Lighter and Stiffer

What might be helpful to the reader in becoming educated in racket construction is the value and relative performance of various design components.

Basically, rackets are designed to meet three distinctive needs:

1. *Weight*
2. *Balance*
3. *Stiffness*

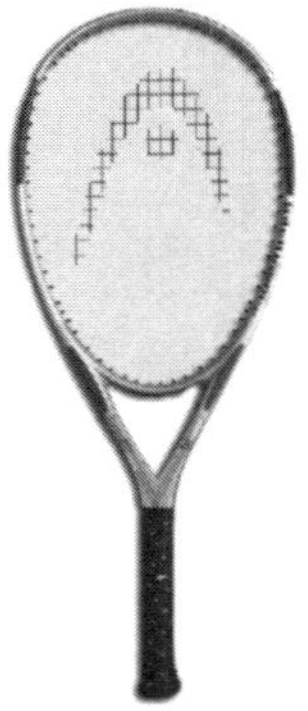

Figure 10
The Head "Intellifiber" racket technology. Using piezoelectric fibers to convert vibration shock to electrical impulses, this racket actually changes its characteristics upon impact with a ball.

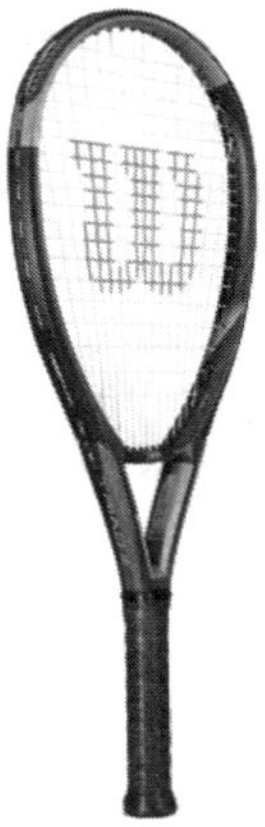

Figure 11
The Wilson "Triad," a three-piece racket designed to reduce stress to the arm while providing controllable power.

Weight

The weight of the racket deals with the overall mass the racket has. Heavy rackets are usually designed for players who are not only strong, but also have swing patterns that can benefit from a heavier racket. Older players who swing with short, compact swings will find heavier rackets not only very uncomfortable, but also hazardous to their health! Hitting a ball off-center or late can create real pain in some players who are not physically capable of using such heavy rackets.

The range of racket weights start on the lighter end around 9 ounces. Rackets considered heavy run around 12 to 14 ounces. Many "ultra light" frames can weigh in at 7.5 and 8 ounces.

Balance

The balance of a racket deals with where the weight of the racket is distributed. In other words, is the racket "head heavy" or "head light"? A racket can be relatively light but "feel" heavy because it is a head-heavy racket.

Players who tend to play the base line usually like head-heavy rackets. This is because groundstrokes are hit using a full swing. This allows the player to create greater inertia with a head-heavy racket and apply more force to the ball in the process.

Net players usually like a head light racket for mobility in quick movements to the ball in close quarters.

Stiffness

A racket that is stiff can transfer more power to the ball. Instead of the racket bowing at contact and absorbing some of the rebound power, stiff rackets convert all the power of the swing with the rebound power of the moving ball to the ball itself.

This is one of the big changes in racket technology in the past ten or fifteen years. Rackets today are becoming lighter AND stiffer without sacrificing strength or durability of the frame. Players today can generate seemingly great racket head speed with these ultra light rackets and convert that speed to great power. With players being able to swing harder, the ability to hit with more spin creates the opportunity to hit with more controlled power. Hence, the modern game of today is faster and more powerful than in the history of the sport.

The problem with stiff rackets is that the player usually has to sacrifice some touch and control in exchange for the added power. The balance for manufacturers today is to provide the power desired within a player's demand for control. This is why many racket manufacturers today carry a line of 15 to 20 models in their "high-performance" line of rackets.

Another interesting technology is being introduced by Head Manufacturing. Head has come up with a racket that uses "Piezoelectric" material that they call "Intellifiber." This material transforms the mechanical energy from the ball's impact into electrical energy. (See Figure 10) This energy then is used to stiffen the racket at key points within the very same piezoelectric fibers that stimulated the electrical impulse. (Piezoelectric fibers create a pulse of electrical energy created from the shock of the ball's impact on the racket.) These piezoelectric fibers contract within one millisecond and stiffen the racket frame prior to the ball leaving the racket. In one of their rackets, this electrical impulse is boosted through a microcomputer chip. This boost, depending on the overall force of the ball on the strings increases the electrical signal back to the piezoelectric fibers. This boosted signal increases the stiffness of the racket by some 40%.

Wilson Racquet Sports has designed a three-piece racket that completely separates the string portion of the racket head from the grip portion. These rackets called "Triad" (See Figure 11) have a shock-absorbing rubber-like material called "Isosorb" between the two parts of the racket. Such a system creates a method of reducing the shock of contact of the ball being transferred to the arm. Integrating this three-piece racket design with their already popular "Hammer Technology," Wilson hopes to provide true comfort with extreme power and control...all in one racket!

As you can see, racket technology continues to provide the consumer with the "next newest thing!" Players will want to try many rackets to find the perfect balance between power, weight, and control.

Bottom Line

All the racket technology or string innovations in the world won't magically make you play incredible tennis! This must be understood completely. All these improvements can do is change the feel of a shot by the player. A player who uses questionable form can improve the feel of a shot but not the technique through such equipment improvements. Oftentimes, a player tries a new racket and immediately gains a level of confidence that can sometimes propel the player to have momentary success within such questionable form. This success is subjective to the player's belief that the racket is responsible for the player's success. This belief allows the player to simply "aim and hit," the very concept that I talked about in Chapter 13 on Mental Tennis. However, these results are more often than not, short-lived. Players soon make the eventual errors that such questionable form usually results in. Questionable form usually diminishes the error room as well diminishes the consistency that is critical to improvement as well as progression. When the player recognizes they are still very vulnerable to errors, especially those due to improper form, the bubble is burst and the player returns to the level of play that is most recognizable among those who use questionable form.

When a player develops proper form and stroke mechanics, then they can not only recognize playing characteristics of various rackets and strings, but they can make use of the subtle advantages particular rackets and/or string provides.

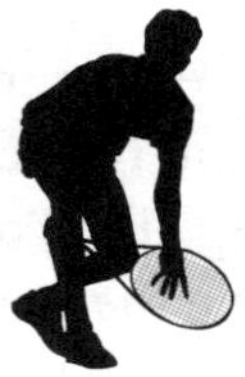

Glossary within the "Advanced Foundation"

There have been hundreds of books printed with the general terminology and "lingo" of tennis printed for students of all abilities. Because Tennis Mastery is written for all levels of players as well as for tennis teaching professionals, I feel that some terms—as they relate specifically to the game—are often misunderstood or not known at all. In addition to the generally accepted meaning or concept, I have added additional information that will help the reader fully understand each word or concept.

Ace: An outright winning serve, hit in such a way that the receiver can not make contact with the ball.

Adjustment Period: Time necessary for a player to accept a certain degree of frustration and inconsistency, (as well as discomfort) while playing and practicing with new strokes or technique.

Advanced Foundation: A system or methodology that does not teach tennis in a transitory manner. Players are taught techniques that are part of the advanced methods found within skilled play.

Advantage: The point following "Deuce" meaning the person who has the "advantage" will win the game being played. Usually spoken in as an abbreviated single syllable "Ad," the word is followed by the either "In" or "Out" depicting who has the advantage: "ad in" if the server has the advantage, "ad out" if the receiver has the advantage.

Alley: The 4'-foot-wide area on the side of each court that is bounded by the singles sideline and the doubles sideline. This area is used only during doubles play following the serve.

Angle of Reflection: The direction a ball will reflect off the hitting surface of a racket.

Angle Volley: The intentional placement of a volley that moves more parallel with the net. (As opposed to a deeper volley which will move more perpendicular to the net.)

Angular Momentum: (Also called rotational momentum) This is any force that is gained through rotational movements of the body, arm, or racket. These movements are usually circular in their movement pattern.

Approach shot: Any shot that a player uses to approach the net on. Usually a drive, hit sometimes with underspin, sometimes with topspin, but generally hit firm and deep into the opponent's court.

ATP: Association of Tennis Professionals: The men's organization of touring pros, comparable to a worker's "union." Established in 1972, it maintains control of the men's world-wide circuit, with the exception of the four "Grand Slam" events. (The Australian, French, Wimbledon, and the U.S. Open.)

Backhand: The stroke that is hit from the opposite side as the forehand or the serve. (Left side of the body for a right-hander.) The backhand can be hit with one or two hands.

Bagel: Slang for a player winning a 6 – 0 set.

Band-aid Repair: Short-term fix for situational strokes that are or have flawed components.

Baseline: The court's back line, connecting the two singles sidelines.

Baseliner: A player who favors playing the back part of the court hitting groundstrokes.

Brake Step: A release of the back leg after contact is made, allowing it to swing around to the side of the player. This leg and foot are then used to brake the player's momentum in one direction and helps them push back into a neutral position in anticipation of the next shot.

Break point: The point when the score is "Ad out." The receiving player has the advantage and, if successful in winning the point, will "break" serve.

Brush: The action of the strings on the ball when a player intentionally wants to impart spin on the ball. Brushing up, brushing across, brushing under, are the three distinct patterns of racket movement to create the three types of spin: Topspin, sidespin, and slice.

Carioca Step: This is the movement of a player's back leg going behind the front leg while the player is moving forward. (Sometimes referred to as a "grapevine step.") This allows a player to remain sideways with the hips and upper body even while still moving forward towards the net.

Choking: Usually due to pressure or importance of a match, a player can't perform up to their potential. Generally, all players feel pressure in match play. However, the player who is better prepared and is "mentally tough" works through this pressure and performs favorably.

Chip and Charge: A tactic where a player will hit a slice "approach shot" and follow this ball into the net.

Closed Stance: The idea of turning sideways to the net and stepping across yourself with your front foot.

Comfort Zone Syndrome: The situation when players who go back to flawed—but familiar—stroke patterns in competition because they are more comfortable.

Crosscourt: A diagonal shot that is hit from right to left or left to right.

Davis Cup: Men's international team competition consisting of two singles players who play a round robin with each match a best-of-five set match, and one doubles match, also played as a 3 of 5 set match. The team play pits countries against countries in an often intense and highly charged match. (These matches are often called "ties.")

Default: Termination of a match with the outcome determined in a way other than actual competition. This can be done in one of three ways: Walkover: A match that has not begun due to one player either not showing up or an unwillingness to begin at the appointed time. Retirement: A player quits a match that has already begun. Disqualification: Violation of rules that leads to expulsion by a tournament judge or director.

Deuce: A game where either player needs two point to win the game. Usually deuce is called at "40-all" or when the player who has had the "Advantage" loses the next point.

Dink: Any intentionally soft shot hit, usually by players who are afraid to miss with any essence of power. A dink is not considered a "drop shot" however a dink usually does end up landing short in the opponent's court. A "Dinker" is someone who primarily relies on dink shots when playing opponents. The dink shot seldom has much spin and relies on gravity and simple trajectory as means of getting the ball to land in the court.

Drop Volley: A volley in which the player intentionally softens the rebound of a ball off his racket and makes the ball land very short on the other side of the net.

Double Fault: When the server faults with both serves resulting in losing the point without the opponent making any play on the ball.

Down-the-line: and shot that is hit parallel and near the singles or doubles side lines.

Drop Shot: A ball hit soft and with underspin that is aimed barely to clear the net and designed to die on the opponent's side of the court.

Fault: Failing to put the ball into play on the serve. Two faults in succession results in a "double fault."

Federation/Fed Cup: The annual women's international team competition equivalent to Davis Cup for men.

Fifteen: The first point won in any game. This score is often spoken as "five" when said in conjuntion with the other player's score, such as: "five-thirty" (for 15 – 30) or "five-all" (for 15-all) etc.

Flushing Meadow: FSite of the U.S. Open in New York City. It has been home of the Open since 1978 and is named the USTA National Tennis Center.

Foot Fault: An intrusion by the server into the court or onto the baseline prior to making contact with the ball on the serve.

Forehand: The stroke hit from the right side of the player for a right-hander.

Forrest Hills: Prior to the U.S. Open being played at Flushing Meadows, Forrest Hills was home of the U.S. National Championships, (later called the U.S. Open after 1968.) While the event was actually played at the West Side Tennis Club, the tournament was referred to as Forest Hills, the residential section of Queens, New York, where the club was located.

Forty: The score of one player who has won three points in one game.

Game: The first player to win four points, unless the score is "deuce" where one player must win the next two points. The points of a Game are known as: 15, 30, 40, and Game. A player must win 6 games by a margin of two games to win a set. A match is a contest of two-out-of-three sets or three-out-of-five sets.

Grand Slam: Referred usually as a player winning the four major championships (Australian, French, Wimbledon, and U.S. Open) all in the same year. These four major events are considered the Grand Slam Events.

Gravity-Reliant Player: This is a player who uses only the force of gravity to keep a ball in play. Because of a limited ability to apply spin to facilitate a ball's ability to drop into the court, a gravity-reliant player is limited to trajectory and soft pace. These players are often called "Dinkers" or "Pushers."

Grip: The method of holding the racket when playing tennis. (Also refers to the wrapping around the handle of a racket, usually of synthetic or leather material.) There are five basic grips: Eastern Forehand, Continental, Eastern Backhand, Semi Western, and the Western.) The grip can be one or two-hands on the racket (as in a two-handed forehand or two-handed backhand).

Groundstroke: A stroke hit after the ball bounces, usually from or near the backcourt. (Often referred to as "groundies" in tennis slang.)

Gut: Type of tennis string that is not synthetic and comes from the intestines of lamb, cows or other animal. Usually considered the best playing string for tennis.

Hacker: Usually refers to someone that does not possess skilled or highly refined tennis strokes. A hacker usually uses unconventional strokes or technique.

Half-Volley: A stroke where the ball is hit immediately following the bounce. Most often, a player approaching the net executes a half volley near mid court. The shot is more distinctive of a short groundstroke than a volley in that the player uses a short upward stroke with a closed racket face.

Hard Courts: Courts usually constructed of concrete or asphalt and coated with an acrylic coating to give the court its texture. Unlike clay or grass courts, hard courts are exactly that…hard.

I-Formation: An unorthodox doubles alignment which places the net man near the center of the court and his partner serving also from near the mid point along the baseline. The purpose is to force opponents to hit a down-the-line return as opposed to the conventional crosscourt return usually attempted against a normal doubles formation.

ITF: International Tennis Federation: Since 1913 it ahs been the world governing body of tennis. While it does not have a great deal of control over professional tennis, it does govern the four major tennis tournaments as well as such international events as Davis Cup, Federation Cup, and Olympic competitions.

Key Position Points: Stroke reference points that a player can associate his specific body, body parts, or racket to in relation to the ball, the player or the court. Example: Keeping the hitting elbow close to the body at contact on a two-handed backhand.

Kick Serve: A serve that is hit more up the inside or back of the ball than a traditional slice or flat serve. This serve will produce a spin that has its axis of rotation almost horizontal.

Kinetic Chain: The chain of body segments that lead up to contact. Usually starting with the feet and legs, the kinetic chain incorporates the actions of each body segment up to the forearm, hand and wrist.

Let: This is called as a signal for a replay. Usually when the serve clips the top of the net and lands in the correct service box, a Let is called. (To replay the serve.) This has been abandoned in collage tennis where players must play any serve that lands in the correct service box regardless of whether the ball has touched the net. A Let is also called when a point is interrupted or interfered with (such as a ball rolling onto the court from an adjacent court).

Linear Learning: Learning form that is associated with skilled play from the start. Players do not have to make necessary changes to reach skilled play within Linear Learning.

Linear Movement: Any movement where force is applied in a single linear direction. These movements include pushing, lunging, and jumping type movements. Linear are less efficient than angular movements but tend to be more controllable.

Lob: A high, arching shot that is meant to either clear a net player or hit as a defensive shot allowing the player who hit the lob time to regain position in the court.

Loop Swing: A backswing that starts high over the shoulders and loops down before starting up to hit a topspin stroke.

Love: A score of zero, such as 15 – love. (One player has won one point, the other player has not won a point.)

Masters: The climax of the tennis year with an eight-man Masters playoff among the top eight finishers in the Grand Prix.

Match: The overall contest between players. A match is usually the best two-out-of-three sets. Or, as in international play such as Davis Cup or Grand Slam events, men will play the best of 5 sets.

Match Point: Any point where a player only needs to win one point to win the match.

Mental Toughness: A conditioned and positive response to adversity.

Mixed Doubles: Doubles featuring one male and one female partner on both teams.

Momentum Shifts: Rallies or shots that cause a significant shift in match momentum.

Moonball: A high, floating groundstroke used from the baseline in a rally. While it may resemble a lob, a moonball is not hit when an opponent is at the net. Instead, it is usually used to slow down the pace of a point.

Net: The barrier running across the court from each net post. The net should be exactly 3 feet high at the center point and 3 feet, 6 inches high at the net post.

Net Cord: This refers to a shot during rally that clips the top of the net and still goes over the net. It also refers to the band or the cable that supports the net along the top.

Net Judge: An official that is seated at one end of the net who detects when a ball has touched the net during a serve. He or she will rest their hand or fingers on the net cord to feel if the serve touched the net. If so, the net judge will yell "NET" and the serve is replayed as a Let if the serve still landed in the proper service box.

No-ad: This is a type of scoring that eliminates the deuce and makes each game end when a player has won four points. Instead of the traditional scoring of love-15-30-40-game, No-ad uses a 0-1-2-3-game scoring sequence for each point. At 3-all (which would be 40-all in traditional scoring) the next point wins the game. The receiving player or team has the choice of which court to receive the 3-all point.

NTRP: A player's ratings system developed by the USTA as a more differentiated mode of ranking competitors. Starting at 1.0 (beginner) and incrementally increasing by .5 levels to a high of 7.0 (professional), players can examine core abilities and determine their rating. While being a subjective method of rating (since players can be ranked higher in some areas of the game than in others), the NTRP does provide a more defined method of determining player abilities (than in the previous A-B-C-D methods).

Open Stance: A position of the feet at contact that maintains the player's body open or facing the net.

Overhead: A stroke that is hit over the head (like a serve) during a rally. These are sometime called "smashes" if hit offensively close to the net.

Passing Shot: This is a stroke (other than a lob) that an opponent will try to hit past a player who has come to the net.

Pinpoint Stance: A serving stance that brings both feet close together during the toss for the serve.

Platform Stance: A two-footed stance on the serve that balances the body between both feet. This stance maintains a separation of the two feet during the serve.

Poach: The act of a net player crossing in front of his partner in an attempt to hit a winning volley.

Point: The smallest unit of scoring in tennis. The first point of a game is called 15, the second point is 30, and the third point won is called 40.

Practice Foundation: Coordinated on-court practice routine based on the Advanced Foundation.

Pronation: The action of the forearm turning out as the racket makes contact. This action, done correctly, provides for a significant amount of racket head speed.

Pusher: This type of player uses soft, limiting strokes to keep the ball in play. Today, a pusher is usually called a dinker. Usually because of limited ability to hit proper strokes, or hit with reliability, a pusher or dinker simply uses gravity, trajectory, and limited power, to keep the ball in play.

Rally: An exchange of shots during a point.

Ready Position: An attentive stance that allows the player to be optimally ready to receive a shot from an opponent.

Recovery Step: A step used after contact that allows a player to recover their bodies directional movement and / or balance. Two recovery steps include the "Brake Step" and the "Reverse Pivot".

Reverse Pendulum: The rotational action of the arm swinging overhead because of a fixed position at the shoulder.

Reverse Pivot: This is a recovery step that allows a player who is moving or falling backwards, away from the net, to add power to a shot as well as quickly recover from this defensive position.

Second Serve Advantage: When a player possesses a quality second serve, the underlying confidence of this second serve allows a player to take a more aggressive approach to his first serve. A player with a weak second serve does not have this luxury.

Seeding: The deliberate placement of strong players known to a tournament. This is so these players will not meet in earlier rounds.

Service or Serve: The act of hitting the first ball of a rally at the start of each point. The serve must be hit from one side of the baseline diagonally over the net and into the opponent's service box. The serve can be hit using any motion, (underhand or overhand).

Service Break: When an opponent wins the opposing player's service game.

Service Courts: These are the two boxes that make up the forecourt on either side of the net. The serve must be hit into the appropriate diagonal box.

Service Winner: An unreturnable serve. (Not an ace which is an untouchable serve.)

Set: When a player or team has won a minimum of six games with a difference of at least two games, they have won the set. Most matches are considered winning 2 of 3 sets or 3 of 5 sets in some men's tournaments.

Set Point: When one player only needs to win the next point to win the set.

Sitter: An easy ball that a player can attack for an easy put-away.

Slice: Underspin slice is when the racket hits the underside of the ball imparting backspin on the ball in relation to its forward movement. Sidespin slice (usually associated with the serve) is when the racket hits along the equator of a ball whose axis is vertical.

Spin: Rotation of the ball created when the racket does not hit the ball perfectly flat. (Virtually every shot in tennis will have some aspect of spin.) Three main categories of spin: Topspin, underspin, and sidespin.

Spin Advantage: Hitting a ball that has spin with a stroke that does not change the rotation direction of the ball.

Split-Step: A momentary pause in a player's movement that provides for balance. This usually includes the feet splitting apart and the player stopping any directional movement so as to react correctly to any shot that their opponent may hit.

Tanking: A player acting he or she doesn't care about winning or losing.

Targeting: The act of having actual targets on the court to practice hitting specific shots at.

Tennis Mastery: Tennis Mastery is the summation of all the elements a player must acquire to compete successfully at any level, against any opponent, under all conditions, and within all circumstances.

Tennis Mechanics: While strokes and stroke production are the staple, tennis mechanics also includes footwork, hand-eye coordination, and shot-making skills and execution.

Thirty: The second point in a game.

Throat: The portion of the racket that is below the hoop (where the strings are) and the grip.

Tiebreaker: An "overtime" end to a set that is usually tied at 6 games all. Instead of playing the set out (where one player must have a 2 game advantage to win), the set is decided by tiebreaker. Developed by Jimmy Van Alen, it was originally called a "9-point tie-breaker." (First one to five, at four all, the next point one the set.) This was often called "sudden death" as a set could be determined by only one point if the set was indeed tied at 4-points all. A revision by the ITF, devised by Peter John, the current 12-point tiebreaker was developed. This made it so that one player or team had to have a minimum of 7 points won in the tiebreaker and a margin of two points. One of the longest tiebreakers on record was a 26 – 24 breaker won by Jan Gunnarson and Michael Mortensen over John Frawley and Victor Pecci at Wimbledon in 1985.) Of the four major championships, the U.S. Open is the only Grand Slam event that settles all sets tied at 6-games all by a tiebreaker. The other three slams play the final set out without a tiebreaker.

Format: One side will server the first point from the deuce court followed by each side serving two points starting from the ad court. Players change ends of the court every 6 points. In doubles, players must follow serving order of the set the tiebreaker is deciding. The first team/player to reach 7 points with a margin of 2 points wins the tiebreaker and the set. The set is scored 7 – 6.

Topspin: A ball that has its spin forward in the direction it is traveling in the air. Due to air friction and air pressure, a ball with topspin will drop faster than a ball with similar velocity from the same height.

Topspin Volley: Hitting a volley as a topspin groundstroke. Instead of blocking and slicing the volley, a topspin volley is hit with a low to high swing pattern that is nearly identical to any topspin groundstroke.

Transitional Learning: Learning tennis by first being introduced to "beginner methods" that will need to be specifically changed if the player hopes to reach skilled levels of play.

Turn: This is when the player will take their racket back not by the arm but by the body turning sideways. (Sometimes referred to as a "Unit Turn")

Two-handed Backhand: For a right-handed player, hitting the ball on the left side of the body with two hands. (Most common form is with the dominant hand on the bottom of the grip.)

Two-handed Forehand: Anytime a player uses two hands to execute a forehand stroke.

Umpire: The official in charge of a match, keeping score and calls the score out. The umpire usually is seen sitting in a tall chair at one end of the net.

Unforced Error: When a player misses a shot that was not pressured by a significant shot by an opponent.

U. S. Open: The fourth and final Grand Slam of each year played in New York at Forest Hills.

USTA: The United States Tennis Association (formerly the U. S. Lawn Tennis Association), is the governing organization of tennis in the United States. The USTA operates the U. S. Open and was founded in 1881.

Volley: To hit a ball during a rally out of the air before it touches the ground.

Wimbledon: The game's oldest tennis tournament. Started in 1877 at its inception, Wimbledon was first played at the "old Wimbledon" on Worple Road. Since 1922, the Championships have been played at the All England Lawn Tennis and Croquet Club in the London suburb of Wimbledon.

Winner: A shot hit for an outright point. (As opposed to winning the point on an "unforced error" by your opponent.)

WTA: The Women's Tennis Association, an organization of leading female pros. Founded in 1973 by Billie Jean King.

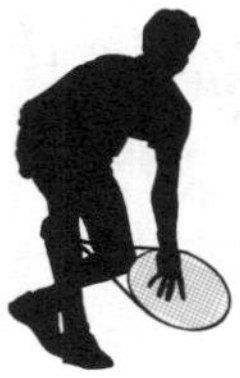

Resources

The following books offer the reader a wealth of additional information that can be useful for players looking to further their tennis education. Many of these books have been helpful to me in writing this book and offer additional teaching concepts that every player can gain from.

Ashe, Arthur & McNab, Alexander, *Arthur Ashe on Tennis.* New York, New York, Avon Books, 1995

Braden, Vic, & Bruns, Bill, *Tennis for the Future.* Boston: Little, Brown, 1977

Braden, Vic, & Bruns, Bill, *Tennis 2000.* Canada,. Little, Brown & Company, 1998

Broudy, Jack W. *The Real Spin on Tennis.* Merrillville, Indiana. ICS Books, 1997

Collins, Bud *Tennis Encyclopedia*, Detroit Michigan, Visible Ink Press 1997

Fein, Paul. *Tennis Confidential.* Dulles, Virgina. Brassey's Inc. 2002

Gallwey, W. Timothy *Inner Tennis*, New York, New York. Random House, Inc. 1976

Gallwey, W. Timothy *The Inner Game of Tennis*, New York, New York. Random House, Inc. 1974, Rev., 1997

Gilbert, Brad & Jamison, Steve, *Winning Ugly.* New York, New York. Fireside Press, 1993

Groppel, Jack L. *High Tech Tennis*, Second Edition, Champaign, Illinois. Leisure Press, 1984

Smith, Stan & Lutz, Bob, *Modern Doubles.* Syracuse, New York. Dix Typesetting Co., Inc., 1975

Tennis Magazine: *Tennis Strokes and Strategies*, New York, New York, Simon and Schuster. 1975

Tourdo, Steve *Unlimited Doubles*. Corte Madera, CA Point Control Technologies, 2000

United States Professional Tennis Association: Tennis: A Professional Guide, New York, New York, Harper and Row Publishers, Inc. 1984

Van Der Meer, Dennis: *Dennis Van der Meer's Complete Book of Tennis*. Ottawa, Illinois, Jameson Books.1986

Yandell, John, *Visual Tennis*, Champaign, Illinois. Human Kinetics. 1999

Rineberg, Dave, *My Seven Years as Hitting Coach for the William Sisters*. Hollywood Florida. Frederick Fell Publishers, Inc. 2001

The National Tennis Ratings Program

(Used with permission by the USTA)

These are the guidelines for the National Tennis Ratings Program (United States). As you will notice, there is no mention of stroke techniques, grips, or stroke patterns. While this system is far more detailed than the ambiguous rating methods such as an "A" "B" "C" system, it does not provide for descriptions that detail the use of specific stroke techniques, grips or stroke patterns. It is understandable since there is no consensus among tennis institutions that a specific stroke technique, grip or pattern is the only way to hit a tennis ball. However, regardless of ability and techniques used, you can rate yourself in these categories and derive a general ability level for yourself.

NTRP 1.0

This player is just starting to play tennis.

NTRP 1.5

This player has limited playing experience and is still working primarily on getting the ball over the net, has some knowledge of scoring but is not familiar with basic positions and procedures for singles and doubles play.

NTRP 2.0

This player may have had some lessons but needs on-court experience; has some obvious stroke weaknesses but is beginning to feel comfortable with singles and doubles play.

FOREHAND: Incomplete swing; lacks directional intent

BACKHAND: Avoids backhands; erratic contact; grip problems; incomplete swing

SERVE/RETURN OF SERVE: Incomplete service motion; double faults common; toss is inconsistent; return of serve erratic

VOLLEY: Reluctant to play net; avoids backhand; lacks footwork

PLAYING STYLE: Familiar with basic positions for singles and doubles play; frequently out of position

NTRP 2.5

This player has more dependable strokes and is learning to judge where the ball is going; has weak coverage or is often caught out of position, but is starting to keep the ball in play with other players of the same ability.

FOREHAND: Form developing; prepared for moderately paced shots

BACKHAND: Grip and preparation problems; often chooses to hit forehand instead of backhand

SERVE/RETURN OF SERVE: Attempting a full swing; can get the ball in play at slow pace; inconsistent toss; can return slow paced serve

VOLLEY: Uncomfortable at net especially on the backhand side; frequently uses forehand racket face on backhand volleys

SPECIAL SHOTS: Can lob intentionally but with little control; can make contact on overheads

PLAYING STYLE: Can sustain a short rally of slow pace; weak court coverage; usually remains in the initial doubles position

NTRP 3.0

This player can place shots with moderate success, can sustain a rally of slow pace but is not comfortable with all strokes; lacks control when trying for power.

FOREHAND: Fairly consistent with some directional intent; lacks depth control

BACKHAND: Frequently prepared; starting to hit with fair consistency on moderate shots

SERVE/RETURN OF SERVE: Developing rhythm; little consistency when trying for power; second serve is often considerably slower than first serve; can return serve with fair consistency

VOLLEY: Consistent forehand volley; inconsistent backhand volley, has trouble with low and wide shots

SPECIAL SHOTS: Can lob consistently on moderate shots

PLAYING STYLE: Consistent on medium-paced shots; most common doubles formation is still one-up, one-back; approaches net when play dictates but weak in execution

NTRP 3.5

This player has achieved stroke dependability and direction on shots within reach, including forehand and backhand volleys, but still lacks depth and variety; seldom double faults and occasionally forces errors on the serve.

FOREHAND: Good consistency and variety on moderate shots; good directional control; developing spin

BACKHAND: Hitting with directional control on moderate shots; has difficulty on high or hard shots; returns difficult shots defensively

SERVE/RETURN OF SERVE: Starting to serve with control and some power; developing spin; can return serve consistently with directional control on moderate shots

VOLLEY: More aggressive net play; some ability to cover side shots; uses proper footwork; can direct forehand volleys; controls backhand volley but with little offense; difficulty in putting volleys away

SPECIAL SHOTS: Consistent overhead on shots within reach; developing approach shots, drop shots, and half volleys; can place the return of most second serves

PLAYING STYLE: Consistency on moderate shots with directional control; improved court coverage; starting to look for the opportunity to come to the net; developing teamwork in doubles

NTRP 4.0

This player has dependable strokes on both forehand and backhand sides; has the ability to use a variety of shots including lobs, overheads, approach shots and volleys; can place the first serve and force some errors; is seldom out of position in a doubles game.

FOREHAND: Dependable; hits with depth and control on moderate shots; may try to hit too good a placement on a difficult shot

BACKHAND: Player can direct the ball with consistency and depth on moderate shots; developing spin

SERVE/RETURN OF SERVE: Places both first and second serves; frequent power on first serve; uses spin; dependable return of serve; can return with depth in singles and mix returns in doubles

VOLLEY: Depth and control on forehand volley; can direct backhand volleys but usually lacks depth; developing wide and low volleys on both sides of the body

SPECIAL SHOTS: Can put away easy overheads; can poach in doubles; follows aggressive shots to the net; beginning to finish point off; can hit to opponent's weaknesses; able to lob defensively on setups; dependable return of serve

PLAYING STYLE: Dependable ground strokes with directional control and depth demonstrated on moderate shots; not yet playing good percentage tennis; teamwork in doubles is evident; rallies may still be lost due to impatience

NTRP 4.5

This player has begun to master the use of power and spins; has sound footwork; can control depth of shots and is able to move opponent up and back; can hit first serves with power and accuracy and place the second serve; is able to rush the net with some success on serve in singles as well as doubles.

FOREHAND: Very dependable; uses speed and spin effectively; controls depth well; tends to overhit on difficult shots; offensive on moderate shots

BACKHAND: Can control direction and depth but may break down under pressure; can hit power on moderate shots

SERVE/RETURN OF SERVE: Aggressive serving with limited double faults; uses power and spin; developing offense; on second serve frequently hits with good depth and placement; frequently hits aggressive service returns; can take pace off with moderate success in doubles

VOLLEY: Can handle a mixed sequence of volleys; good footwork; has depth and directional control on backhand; developing touch; most common error is still overhitting

SPECIAL SHOTS: Approach shots hit with good depth and control; can consistently hit volleys and overheads to end the point; frequently hits aggressive service returns

PLAYING STYLE: More intentional variety in game; is hitting with more pace; covers up weaknesses well; beginning to vary game plan according to opponent; aggressive net play is common in doubles; good anticipation; beginning to handle pace

NTRP 5.0

This player has good shot anticipation; frequently has an outstanding shot or exceptional consistency around which a game may be structured; can regularly hit winners or force errors off of short balls; can successfully execute lobs, drop shots, half volleys and overhead smashes; has good depth and spin on most second serves.

FOREHAND: Strong shot with control, depth, and spin; uses forehand to set up offensive situations; has developed good touch; consistent on passing shots

BACKHAND: Can use backhand as an aggressive shot with good consistency; has good direction and depth on most shots; varies spin

SERVE/RETURN OF SERVE: Serve is placed effectively with the intent of hitting to a weakness or developing an offensive situation; has a variety of serves to rely on; good depth, spin, and placement on most second serves to force weak return or set up next shot; can mix aggressive and off-paced service returns with control, depth, and spin

VOLLEY: Can hit most volleys with depth, pace, and direction; plays difficult volleys with depth; given opportunity, volley is often hit for a winner

SPECIAL SHOTS: Approach shots and passing shots are hit with pace and a high degree of effectiveness; can lob offensively; overhead can be hit from any position; hits mid-court volley with consistency; can mix aggressive and off-paced service returns

PLAYING STYLE: Frequently has an outstanding shot or attribute around which his game is built; can vary game plan according to opponent; this player is 'match wise,' plays percentage tennis, and 'beats himself' less than the 4.5 player; solid teamwork in doubles is evident; game breaks down mentally and physically more often than the 5.5 player

NTRP 5.5

This player can execute all strokes offensively and defensively; can hit dependable shots under pressure; is able to analyze opponents' styles and can employ patterns of play to assure the greatest possiblity of winning points; can hit winners or force errors with both first and second serves. Returns of serve can be an offensive weapon.

NTRP 6.0

This player has mastered all the above skills, has developed power and/or consistency as a major weapon; and can vary strategies and styles of play in a competitive situation. This player typically has had intensive training for national competition at junior or college levels.

NTRP 6.5

This player has mastered all of the above skills and is an experienced tournament competitor who regularly travels for competition and whose income may be partially derived from prize winnings.

NTRP 7.0

This is a world class player.

Advancement Foundation Rating System *(A key to identify progressive improvement within the Advanced Foundation.)*

Level	Volley	Serve	Forehand Groundstroke	Backhand Groundstroke	Overhead
1.0	Can bounce the ball on ground with the Continental grip; Uses Continental grip; is able to make contact on the forehand; has trouble holding elbow straight on backhands.	Is learning to hit the right side of the ball and impart slice spin using the Continental grip; ball tends to spin too much and land too far to the side	Can swing with one or two hands from low to high with out the ball; consistently can brush up ball with minimal control. Can identify the Eastern Forehand grip.	Can mimic the two-handed backhand motion; brushes up on the ball when hit however has minimal control. Learning to maintain balance; back leg tends to swing around too much.	Is trying to use the Continental grip; hits too much slice on the overhead or misses the ball; player tends to face the net too much during swing.
2.0	Coordinates the step at contact; stays sideways at contact and is holding the racket firm; elbow is starting to stay straight on backhand; minimal backswing.	Able to stay sideways to contact; racket head is leading over the hitting hand at contact; serve starting to land in court; still hits ball too far left.	Steps into ball with closed stance; uses straight back swing keeping racket head pointed down to contact; Starting to use off hand and arm on shoulder turn; learning to catch racket with off hand on follow-through.	Beginning to have repetition on backhand swing; has trouble moving up to short balls and maintaining two hands on racket; can move to the left and use proper footwork with closed stance on balls that are not too far away; holding the follow-through for a moment.	Player points at ball in the air with off hand then is bringing arm to chest at contact; beginning to make flatter contact with the Continental grip by pronating correctly; is able to direct most overheads to the left; has trouble turning enough to hit normal stroke to the right.
3.0	Is able to reproduce the volley consistently on both sides; elbow is held firm through the backhand; able to hit low volleys with firm short slice motion and control; can hit angle volleys on both sides	Is able to direct slice and semi-topspin serves into general areas; gaining pace on serve; starting to lean forward over toss shoulder at contact; pronates correctly	Creating a full upper-body turn on the backswing; is creating a slight loop pattern; is able to maintain balance through swing; keeps feet down after contact; hitting slice strokes with some control	More aggressive swing pattern with a slight loop; creates extra topspin when needed; maintains feet through follow-through; is able to brush up and around the outside of the ball as well as up the back of the ball; can hit sharp crosscourt angles as well as depth; can slice the backhand with some control	Full overhead swing pattern with consistent contact; keeps back foot back after contact; is able to hit reverse overheads to the right side of court with no change is grip or stroke; starting to "scissors-kick" on deeper overheads;
4.0	Player can direct low and high volleys with firm slice to all parts of the court; has no trouble with low volleys; can volley effectively from deeper parts of the court; reacts to fast shots with proper form	Offensive second serve with high ball rotation; can swing harder on second serves; is able to hit kick serves and flat serves with high ball velocity; seldom double faults	Can hit open or closed stance forehands; can create greater topspin by adjusting grip to semi-western; can hit inside out forehands with depth and some angle; can hit aggressive passing shots; can drive slice strokes	Is able to take ball on rise and hit either drives or sharp dipping angles; can hit effective slice strokes with depth and topspin passing shots; able to hit consistent depth with power	Hitting full overheads from all parts of the court; able to hit _ speed overheads from behind the baseline accurately; is able to hit full overheads while moving side to side
5.0	Can hit offensive volleys from all parts of the court; hits angle volleys off difficult balls; has no trouble with hard hit, low balls; poaches at opportune times; can hit topspin swinging volleys and flat volleys under control	Can hit aces from both the ad and deuce sides; can direct second serves with effective depth and speed; usually holds serve in all matches	Hits winners from the back court; can vary the angle and pace of the forehand; can hit excessive topspin when needed; can hit topspin lobs with accuracy	Hits winners from the back court; can vary the angle and pace of the backhand; can hit excessive topspin when needed; can hit topspin lobs with accuracy	Can hit overheads from any part of the court to any part on opponent's side; can hit powerful and deadly overheads

6.0 – 7.0 Players at these levels can hit all shots and compete with all top-level players. Rating comes from competitive results.

David W. Smith's

Tennis Mastery

A REVOLUTIONARY APPROACH TO TENNIS

About the Author

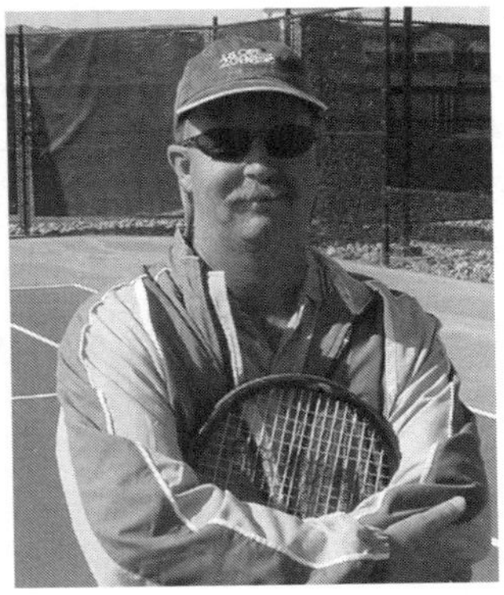

For over 35 years, David Smith has been a tennis coach and teaching professional. As a coach, David has a personal team win-loss record of over 800 League & Regional wins against less than 25 losses over a 22 year coaching career in California and Arizona. Over the past three decades, he has trained over 3000 players including hundreds of state, national and/or world-ranked players. This vast experience has opened his eyes to what systems work and what systems leave players far below their potential. David's Advanced Foundation platform is the culmination of discovering proven components and learning the best methods in which players can learn these elements.

David speaks at conferences, clubs and resorts, discussing his Advanced Foundation and his methods of developing perennial team championships and individual champions. His second book, COACHING MASTERY has become a coaching "handbook" for thousands of coaches, tennis instructors and tennis parents.

David is a Dunlop Mastery Professional and is on the Dunlop Speaker's Bureau. In 2002, David won the "Speaker of the Year" award at both the California and Intermountain USPTA Divisional conferences. He has served as a board member of the Intermountain USPTA Division and has spoken at World USPTA Conventions.

In the past ten years, David has published over 200 tennis articles including feature articles for USPTA's ADDvantage Magazine and Belgium's "Tennis & Coach."

David is perhaps best known for his contributions to tennis as Senior Editor for TennisOne.com, one of the world's top-rated tennis instructional web sites.

David is married to Dr. Kerri Smith, a pediatrician, and they have two children, Kyla, eleven, who has been featured in several tennis development articles, and Keaton who is six years of age at the printing of this Second Edition. David and his family live in picturesque St. George, Utah.

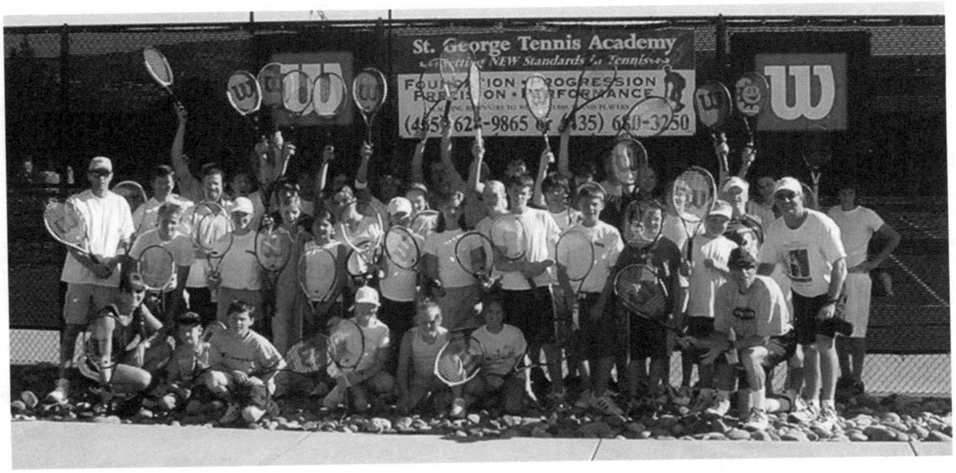

St. George Tennis Academy • St. George, Utah